Biomechanics of Spine Stabilization

Biomechanics of Spine Stabilization

Principles and Clinical Practice

EDWARD C. BENZEL, M.D., F.A.C.S.

Professor and Chief
Division of Neurosurgery
University of New Mexico School of Medicine
Albuquerque, New Mexico

McGRAW-HILL, INC.
Health Professions Division
New York   St. Louis   San Francisco   Auckland   Bogotá
Caracas   Lisbon   London   Madrid   Mexico City   Milan
Montreal   New Delhi   San Juan   Singapore   Sydney   Tokyo   Toronto

This book is dedicated to my foundation and source of strength, Mary Benzel

1234567890 KGP KGP 987654
ISBN 0-07-005091-0

This book was set in Berkley Old Style Medium by University Graphics, Inc. The editors were Jane Pennington and Steven Melvin; the production supervisor was Robin White; the index was prepared by Alexandra Nickerson; the cover designer was Nicoletta Barolini. Arcata Graphics/ Kingsport was printer and binder. The book is printed on acid-free paper.

Illustrated by Michael Norviel.

Library of Congress Cataloging-in-Publication Data

Biomechanics of spine stabilization / editor, Edward C. Benzel. — 1st ed.
    p. cm.
    Includes bibliographical references and index.
    ISBN 0-07-005091-0
    1. Spine—Instability—Surgery.   2. Spinal implants.   3. Spine
—Mechanical properties.   I. Benzel, Edward C.
    [DNLM: 1. Biomechanics.   2. Spinal Injuries—surgery.   3. Spinal
Diseases—surgery.   4. Orthopedic Fixation Devices. WE 725 B6145
1994]
RD771.I58B55   1994
617.3'750592—dc20
DNLM/DLC
for Library of Congress   93-44002

CONTENTS

FOREWORDS

Over the past two decades there have been major advances in the treatment of spinal disorders including anterior decompression of the neural structures as well as various forms of spinal stabilization by utilization of implants.

Historically, laminectomy alone, which was used for years to treat certain spinal disorders such as tumors and trauma, created increased instability and, in some cases, increased neural deficit. Part of the problem of the past has been a lack of understanding by the surgeon of the biomechanics of the spine in relationship to its osseous architecture and neural structures.

This treatise beautifully describes and illustrates the basic principles of the biomechanics of the spine in relation to the normal anatomy, kinematics, deformity, and spinal as well as neural injury. Important basic principles are described including the fact that neurons can withstand neural compression and remain functional, the spinal cord can become ischemic with mechanical deformation, and total restoration of normal spinal alignment is not absolutely necessary if decompression of the spinal cord and stabilization are accomplished.

Dr. Benzel is a unique person in that he combines the expertise of an engineer and the wide experience of a spine surgeon. This text will have a major impact on the world of neurosurgery, orthopaedics, and spinesurgery because it will educate those surgeons who treat complex disorders and trauma of the spine. Most importantly it will produce better collaboration between the neurosurgeon, the orthopaedist, and the engineer to enhance patient care.

Henry H. Bohlman, M.D.
Professor, Orthopaedic Surgery
Case Western Reserve University School of Medicine
Chief, Traumatic & Reconstructive Spine Surgery
University Hospitals of Cleveland
Chief, Acute Spinal Cord Injury Service
Veterans Administration Medical Center

During the last two decades, surgery of the spine has changed dramatically. These changes primarily reflect the development of better techniques of diagnosis and anesthesia, as well as new fusion procedures that are often supplemented with instrumentation. Stabilizing the spine or correcting a deformity with instrumentation and bone

mandates that the spinal surgeon understand the biomechanics of both the normal and the injured spine. This volume by Dr. Edward Benzel bridges the gap that has existed between the physics of biomechanical research and the clinical arena. As such, the book will help spinal surgeons to plan treatments for the injured spine based on sound biomechanical principles—principles that will influence the surgeon's choice of the surgical approach, type of fusion, and type of instrumentation. By integrating the complexities of the biomechanics of the spine into a clinically relevant treatise, Dr. Benzel's book will be a valuable resource for every practicing spinal surgeon and an invaluable learning source for those who aspire to the profession.

Volker K. H. Sonntag, M.D.
Division of Neurological Surgery
Barrow Neurological Institute St. Joseph's Hospital
Phoenix, Arizona

There has been considerable activity in the surgical management of spinal disorders during the past two decades. This has resulted in significant improvements in all facets of the field, particularly regarding stabilization. Developments in spinal instrumentation have provided the ability to achieve rigid segmental fixation while at the same time immobilizing fewer segments of the spine. Successful patient outcomes are influenced by a surgeon's familiarity with a given implant, knowledge of appropriate indications for stabilization and fusion, and biomechanical operatives.

There are presently a number of ways to gain exposure to these systems at the residency, fellowship, and continuing medical education levels. A growing number of residency programs provide in-depth exposure to spinal instrumentation and fusion. Additionally, there are increasing fellowship opportunities available to both neurosurgeons and orthopaedic surgeons enabling a concentrated period of study in this area. Finally, numerous "hands-on" and didactic courses give today's practicing surgeons an introduction to the principles and techniques of modern stabilization and fusion.

The fundamental problem confronting spine surgeons is that indications for fusion are often controversial. Much of the uncertainty relates to the absence of a precise, widely accepted definition of spinal stability. This is especially true in the area of degenerative lumbar spine disease. It is hoped that prospective fusion studies that are beginning to take place will enhance our understanding of what truly constitutes an unstable spine and will thereby facilitate predicting which of these situations will benefit from fusion.

Once it has been determined that clinical instability exists and that a fusion is necessary, a treatment strategy has to be designed. Is internal fixation desirable? If so, which of the many available techniques is best suited for the job? What would the optimal design configuration of this device be? For these questions to be satisfactorily answered there needs to be a solid biomechanical foundation. Only after the forces creating an instability are identified can a logical plan to correct these forces be planned.

Biomechanics of Spine Stabilization is dedicated to explaining clearly and concisely these clinically relevant mechanical issues. It is well written and illustrated, remaining focused on the most pertinent topics of spinal stabilization and fusion. The book is exciting because it addresses important issues that previously have not been well described. These features make it a cover-to-cover "must read" book for anyone who is involved with the care of the patient with an unstable spine. The book represents an extremely important contribution in the area of spine stabilization particularly during a time when the field's technological advances have developed at an explosive pace.

It is a testimony to Dr. Benzel's insight to recognize the need for a contemporary spinal biomechanics book, and to his discipline and intellect to accurately simplify such a complex topic. The text is extremely valuable and will be instructional for generations to come. This monumental effort has again demonstrated Dr. Benzel's unwavering commitment to teaching fellow surgeons, so that they may ultimately provide optimal care to their patients.

Charles B. Stillerman, M.D.
Director of Spine Surgery
Department of Neurosurgery
University of Southern California
School of Medicine
Los Angeles, California

PREFACE

Spinal stabilization may be achieved by a variety of methods. Each is associated with method-specific nuances, complications, and advantages. Each, in addition, is accompanied by biomechanical principles that establish the guidelines that direct decision-making and, ultimately, clinical outcome. This book presents the biomechanical foundation upon which clinical spine stabilization decisions are based. Without an understanding of this foundation for clinical decision-making, the surgeon is ill-equipped to optimize patient outcome. This information is of particular importance in this era of rapidly evolving advances in technology with its accompanying emphasis on technology transfer to the clinical arena.

It is emphasized that *the goal of all spinal stabilization techniques is to establish and maintain a nonpathological relationship between the neural elements and the surrounding bony and extrinsic soft tissue in a biomechanically favorable environment.* A perfectly aligned spinal column is not necessary if no neural impingement or deformation is present and if the spinal arrangement is such that the chance for the progression of spinal deformity is essentially nil. These points are repetitively addressed in this book.

This text has been designed to offer the practicing spine surgeon, resident in training, biomechanical engineer, instrumentation designer, and instrumentation manufacturer a foundation of knowledge regarding clinically applicable spinal instrumentation biomechanics. Without this, the design and surgical application of spinal implants (including the determination of surgical indications) may very well be misguided.

Since the vast majority of spinal implant failures are not actual device failures, but are instead errors made by the surgeon regarding improper construct selection and inappropriate patient selection, this text focuses upon clinically relevant structural considerations and force applications. This approach encourages the reader to "think" in terms of biomechanical principles first, followed by the consideration of specific technique applications. Since biomechanical principles are emphasized, specific construct types may be discussed in several locations within this volume; each time in the context of differing biomechanical principles.

A precise definition of terms is imperative to the understanding of any discipline. The discipline of spine surgery is no exception. Therefore, a glossary of biomechanical terminology is provided at the end of the text.

I am a surgeon and an educator. This book, thus, reflects my clinical orientation and bias. Biomechanical principles are addressed only with respect to their clinical applicability. With this in mind, this text begins with the essentials, proceeds gradually toward the development of an understanding of biomechanical principles, and, finally, provides a basis for clinical decision-making. The essentials are covered in chapters addressing anatomy, physical principles, and spinal stability and instability. Clinical correlates of these principles are developed in chapters addressing degenerative and inflammatory diseases, trauma, spine deformities, neural element injuries, surgical approaches, and the destabilizing and stabilizing effects of spinal surgery. The biomechanical principles involved with spinal stabilization are then addressed with attention paid to the general principles involved with spinal implants and their clinical application. Finally, this essential information is incorporated into the clinical decision-making process by discussions centered about the desired qualitative attributes of spinal implants with accompanying discussions regarding complex instrumentation constructs and force applications, spinal orthotics, and the surgical indication decision-making process.

Illustrations are liberally utilized to create mental images of critical anatomical, biomechanical, and clinical points. In this vein, this text can be perused by scanning the figures and figure legends. A more in-depth understanding could then be selectively achieved by delving into the appropriate aspect of the text and appropriate references.

Applicability and practicality are emphasized. It is in this sense that (1) the practicing surgeon can effectively employ information found herein to his or her patients by designing logical and sound treatment strategies, (2) the resident in training can readily understand the foundations on which surgical procedures and clinical decisions are based, and (3) the engineer and the instrumentation designer and manufacturer can appreciate the dilemmas and difficult decision-making predicaments commonly faced by clinicians. It is therefore hoped that this book can function both as a text for the methodical acquisition of information and as a reservoir of information, to be utilized on an as needed basis, for a variety of clinical and instrumentation and construct design applications. The intent of the author is to provide a comprehensive, yet practical, approach to the understanding of this important and often underrated aspect of clinical medicine; i.e., the biomechanics of spine stabilization.

The author acknowledges those who provided the ideas, the counsel, the emotional support, the technical and editorial advice, and the creative and skillful artistic interpretation. Without them this work would not have been possible: Nevan Baldwin; Perry Ball; Mary Benzel; Bruce McCormack; Michael Norviel.

Part I

Overview of Fundamental Concepts

Biomechanically Relevant Anatomy and Material Properties of the Spine and Associated Elements

ANATOMY

The vertebral column complex consists of ventrally located vertebral bodies and intervening intervertebral disks that collectively assume most of the axial load-bearing responsibilities of the spine. The pedicles connect the ventral and dorsal components of each spinal segment. The laminae provide a roof for the spinal canal; the facet joints limit rotation, flexion, extension, lateral bending, and translation. The muscles and ligaments provide for, and limit, torso movement. They also provide for some axial load-bearing. Each of these spinal components will be discussed separately.

Many of the figures in this chapter depict summations of information gleaned from a number of sources. Occasionally the data from these sources vary widely. Average data, therefore, are presented in a figure format in order to depict general trends as well as appropriate data points. Because of gaps in the available information, some figures depict extrapolated data, where appropriate.

The Vertebral Body

Both the width and the depth of the vertebral bodies increase as one descends in a rostral-to-caudal direction (Fig. 1-1).[1-4] The vertebral body height also increases in a rostral-to-caudal direction, with the exception of a slight reversal of this relationship at the C6 and lower lumbar levels (Fig. 1-2).[1-4] The height of the C6 vertebral body is usually less than those of the C5 and C7 bodies, and the heights of the lower lumbar vertebral bodies are usually less than that of the L2 vertebral body. In the cervical spine, the uncinate process projects from the cephalo-dorsal-lateral aspect of each vertebral body (C3 through C7) (Fig. 1-3). The uncovertebral joint allows an articulation of this process with the caudal-dorsal-lateral aspect of the vertebral body above. This is essentially an extension of the intervertebral disk that plays a role in the coupling phenomenon (see Chap. 2) and in rotation.[5]

The progressive increase in size of the vertebral bodies as one descends the spine correlates with strength, or stress-resisting ability. The decreased incidence of spine fractures observed in the lower lumbar spine is related, at least in part, to the increased strength of the vertebrae in this region. This correlates with the axial load-resisting ability of the spine (Fig. 1-4).[4,6-9]

The shape of the vertebral body varies from region to region. Although its shape is generally that of a cylinder, the dorsal aspect of the vertebral body (the surface facing the spinal canal) is concave dorsally (Fig. 1-5). This is particularly significant in ventral spinal operations where screw purchase of the dorsal vertebral body cortex is critical. Misinterpretation of the lateral x-ray may lead to neural impingement by the screw.

The Facet Joints

The facet joints, in and of themselves, do not substantially support axial loads unless in an extension posture. They are apophyseal joints that have a loose capsule and a synovial lining. In the cervical spine, the facet joints are primarily oriented in a coronal plane (Fig. 1-6A).[4] The orientation of the facet joints changes significantly as one descends the thoracic and lumbar spine (Fig. 1-6B and C). The angle (from midline) increases from L1 to L5 (Fig. 1-6D).

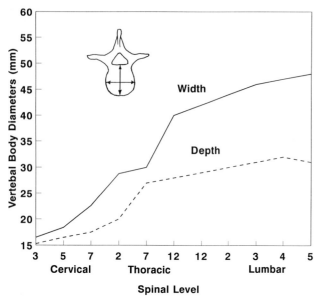

FIGURE 1-1 Vertebral body diameters versus spinal level. The width *(solid line)* and depth *(dashed line)* of the vertebral bodies are depicted separately. *(From J. Berry et al.,[1] M. Panjabi et al.,[2] M. Panjabi et al.,[3] A. White and M. Panjabi.[4])*

The facet joint surfaces of vertebral bodies C3 through C7 face the *instantaneous axis of rotation (IAR;* the axis about which a vertebral segment rotates) and are not particularly restrictive of gliding movements. The cervical spine facet joint's abilities to resist flexion and extension, lateral bending, and rotation are relatively diminished because of

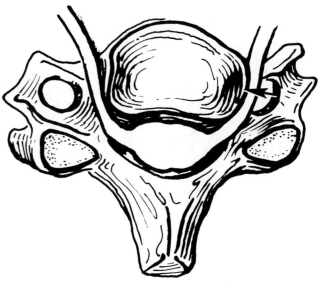

FIGURE 1-3 The uncinate process *(arrow)* and its relationship to the rostral-dorsal-lateral aspect of the vertebral body and exiting nerve root.

this coronal plane orientation. Thus, such movement is substantial in this region (Fig. 1-7).[4,10,11]

In the lumbar region, however, the facet joints are oriented in a sagittal plane (Fig. 1-6).[4,12,13] Their ability to resist flexion or translational movement in this region is minimal, whereas their ability to resist rotation is substantial (Fig. 1-7).

The nearly coronal facet orientation at L5-S1 may be a factor in the relatively decreased incidence of subluxation,

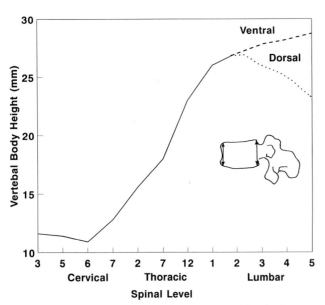

FIGURE 1-2 Vertebral body height versus spinal level. The dorsal height *(dotted line)* and ventral height *(dashed line),* where significantly different, are depicted separately. *(From J. Berry et al.,[1] M. Panjabi et al.,[2] M. Panjabi et al.,[3] A. White and M. Panjabi.[4])*

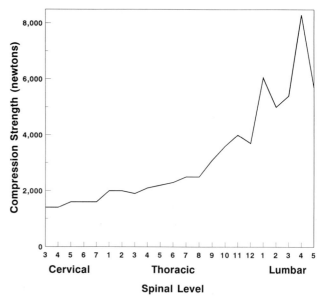

FIGURE 1-4 Vertebral compression strength versus spinal level. *(From A. White and M. Panjabi,[4] G. Bell et al.,[6] J. Macintosh and B. Nikolai,[7] O. Perry,[8] O. Perry.[9])*

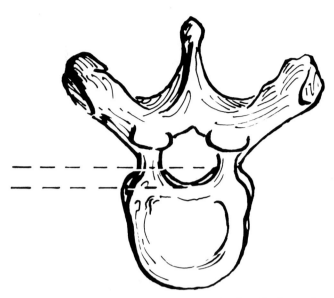

FIGURE 1-5 Vertebral body shape. Note the dorsally directed concavity. This may present problems in the interpretation of lateral radiographs. A lateral radiograph "sees" the dorsal aspect of the vertebral body at the level of the upper dashed line. In the mid-sagittal plane, however, the dorsal aspect of the vertebral body (and dural sac) is at the level of the lower dashed line.

in the presence of intact facet joints, at the lumbosacral joint; that is, in degenerative spondylosis, subluxation is more common at L4-L5 than at L5-S1 in spite of the relative vertical orientation of the L5-S1 disk interspace.

The facet joints absorb a greater fraction of the axial load-bearing if the spine is oriented in extension (see below). This varies with the type of load.[14]

The Lamina, Spinal Canal, and Spinal Canal Contents

The lamina provides dorsal protection for the dural sac and a foundation for the spinous processes, which serve as solid attachment sites for muscles and ligaments. Forces applied via the spinous processes cause movement of the spine.

The tracts within the spinal cord in the cervical and thoracic regions and the nerve roots within the lumbar region are somatotopically oriented. This orientation is consistent. In the region of the spinal cord the corticospinal tracts are

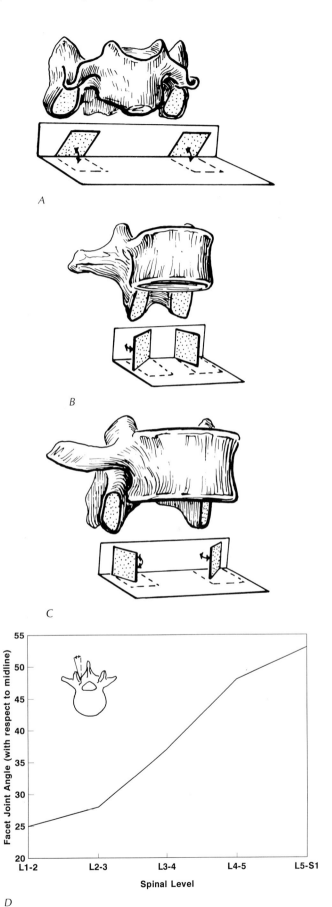

FIGURE 1-6 Facet joint orientation. *A.* The relative coronal plane orientation in the cervical region. *B.* The intermediate orientation in the thoracic region. *C.* The relative sagittal orientation in the lumbar region. *D.* The facet joint orientation changes substantially in the lumbar region; here the facet joint angle (with respect to midline) is depicted versus spinal level. *(From A. White and M. Panjabi,[4] J. Van Schaik et al.,[12] A. Ahmed et al.,[42] J. Taylor and L. Twomey.[43])*

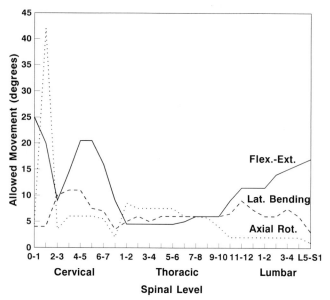

FIGURE 1-7 Segmental motions allowed at the various spinal levels. (Combined flexion and extension, *solid line*; unilateral lateral bending, *dashed line*; unilateral axial rotation, *dotted line*.) (*From A. White and M. Panjabi,[4] H. Lin et al.,[10] M. Panjabi et al.[11]*)

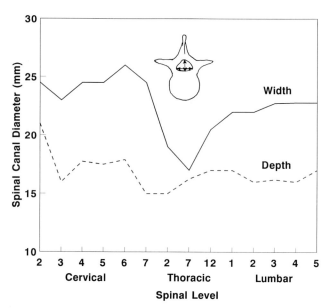

FIGURE 1-9 Spinal canal diameter versus spinal level. The width (*solid line*) and depth (*dashed line*) of the canal are depicted separately. (*From J. Berry et al.,[1] M. Panjabi et al.,[2] M. Panjabi et al.,[3] A. Reynolds et al.[16]*)

somatotopically arranged so that hand function is located most medially, while foot function is located laterally. The spinothalamic tract is arranged so that hand sensation is located most medially and ventrally, while sacral sensation is located most dorsally and laterally. The posterior columns are similarly arranged in a somatotopic manner. In the lumbar region the nerve roots are arranged so that the lower sacral segments are located most medially, and the exiting upper lumbar segments most laterally (Fig. 1-8).[15]

The spinal canal dimensions, and hence the extramedullary space in the nonpathological spine, are generous. In the upper cervical region they are the most generous, and in the upper thoracic region the least so. In the lumbar region, both the epidural and the intradural space are, in general, capacious (Figs. 1-9 and 1-10).[1-3,16] In the case of a preexisting spinal stenosis, however, the factor of safety may be small. This is important when one is considering a spinal

instrumentation application that might impinge on the neural elements—that is, a sublaminar placement.

The lumbar spinal canal's depth does not change significantly as one descends from the upper to the lower lumbar region, but its width increases (Fig. 1-9). The lumbar and sacral canal's cross-sectional area is generous. It contains the cauda equina, which is relatively resistant to neurological insults (compared with the spinal cord proper). Therefore, posttraumatic neural element injury in the lumbar region is less common than that associated with comparable spinal column deformation elsewhere in the spine.

The shape of the spinal canal itself varies along the length of the spine. In the cervical, thoracic, and upper lumbar regions the shape of the spinal canal is that of a "ballooned" triangle. Toward the lumbosacral junction, however, it assumes a "Napoleon's hat–like" (bicorne) configuration (Fig. 1-10).[12]

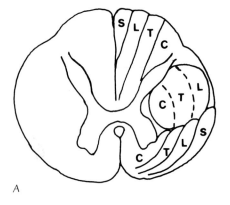

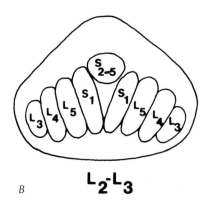

A *B*

FIGURE 1-8 *A*. Diagrammatic axial section of the spinal cord demonstrating the somatotopic orientation of spinal tracts. *B*. Diagrammatic axial section of the spinal canal at the level of the mid-lumbar spine. Note the orientation of the neural elements (depicted in clusters)—the lower elements are situated most medially and those preparing to exit the spinal canal most laterally.

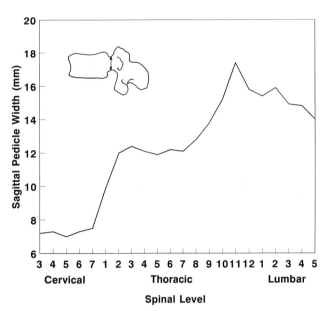

FIGURE 1-10 A diagrammatic representation of the respective shapes and sizes of a typical spinal canal in the cervical (*A*), thoracic (*B*), and lumbar (*C*) regions. (*From J. Van Schaik et al.*[12])

The Pedicle

The pedicles of the cervical spine are shorter and proportionally of greater diameter than those of other regions of the spine. The transverse pedicle width decreases gradually from the cervical to the midthoracic region and then increases as one descends in the lumbar spine (Fig. 1-11).[2,17,18] The pedicle height (sagittal pedicle width) increases gradually (except at C2) from the cervical to the thoracolumbar region and then decreases as one descends in the lumbar spine (Fig. 1-12).[2,17,18] This relationship is favorable for transpedicular screw placement in the lumbar spine, since pedicle width is more important than height in this regard. A small variation in pedicle height (sagittal pedicle width) in the lumbar region is not clinically significant, because of the already generous dimension (Fig. 1-12).[17,18]

The transverse pedicle angle decreases from the cervical spine to the thoracolumbar region and then increases as the lumbar spine is descended (Fig. 1-13).[2,17,18] This necessitates a wider angle of approach for the placement of pedicle screws in the low lumbar spine. An appreciation of vertebral anatomy is similarly important when pedicle screws are to be placed in the sacral region.[19] There is, however, usually a greater margin of safety in screw placement.

FIGURE 1-12 Sagittal pedicle width versus spinal level. (*From M. Panjabi et al.,*[2] *M. Krag et al.,*[17] *M. Zindrick et al.*[18])

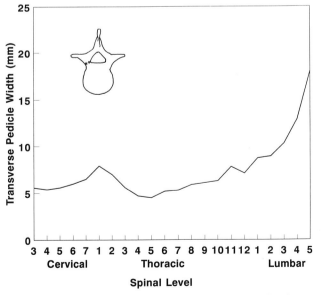

FIGURE 1-11 Transverse pedicle width versus spinal level. (*From M. Panjabi et al.,*[2] *M. Krag et al.,*[17] *M. Zindrick et al.*[18])

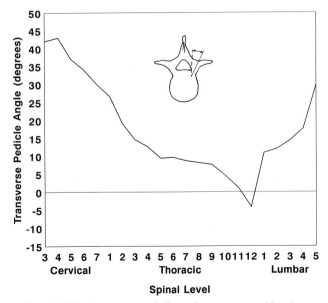

FIGURE 1-13 Transverse pedicle angle versus spinal level. (*From M. Panjabi et al.,*[2] *M. Krag et al.,*[17] *M. Zindrick et al.*[18])

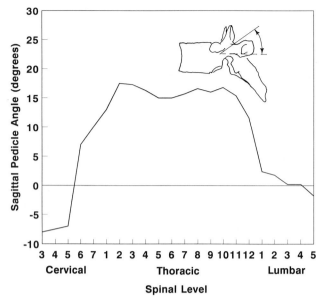

FIGURE 1-14 Sagittal pedicle angle versus spinal level. *(From M. Panjabi et al.,[2] M. Krag et al.,[17] M. Zindrick et al.[18])*

Also important, particularly regarding pedicle screw placement in the upper lumbar and thoracic spine—where the margin of safety is less than in the low lumbar region— is the sagittal pedicle angle (Fig. 1-14).[2,17,18] In the upper lumbar and thoracic spine this angle becomes relatively steep.

The Intervertebral Disk

The intervertebral disks are composed of a nucleus pulposus and an annulus fibrosus that provide support, absorb shock, and both allow and resist movement. Their ability to resist axial stresses is substantial but decreases with age.[13] The addition of flexion, extension, or lateral-bending force vectors, however, causes significant deformity of the disk interspace and fosters disk bulging and herniation. The disk itself is surrounded by an endplate that resists herniation of the disk into the vertebral body (Schmorl's node).

The annulus fibrosus is composed of several layers of radiating fibers attached to the cartilaginous endplates (inner fibers) and to the cortical bone on the walls of the vertebral body (Sharpey's fibers). These components incompletely resist deformation (Fig. 1-15). Note that disk bulging occurs on the concave side of a bending of the spine (Fig. 1-15C). This correlates with osteophyte formation. Disk bulging, however, is not to be confused with disk herniation. The former is caused by distortion of the annulus fibrosus by compression; the latter is caused by migration of the nucleus pulposus from its normal location.

In contrast to the direction of disk (annulus) bulging (i.e., toward the concavity of a spinal bend), the nucleus pulposus moves in the opposite direction (Fig. 1-15D).[20] Flexion, therefore, causes bulging of the annulus fibrosus ventrally.

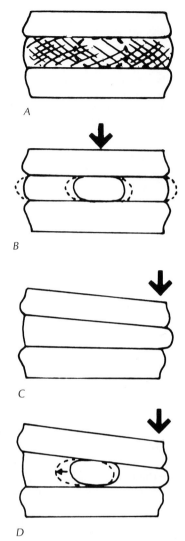

FIGURE 1-15 The intervertebral disk. The fibers of the annulus fibrosus are oriented radially and in opposite directions throughout several layers. *A.* The nucleus pulposus *(dashed outline)* is contained (in nonpathological situations) by the annulus fibers. *B.* The bearing of an axial load results in an even distribution of forces. *C.* An eccentrically borne load results in annulus fibrosus bulging on the concave side of the resultant spinal curve, while annulus fibrosus tension is present on the convex side of the curve. *D.* The nucleus pulposus, however, tends to move *opposite* the direction of the annulus fibrosus bulge when an eccentric load is borne *(solid to dashed outline).*

It also causes the tendency of the nucleus pulposus to migrate dorsally. Significant strains are placed on the annulus fibrosus by physiological loads.[21]

The Transverse Process

The transverse processes provide sites for attachment of the paraspinous muscles. As moment arms for attached muscles, they allow leverage for lateral bending. They are easily fractured, because of their relatively small size and poor vascularization. This is particularly so in the lumbar region, where applied forces are often substantial.

The transverse processes arise from the junction of the pedicle and the lamina. In the mid- to lower thoracic region they are reasonably substantial and project in a lateral and slightly upward direction. Their projection from the spine is roughly at the same anteroposterior plane as the facet joints and dorsal aspect of the pedicles. In the lower thoracic region the transverse processes become more atretic, and thus are less useful for hook placement.

In the lumbar region the transverse processes project from the spine in a more ventral and anteroposterior position. They become more substantial and thus are able to become sites for bony fusion. Their utility for this purpose, however, is limited by their relatively poor blood supply and their often-less-than-optimal robustness.

The upper six cervical vertebrae usually transmit the vertebral artery through the foramina transversarium. The foramina transversarium is juxtaposed to the uncovertebral joint.

The Spinous Processes

The spinous processes in general are directed dorsally and caudally. The spinous processes of C3 through C6 are usually bifid. In the cervical spine the spinous processes lengthen as one travels downward. In the cervical and upper to mid-thoracic spine, they project more caudally than in the thoracolumbar and lumbar regions. This caudal projection often dictates the resection of the overhanging spinous process (and interspinous ligament) in order to gain access to the interlaminar space in the thoracic region.

The Ligaments

A variety of well-studied spinal ligaments provide varying degrees of support for the spine. These include the interspinous ligament, the ligamentum flavum, the anterior and posterior longitudinal ligaments, and the capsular ligaments. Their strength characteristics vary from ligament to ligament and from region to region (Fig. 1-16).[4,13,22–30]

The effectiveness of a ligament depends on its morphology, and particularly on the moment arm through which it acts.[31] In order to appreciate the contribution of an individual spinal ligament to the integrity of the spine, one must consider the length of the lever arm (Fig. 1-17A) as well as the strength of the ligament. The length of the lever arm is the perpendicular distance between the force vector (the force and its direction, as applied by the ligament) and the IAR. A very strong ligament that functions through a relatively short lever arm may contribute less to stability than a weaker ligament working through a longer lever arm, on account of the latter's greater mechanical advantage.

Although the *interspinous ligament* is not substantial, its attachment to a bone with a relatively long lever arm (spi-

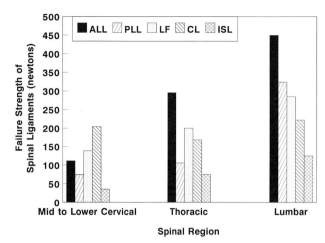

FIGURE 1-16 Failure strength of spinal ligaments versus spinal region. (ALL = anterior longitudinal ligament; PLL = posterior longitudinal ligament; LF = ligamentum flavum; CL = capsular ligament; ISL = interspinous ligament.) *(From A. White and M. Panjabi,[4] A. White and M. Panjabi,[13] J. Chazal et al.,[22] V. Goel and G. Njus,[24] J. Myklebust et al.,[25] A. Nachemson and J. Evans,[26] M. Panjabi et al.,[27] M. Panjabi et al.,[28] I. Posner et al.,[29] H. Tkaczuk.[30])*

nous process) allows the application of a significant flexion-resisting force to the spine (by virtue of the significant distance between the IAR and the point of attachment of the ligament to the spinous process). In this case the lever arm (moment arm) is the perpendicular distance from the point of attachment of the ligament (spinous process) to the IAR of the affected vertebral body (Fig. 1-17B). Note that the interspinous ligament may be absent at the L5-S1 level and deficient at the L4-L5 level.

The *ligamentum flavum* is a stronger ligament, but offers less flexion resistance on account of its more ventral site of attachment. Its moment arm, therefore, is much shorter than that of the interspinous ligaments. That is, its point of attachment is closer to the IAR of the vertebral body than that of the interspinous ligament (Fig. 1-17B). It is a discontinuous ligament that extends from C2 to S1. It is deficient in midline; that is, a longitudinal midline cleavage plane exists. This facilitates surgical entrance into the epidural space. The ligamentum flavum has the highest percentage of elastic fibers of any human tissue. It is also, except in extreme extension, not lax. These two factors minimize the chance of buckling during extension, which might result in dural sac compression.

The *anterior longitudinal ligament* is a relatively strong ligament attached to the vertebral body edges (and not so firmly attached to the annulus fibrosus) at each segmental level of the spine. Its position, usually anterior to the IAR, provides resistance to extension (Fig. 1-17B). Its most rostral aspect attaches to the clivus, and its most caudal aspect to the sacrum.

The *posterior longitudinal ligament* is not as strong as the anterior longitudinal ligament. Its location, dorsal to the

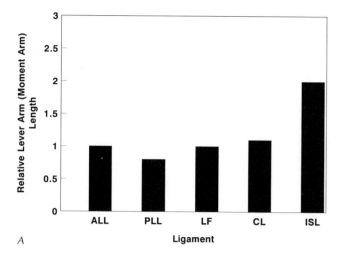

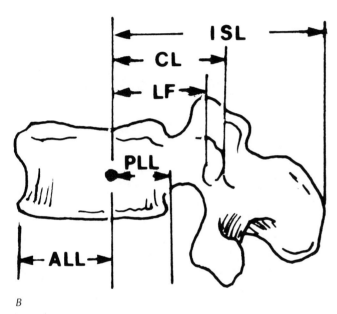

FIGURE 1-17 *A.* The relative lever arm (moment arm) length of ligaments causing flexion (or resisting extension). *B.* The ligaments and their effective moment arms. Note that this length depends on the location of the IAR. An "average" location is used in this illustration. (Dot = IAR; ALL = anterior longitudinal ligament; PLL = posterior longitudinal ligament; LF = ligamentum flavum; CL = capsular ligament; ISL = interspinous ligament.)

IAR, combined with a short moment arm, causes it to weakly resist flexion (Fig. 1-17). Its relative lack of strength, combined with its mechanically disadvantageous position, does not allow it to provide consistent anteropulsion of retropulsed bone and/or disk fragments with the application of distractive forces. As opposed to the anterior longitudinal ligament, the posterior longitudinal ligament is predominantly attached to the disks (annulus fibrosus). The posterior longitudinal ligament extends from the clivus rostrally (tectorial membrane) and extends caudally to the coccyx.

The ligament widens substantially in the region of the disk interspace (Fig. 1-18). Its relatively narrow width is partly responsible for the tendency of the posterolateral region of the disk to be the most common location for herniation. The mechanism of sudden disk prolapse has been shown to be an axial load applied to a spine in a flexed and rotated (away from the side of the prolapse) position.[32]

The *capsular ligaments,* particularly in the cervical spine, play a large part in the maintenance of spinal stability. The length of their lever arm (Fig. 1-17) is modest, but their strength, compared to the stresses placed upon them, is relatively high.

The concept of the *neutral zone,* as outlined by Panjabi, is essential to the understanding of both the importance and the limitations of spinal ligaments with respect to spinal stability.[33] The neutral zone is the component of the physiologic range of motion associated with significant flexibility and minimal stiffness at low loads; that is, minimal or no ligament tension. The *elastic zone* consists of the rest of the physiologic range of motion (Fig. 1-19). The neutral zone can be increased by stretching exercises, which increase the length of contracted ligaments, thus increasing the physiologic range of motion and flexibility. The neutral zone is similarly increased in cases of ligamentous injury where the

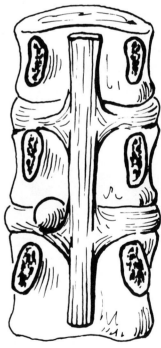

FIGURE 1-18 The posterior longitudinal ligament is narrow in the region of the vertebral body and attached laterally (at the level of its widest point) in the region of the disk interspace. The most common site of disk herniation is the dorsal paramedian region of the intervertebral disk. This injury has been reproduced by flexion, lateral bending (away from the side of the prolapse), and the application of an axial load. (*From M. Adams and W. Hutton.*[32])

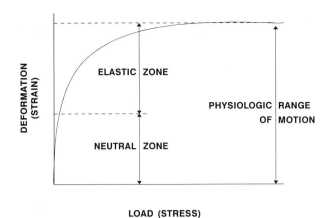

FIGURE 1-19 A typical load deformation curve depicting the neutral and elastic zones (deformation, or strain, versus load, or stress).

ligament has been pathologically increased in length; in such cases the flexibility of the spine is pathologically increased. Under unloaded conditions the spine is lax (i.e., floppy) within the neutral zone. Assumption of the upright posture, however, is not possible if the spine remains floppy. Continuous muscular influences compensate for this by limiting intervertebral movement, thus decreasing the size of the neutral zone and increasing stability.

Spine surgery is usually destabilizing. The extent of destabilization, however, can usually be controlled if fundamental principles are followed.[34]

The Muscles

Muscles move the torso by affecting the spine either directly or indirectly. The morphology[7] and geometry[35] of these muscles have been studied extensively. The erector spinae muscles cause spinal extension and lateral bending via their bony attachments. The psoas muscle contributes to flexion. The rectus abdominis muscle causes spinal flexion without direct spinal attachments; it is a strong torso flexor, because of its long moment arm (from the anterior abdominal wall to the IAR).[35] It is an important spinal support muscle and should be considered in the rehabilitation process.

The continuous influence of muscles on spinal stability, by their limiting the size of the neutral zone (Fig. 1-19), cannot be overemphasized. Chronic pain syndromes associated with muscle imbalance and overload are common. Furthermore, biomechanical studies involving cadavers are uniformly complicated by the inability to accurately mimic the stabilizing contributions of continuous muscular influences.

The rib cage, although not a component of the spinal column, plays a major role in spinal stability. The maintenance of the bony shell and an intact sternum is vital to this role. The stabilizing effect of the rib cage is greatest in extension and least in flexion.[36]

Bone

As previously stated, the vertebral body is the component of the spine that bears the majority of an axial load. The vertebral bodies' dimensions are proportional to the loads they support (Figs. 1-1, 1-2, and 1-4).

The ratio of cortical to cancellous bone (bone density) affects weight-bearing potential. It is greater in the pedicles than in the vertebral bodies, and greater in small pedicles (thoracic and upper lumbar) than in larger pedicles (sacral). Bone density correlates with screw-pullout resistance. Hence, pedicles resist pullout better than vertebral bodies, and small pedicles better than large pedicles. The low bone density of the sacrum translates into significant problems with pedicle screw pullout in this region. Furthermore, osteoporosis significantly decreases bony integrity. A 50-percent decrease in the mass of osseous tissue (usually via ash content loss) results in a reduction of strength to 25 percent of the original.[4]

CONFIGURATION OF THE SPINE

Under normal conditions the cervical and lumbar regions of the spine assume a lordotic posture. A kyphotic posture, as exists in the thoracic and thoracolumbar regions, predisposes the spine to exaggerated stresses. These exaggerated stresses are related to an increased bending moment (see Chap. 2). Thus the intrinsic configuration of this region of the spine substantially determines the type of spinal column injury that is likely to be incurred. For example, at the thoracolumbar junction, the lower terminus of the thoracic kyphosis (along with the absence of the protective support of the rib cage and the absence of the more massive lower lumbar vertebral body support) fosters vertebral column injury. The intrinsic bending moment allowed by the kyphosis, the lack of intrinsic protection (relative), and the abrupt change in mechanics results in focally increased amounts of strain and in an increased incidence of compression fractures in this region. The incidence of fractures peaks similarly in the midcervical region (Fig. 1-20).[37,38]

In the lower lumbar region, the more massive vertebral bodies offer substantial support. The intrinsic lumbar lordosis essentially eliminates the bending moment that is observed when stresses are placed upon the spine at the thoracolumbar junction. In the absence of a significant bending moment, pure axial loads are commonly presented to the spine; therefore, burst fractures are more common in this location. However, fractures in general are less frequent than in other parts of the spine.

At the lumbosacral junction, the angle of the sacrum in relation to the L5 vertebral body (the lumbosacral joint angle) may substantially affect pathological processes, both traumatic and degenerative. Furthermore, this joint, which

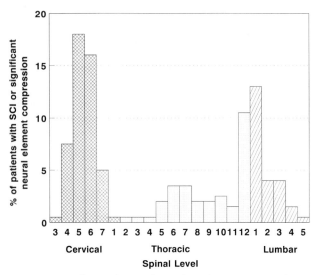

FIGURE 1-20 The incidence of spinal cord injury (or significant neural element compromise), following trauma, versus spinal level. (*Hatched line,* cervical; *dotted line,* thoracic; *diagonal line,* lumbar.) (*From E. Benzel and S. Larson,*[37] *E. Benzel and S. Larson.*[38])

is exposed to significant axial stresses, must resist substantial translational forces. The greater the lumbosacral joint angle, the greater the applied translational forces. The ability to resist these forces is diminished by the vertical joint orientation, the orientation of the facet joints, and the

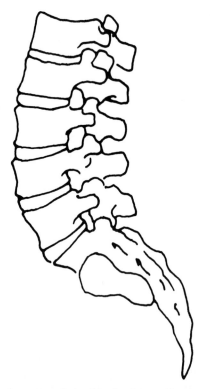

FIGURE 1-21 Orientation of the lumbar and lumbosacral joints. Note that as the spine is descended the joint angle becomes more nearly vertical. (*From J. Van Schaik et al.*[12])

strength characteristics of the ligaments. Spondylolisthesis may ensue. Patients with exaggerated lumbar lordoses are especially prone to the sequelae of these stresses (Fig. 1-21).

REGIONAL CHARACTERISTICS

The Upper Cervical Spine and Craniocervical Junction

The upper cervical spine deserves special attention, because of its unique anatomic arrangement. C1 has no centrum; this allows the intrusion of the odontoid process of C2 between C1's two lateral masses. The odontoid process articulates with the dorsal aspect of the ventral portion of the ring of C1 and with the transverse ligament of the atlas by separate synovial joints.

The lateral masses of C1 articulate with the occipital condyles and C2 by kidney-shaped articulations. The superior facet of C1 faces in a rostral and medial direction, while the inferior facet faces in a caudal and medial direction. This unique wedgelike configuration results in a lateral transmission of force vectors resulting from axial loads [C1 burst (Jefferson) fracture]. The transverse ligament of the atlas attaches to the tubercles on the medial aspect of the ring of C1. This anatomic arrangement, along with the anterior aspect of the ring of C1, allows the containment of the intruding odontoid process. The short and strong transverse processes allow the attachment of the rotators of the upper cervical spine. The anterior ring of C1 is strong—that is, it is made of dense cortical bone. This has an important bearing on the integrity of C1 following laminectomy or posterior arch fractures. A circumferentially intact ring of C1 is not necessary for the attainment of stability.

C2 has many attributes of the more caudal cervical vertebrae. However, it also has a rostral extension, the odontoid process. The pars interarticularis (not to be confused with the pedicle) is substantial and projects from the lamina in a rostral and ventral direction to attach to the lateral mass. This in turn attaches with the pedicle, which passes medially to the vertebral body. The transitional nature of this vertebra dictates a complicated anatomic configuration. The occipital nerve passes dorsal to the atlantoaxial joint. This must be kept in mind during transfacet C1-C2 screw fixation (Fig. 1-22).

C2 is directly connected to the occiput by the alar and apical ligaments and the tectorial membrane. C1 functions, in a sense, as an intermediate "fulcrum" that "regulates" movement between the occiput and C2.[39] The atlantooccipital joint allows flexion, extension, and a minimal degree of lateral flexion. Minimal rotation is allowed. The atlantoaxial joint allows some lateral bending (which is coupled with rotation).[40] Most cervical rotation, which occurs about the dens, is allowed at this joint. The movements allowed in the craniocervical region are depicted in Table 1-1.[4,5,11]

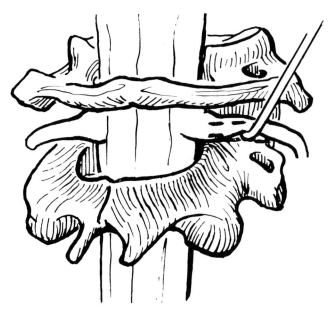

FIGURE 1-22 Anatomy of the dorsal aspect of the occiput-C1-C2 region, with the occipital nerve passing dorsal to the facet joints.

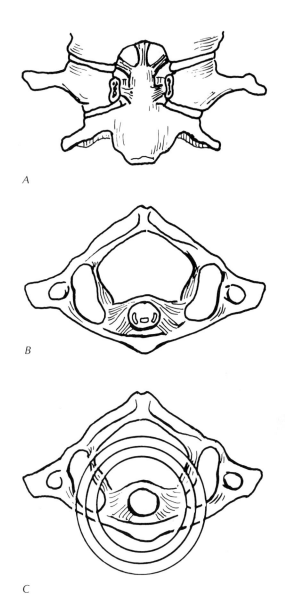

FIGURE 1-23 *A.* The occiput-C1-C2 ligaments as viewed from a ventral orientation with the anterior arch of C1 removed. *B.* The same ligaments viewed from a rostral orientation. *C.* The predominance of rotation of the cervical spine is allowed between C1 and C2 about the odontoid process peg (IAR).

The failure strength of the alar ligament is about 200 N; that of the transverse ligament of the atlas is about 350 N.[23] These ligaments are very strong compared to the loads placed upon them (compare to subaxial ligament strengths—Fig. 1-16). This explains, in part, the relatively low incidence of failure of upper cervical ligaments.

Surgery on the upper cervical spine is complicated by the difficulties associated with calvarial fixation; by the unique anatomy of the upper cervical vertebrae; and by the substantial spinal movement allowed in this region. The anatomic features of the upper cervical spine—especially the articulations of the vertebrae to each other and to the skull—offer little in the way of points of fixation for instrumentation constructs and sites for bony fusion attachment. Furthermore, the unique anatomic arrangement allows movement in all directions and in rotation as well. Although the movement allowed in the upper cervical region is not manifest in all planes and in rotation at *each* spinal level, its sum from occiput to C2 is greater than that seen in any other region of the spine (Fig. 1-23).

TABLE 1-1 Movements allowed in the craniocervical region

Joint	Motion	Range of motion (degrees)
Occiput-C1	combined flexion/extension	25
	lateral bending (unilateral)	5
	axial rotation (unilateral)	5
C1-C2	combined flexion/extension	20
	lateral bending (unilateral)	5
	axial rotation (unilateral)	40

The Mid- and Lower Cervical Spine

The vertebrae of the mid- and lower cervical spine are relatively uniform. A unique characteristic of this region is its lordotic posture. This may aid in spinal cord injury prevention, since most axial loads are imparted symmetrically to the spine, rather than with a significant flexion component (which would cause asymmetrical load application). Since the addition of a flexion component to an axial load greatly increases the chance of vertebral body failure with retropulsion of bone and disk fragments into the spinal canal, the lordotic posture also helps to prevent catastrophic injury.

The orientation of the facet joints in the coronal plane does not excessively limit spinal movement in any direction (or in rotation) except extension. With the cervical spine in extension, however, the spine's ability to resist axial loading is greatest. This may be related to the facts that the facet joints can participate in axial load support most effectively in extension and that, as mentioned above, the likelihood of a flexion component in the injury is small. In this case, the facet joints function in a load-sharing capacity (Fig. 1-24).

The orientation of the facet joints in the cervical spine (in a coronal plane) facilitates spinal instrumentation in certain situations. If the integrity of the facet joints and pedicles has been maintained and the vertebral bodies are able to adequately resist axial loading, translational instability may be effectively managed by the application of a tension-band fixation construct (Fig. 1-25), as discussed in Chap. 23.[41]

The Thoracic Spine

The thoracic spinal cord is shielded from injury by the massive regional paraspinal muscle masses and by the thoracic cage. The narrow spinal canal diameter in the upper thoracic region, however, complicates the issue. The former attributes help to protect the neural elements; the latter attribute contributes to neural injury. This may explain the increased incidence of catastrophic neurological injuries associated with spinal fractures in this region. The increased paraspinal muscle mass protects the spine from failure, thus causing something of an all-or-nothing risk of neural injury; that is, significant kinetic energy is required to fracture the upper thoracic spine, but if such a fracture occurs, the nar-

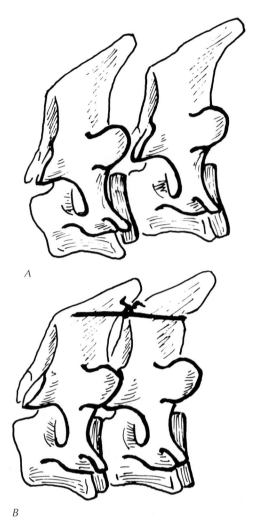

A

B

FIGURE 1-25 In the cervical spine, the orientation of the facet joints can be used to advantage via cerclage wiring techniques. *A.* The compression of two spinous processes together in a tension-band manner prevents subluxation by bringing the superior and inferior facets together. *B.* Since the facet joints are oriented coronally, the close approximation of the superior and inferior facets causes them to abut each other and thus prevent translational deformity. (*From E. Benzel and L. Kesterson.[41]*)

row spinal canal leaves little room to spare for neural element protection (Fig. 1-26).[37] The normal kyphotic posture of the thoracic spine, with its associated predisposition to spinal fracture, amplifies all of these factors.

The Thoracolumbar Junction

The thoracolumbar junction is located at a point of transition that makes it vulnerable to excessive applied force. At this junctional region of the spine, the rib cage no longer offers spinal support and the kyphotic curvature of the spine predisposes the spine to fracture. Furthermore, the vertebral bodies of the spine have not yet achieved the massive size of the mid- to low lumbar vertebrae (with their associ-

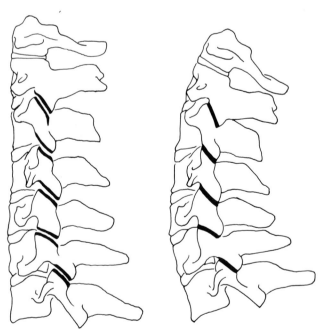

FIGURE 1-24 *A.* In a neutral spinal orientation, the facet joints of the cervical spine are unloaded during moderate axial loading. *B.* In a lordotic orientation (relative extension), however, they are loaded and, thus, subjected to injury during similar loading.

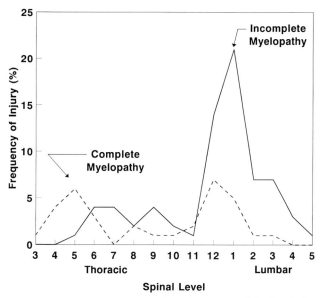

FIGURE 1-26 A representation of the frequency of the level of vertebral injury in patients with traumatic spinal cord injury, contrasting complete myelopathies (no function preserved below the level of injury—*dashed line*) and incomplete myelopathies (some function preserved below the level of injury—*solid line*). Note that in patients with complete myelopathies the curve is shifted to the left. (*From E. Benzel and S. Larson.*[37])

ated increased ability to resist deformity). Therefore, an increased incidence of fractures occurs at this junction (Fig. 1-20).[37]

The transverse processes of the lower thoracic region are often diminutive or rudimentary. This presents problems if instrumentation fixation to the transverse processes is desirable; alternate fixation sites are often necessary.

The Upper and Mid-Lumbar Spine

The vertebral bodies of the upper and mid-lumbar spine are larger and more massive than those at more rostral spinal levels. This, combined with the resumption of a lordotic curvature of the spine in this region, makes this region of the spine relatively resistant to excessive forces. Furthermore, the transition of the spinal cord into the cauda equina (which is more tolerant to trauma than the spinal cord) makes catastrophic spinal injury from trauma less likely (Figs. 1-20 and 1-26).[37]

The Low Lumbar Spine and Lumbosacral Junction

The caudal end of the spinal column is associated with significant logistic therapeutic dilemmas. A frequently observed inability to obtain substantial points of sacral fixation creates a multitude of surgical problems. Similarly, an appropriate bending moment is not often achieved by the instrumentation construct, because of the lack of an adequate length of lever arm below the injury (see below). Fur-

thermore, the relatively steep orientation of the lumbosacral joint exposes the lumbosacral spine to an increased risk of translational deformation (Fig. 1-21).

REFERENCES

1. Berry JL, Moran JM, Berg WS, et al: A morphometric study of human lumbar and selected thoracic vertebrae. *Spine* 1987; 12:362–366.
2. Panjabi MM, Duranceau J, Coel V, et al: Cervical human vertebrae: Quantitative three-dimensional anatomy of the middle and lower regions. *Spine* 1991; 16:861–869.
3. Panjabi MM, Takata K, Coel V, et al: Thoracic human vertebrae: Quantitative three-dimensional anatomy. *Spine* 1991; 16:888–901.
4. White AA, Panjabi MM: *Clinical Biomechanics of the Spine*, 2d ed. Philadelphia; Lippincott, 1990: 1–125.
5. Penning L, Wilmink JT: Rotation of the cervical spine: A CT study in normal subjects. *Spine* 1987; 12:732–738.
6. Bell GH, Dunbar O, Beck JS, et al: Variation in strength of vertebrae with age and their relation to osteoporosis. *Calcif Tissue Res* 1967; 1:75–86.
7. Macintosh JE, Nikolai B: The morphology of the lumbar erector spinae. *Spine* 1987; 12:658–668.
8. Perry O: Fracture of the vertebral end-plate in the lumbar spine. *Acta Orthop Scand* 1957; 25 (suppl): 157–165.
9. Perry O: Resistance and compression of the lumbar vertebrae, in *Encyclopedia of Medical Radiology*. New York; Springer-Verlag, 1974: 215–221.
10. Lin HS, Liu YK, Adams KH: Mechanical response of the lumbar intervertebral joint under physiological (complex) loading. *J Bone Joint Surg* 1978; 60A:41–55.
11. Panjabi M, Dvorak J, Duranceau J, et al: Three-dimensional movements of the upper cervical spine. *Spine* 1988; 13:726–730.
12. Van Schaik JPJ, Verbiest H, Van Schaik FDJ: The orientation of laminae and facet joints in the lower lumbar spine. *Spine* 1985; 10:59–63.
13. White AA, Panjabi MM: The basic kinematics of the human spine: A review of past and current knowledge. *Spine* 1978; 3:12–20.
14. Shirazi-Adl A: Finite element evaluation of contact loads on facets of an L2-L3 lumbar segment in complex loads. *Spine* 1991; 16:533–541.
15. Wall EJ, Cohen MS, Massie JB, et al: Cauda equina anatomy. 1. Intrathecal nerve root organization. *Spine* 1990; 15:1244–1247.
16. Reynolds AF, Roberts A, Pollay M, et al: Quantitative anatomy of the thoracolumbar epidural space. *Neurosurgery* 1985; 17:905–907.
17. Krag MH, Weaver DL, Beynnon BD: Morphometry of the thoracic and lumbar spine related to transpedicular screw placement for surgical spinal fixation. *Spine* 1988; 13:27–32.
18. Zindrick MR, Wiltse LL, Doornik A, et al: Analysis of the morphometric characteristics of the thoracic and lumbar pedicles. *Spine* 1987; 12:160–166.
19. Esses SI, Botsford DJ, Huler RF, et al: Surgical anatomy of the sacrum. *Spine* 1991; 16:283–288.
20. Krag MK, Seroussi RE, Wilder DG, et al: Internal displacement distribution from in vitro loading of human thoracic and lumbar spinal motion segments: Experimental results and theoretical predictions. *Spine* 1987; 12:1001–1007.
21. Broberg KB: On the mechanical behaviour of intervertebral discs. *Spine* 1983; 8:151–165.
22. Chazal J, Tanguy A, Bourges M, et al: Biomechanical properties of spinal ligaments and a histological study of the supraspinal ligament in traction. *J Biomech* 1985; 18:167–176.

23. Dvorak J, Schneider E, Saldinger P, et al: Biomechanics of the craniocervical region: The alar and transverse ligaments. *J Orthop Res* 1988; 6:452–461.
24. Goel VK, Njus GO: Stress-strain characteristic of spinal ligaments. *32d Trans Orthop Res Soc,* New Orleans, 1986: 1–2.
25. Myklebust JB, Pintar F, Yoganandan N, et al: Tensile strength of spinal ligaments. *Spine* 1988; 13:526–531.
26. Nachemson A, Evans J: Some mechanical properties of the third lumbar inter-laminar ligament (ligamentum flavum). *J Biomech* 1968; 1:211–217.
27. Panjabi MM, Hausfeld JN, White AA: A biomechanical study of the ligamentous stability of the thoracic spine in man. *Acta Orthop Scand* 1981; 52:315–326.
28. Panjabi MM, Jorneus L, Greenstein G: Lumbar spine ligaments: An in vitro biomechanical study. *Tenth Meeting of the International Society for the Study of the Lumbar Spine,* Montreal, 1984: 1–3.
29. Posner I, White AA III, Edwards WT, et al: A biomechanical analysis of the clinical stability of the lumbar and lumbosacral spine. *Spine* 1982; 7:374–389.
30. Tkaczuk H: Tensile properties of human lumbar longitudinal ligaments. *Acta Orthop Scand* 1968; 115 (suppl): 1.
31. Panjabi MM, Greenstein G, Duranceau J, et al: Three-dimensional quantitative morphology of lumbar spinal ligaments. *J Spinal Disord* 1991; 4:54–72.
32. Adams MA, Hutton WC: Prolapsed intervertebral disc. A hyperflexion injury. *Spine* 1982; 7:184–191.
33. Panjabi MM: The stabilizing system of the spine. Part II: Neutral zone and instability hypothesis. *J Spinal Disord* 1992; 5:390–397.
34. Cusick JF, Yoganandan N, Pintar FA, et al: Biomechanics of sequential posterior lumbar surgical alterations. *J Neurosurg* 1992: 76:805–811.
35. Tracy MF, Gibson MJ, Szypryt PE, et al: The geometry of the muscles of the lumbar spine determined by magnetic resonance imaging. *Spine* 1989; 14:186–193.
36. Andriacchi TP, Schultz AB, Belytschko TB, et al: A model for studies of mechanical interactions between the human spine and rib cage. *J Biomech* 1974; 7:497–507.
37. Benzel EC, Larson SJ: Functional recovery after decompressive operation for thoracic and lumbar spine fractures. *Neurosurgery* 1986; 19:772–777.
38. Benzel EC, Larson SJ: Functional recovery after decompressive spinal operation for cervical spine fractures. *Neurosurgery* 1987; 20:742–746.
39. Jofe MH, White AA, Panjabi MM: Clinically relevant kinematics of the cervical spine, in The Editorial Committee of the Cervical Spine Research Society (eds): *The Cervical Spine,* 2d ed. Philadelphia; Lippincott, 1989: 57–69.
40. Shapiro R, Youngberg AS, Rothman SLG: The differential diagnosis of traumatic lesions of the occipito-atlanto-axial segment. *Radiol Clin North Am* 1973; 11:505–526.
41. Benzel EC, Kesterson L: Posterior cervical interspinous compression wiring and fusion for mid to low cervical spine injuries. *J Neurosurg* 1989; 70:893–899.
42. Ahmed AM, Duncan NA, Burke DL: The effect of facet geometry on the axial torque-rotation response of lumbar motion segments. *Trans Orthop Res Soc,* Atlanta, 1988:1–10.
43. Taylor JR, Twomey LT: Age changes in lumbar zygapophyseal joints. Observations on structure and function. *Spine* 1986; 11:739–745.

Chapter 2

Physical Principles and Kinematics

INTRODUCTION

Physics is the most fundamental of all sciences. An understanding of the physical principles involved in a discipline such as spine surgery allows one to appreciate actions and reactions, force vectors, and the movements and/or deformations that they cause; and to apply fundamental physical principles to clinical practice.

Kinematics is the study of the motion of rigid bodies. By its nature, it involves the application of physical principles. Thus the disciplines of physics and kinematics cannot be completely separated. Their discussion is necessarily intertwined. A serious attempt has been made herein to minimize discussion of overly technical and clinically unnecessary information. What follows is a distillation of the disciplines of physics and kinematics, intended to emphasize clinically relevant information regarding spinal instrumentation and the pertinent physical principles and laws.

VECTORS, MOMENT ARMS, BENDING MOMENTS, AND AXES OF ROTATION

Forces applied to the spine can always be broken down into component *vectors*. A vector is defined here as a force oriented in a fixed and well-defined direction in three-dimensional space (Fig. 2-1).

A force vector may act on a lever *(moment arm),* causing a *bending moment.* The bending moment applied to a point in space causes rotation, or a tendency to rotate, about an axis. This axis is the *instantaneous axis of rotation (IAR).* In order to establish an easily defined and reproducible coordinate system, the standard Cartesian coordinate system has been applied to the spine. In this system there are three axes: the *x, y,* and *z* axes. About these axes, rotational and translational movements can occur. This results in 12 potential movements about the IAR; two translational movements *along* each of the three axes (one in each direction), and two

rotational movements *around* each of the axes (one in each direction). These potential movements may also be considered in terms of *degrees of freedom;* thus, six degrees of freedom exist about each IAR (Fig. 2-2).

For our purposes, the IAR is the axis about which each vertebral segment rotates at any given instant and is, by definition, the center of the coordinate system (in the plane perpendicular to the IAR) for each motion segment. When a spinal segment moves, there is an axis passing through, or close to, the vertebral body that does not move; this is the axis about which the vertebral body rotates (the IAR). Usually, but not always, it passes through the confines of the vertebral body. Multiple factors, such as degenerative disease, fractures, ligamentous injuries, and instrumentation and/or fusion placement, can affect the position of the IAR (Fig. 2-3).

In a sense, the IAR is a fulcrum. For example, if the spine is flexed, all points ventral to the IAR come closer together and all points dorsal to the IAR move farther apart (Fig. 2-4).

The IAR should be considered dynamic. As spinal movement occurs, the IAR of each involved spinal segment moves. The IAR is derived, in the clinical situation, from dynamic x-rays (i.e., flexion and extension x-rays).

The IAR, however, depends on the method of determination. In the present context the IAR is theoretical. In the unloaded and nonpathological spine, it is assumed to be located within the vertebral body's confines, in the sagittal plane. This assumes that the vertebral body pivots about a point within, ventral, or dorsal to its confines (Fig. 2-5A).

Another theoretical assumption is that flexion or extension, as elicited by adjacent vertebral body flexion or extension about an intervertebral disk, results in the IAR positioned in the region of the intervertebral disk (Fig. 2-5B). Therefore, the location of the IAR depends on the theoretical foundation on which its definition is based and the manner in which it is calculated. The IAR can be determined as by White and Panjabi (Fig. 2-5C).[1] The *center of rotation*

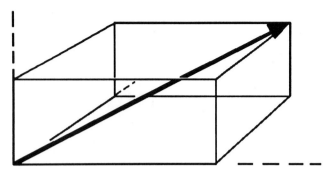

FIGURE 2-1 A force vector in three-dimensional space.

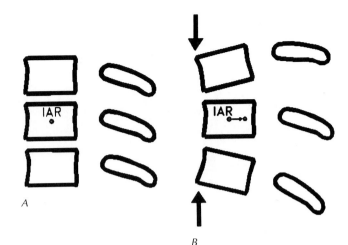

FIGURE 2-3 A depiction of an applied bending moment altering the location of the IAR from the preload situation (*A*) to the postload situation (*B*). Since a ventral bending moment was applied, the IAR, as is often the case, moved dorsally.

(*COR*), as applied by Smith, is similar to the IAR.[2] Its determination and clinical application, however, present problems similar to those encountered with the IAR (Fig. 2-5D).[2,3]

When rotation is superimposed on translation, the resultant component of movement described by the translational movement vector is called the *helical axis of motion (HAM)* (Fig. 2-5E). It is oriented in the direction of the translational movement. A screw motion can be defined, in part, by this parameter. It must be emphasized that *the determination of each of the axes described here is subject to error.*

The concepts of the moment arm and the bending moment are critical to the understanding of spinal biomechanics. The moment arm associated with a spinal implant is defined as that "imaginary lever" that extends from a point (usually the IAR) to the position of application of force to the spine (perpendicular to the direction of the applied force). This is true regardless of the nature of the force's application—whether natural (e.g., from ligaments) or extrinsic (e.g., via instrumentation constructs). The bending

moment (*M*) is defined as the product of the force (*F*) applied to the lever arm and the length of the lever arm (*D*):

$$M = F \times D$$

(where *M* = bending moment, F = applied force, and *D* = the perpendicular distance from the force vector to the IAR) (Fig. 2-6). The bending moment is effectively the torque applied by the force.

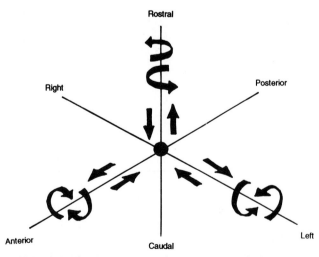

FIGURE 2-2 The Cartesian coordinate system with the IAR as the center. Translation and rotation can occur in both of their respective directions about each axis.

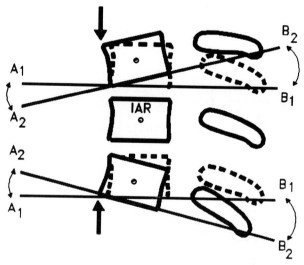

FIGURE 2-4 A depiction of the fulcrum-like nature of the IAR. If spinal flexion occurs, all points ventral to the IAR come closer to each other and all points dorsal to the IAR become farther apart. A_1 and B_1 designate ventral and dorsal points aligned with the vertebral endplates in the neutral position. A_2 and B_2 represent ventral and dorsal points aligned with the vertebral endplates following flexion.

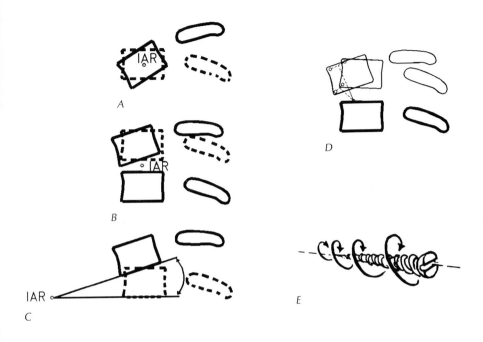

FIGURE 2-5 The determination of the axes of rotation. *A.* The instantaneous axis of rotation (IAR), as applied herein, is the point about which a vertebral body pivots. *B.* The IAR can also be thought of as a point about which two vertebral bodies flex or extend. *C.* The IAR can be determined as by White and Panjabi.[1] *D.* The center of rotation (COR), similar to the IAR, is determined by comparing segmental vertebral positions as illustrated.[2] *E.* The helical axis of motion (HAM). These are all crude methods of describing the center of motion or the axis of motion. Errors of calculation or interpretation can easily occur.

In the pages that follow, some of the discussion and associated illustrations address concepts related to the bending moment. In these illustrations, the bending moment is portrayed by a curved arrow. The maximum bending moment is located at the center of the circle defined by this arrow (i.e., the IAR). (This convention has been applied in Fig. 2-6.)

PARADOXICAL SPINAL MOTION

Paradoxical spinal motion is the unexpected and potentially untoward segmental spinal movement that occurs during the application of flexion, extension, or rotation stresses to the involved spinal segment and adjacent segments. It occurs in two circumstances: (1) in cases of segmental spine instability, and (2) in cases where stabilization techniques (spinal implants or external splints) are used that limit motion between two nonadjacent vertebrae with at least two intervertebral disks located between the termini of the implant or splint (Fig. 2-7). In the case of segmental spine instability, paradoxical movement can occur at adjacent levels. In the case of stabilization techniques, the suspension of vertebral body segments between rigidly immobilized segments allows segmental muscular attachments to effect segmental movement in a paradoxical manner (snaking). *Snaking* is a characteristic type of movement of spinal segments

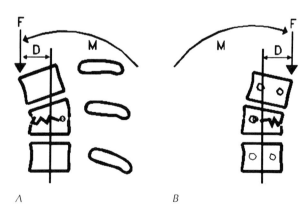

FIGURE 2-6 The bending moment (*M*, depicted by a curved arrow) is the product of the force (*F*) and the length of the moment arm (*D*). The maximum bending moment is located at the center of the circle defined by the radius of the bending moment's arc (i.e., the IAR). *A.* Lateral view. *B.* Anteroposterior view.

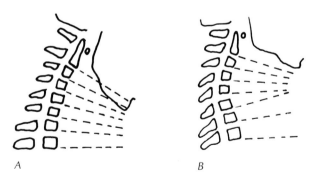

FIGURE 2-7 Paradoxical spinal motion is the phenomenon whereby an intended motion, such as flexion, is accompanied by an unintended motion, such as extension, at one or more motion segments. Paradoxical motion can occur when at least two intervertebral disks are suspended between fixation points (either via external splinting or via spinal instrumentation). *A.* Unobstructed cervical flexion results in uniform segmental flexion in the nonpathological situation. If restriction of movement at the termini of a brace (e.g., halo) is significant, paradoxical spinal motion may occur. *B.* Spinal snaking is a manifestation of the paradoxical spinal motion phenomenon. It is depicted in the case of a rigid external spinal splint.

in response to external force applications; in such movement the sum of movements of individual spinal motion segments is greater than the overall spinal movement observed. In some clinical circumstances it can be objectively assessed.[4] In these cases, it can be quantitated by measuring the overall movement between the rigidly immobilized rostral and caudal components. The result is then subtracted from the sum of the individual intervening segmental movements (the absolute values of each segmental movement are added) (Fig. 2-7).[4]

The paradoxical motion phenomenon may become significant in external spinal splinting or in cases where an instrumented spine is not instrumented at every segmental level. In either case, movement of the suspended spinal segments can occur (between the extremes of the fixation).

MOMENTUM AND NEWTON'S LAWS OF MOTION

Momentum is the product of mass and velocity. Momentum, therefore, is defined in part by *direction;* it demonstrates its vector component in this manner. In order to appropriately appreciate the stresses withstood by the spine, one must understand the fundamental action-reaction phenomenon. An appreciation of the concept of momentum is integral to this process. Let us begin with Sir Isaac Newton's laws of motion, since they describe how objects respond to external force applications.

Newton's first law of motion, the law of inertia, can be stated thus: *If a body is subjected to no net external influence, it has a constant velocity, either zero or nonzero.* As long as there is no force acting on an object, its speed and direction of motion do not change.

Newton's second law of motion, the law of superposition of forces, can be stated thus: *The time rate of momentum of a body is equal in magnitude and direction to the vector sum of the forces acting upon it.* In other words, an object responds to the summation of the forces applied to it.

Newton's third law of motion, the law of conservation of momentum, can be stated thus: *Interactions between objects result in no net change in momentum.* When two objects interact, in a collision, the first body exerts a force on the second. The overall momentum of the two bodies remains constant; that is, any momentum lost by one body is gained by the other. In other words, *for every action there is an equal (in magnitude) but opposite (in direction) reaction.*

FORCE PAIRS

Forces occur in pairs only. When a reflex hammer strikes the patellar tendon, the force exerted by the hammer on the tendon is precisely equal in magnitude to the force exerted by the tendon on the hammer. Similarly, when a force is

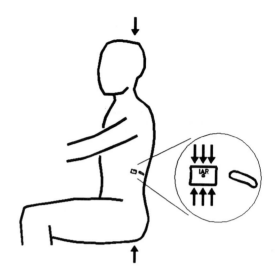

FIGURE 2-8 Forces always occur in pairs. For every action there is an equal but opposite reaction (Newton's third law). If an axial load is applied to a vertebral body, the forces impinging upon the rostral and caudal portions of the vertebral body are equal.

applied to a vertebral body by the application of an axial load, the force applied by the vertebral body on its neighboring vertebral bodies is equal in magnitude, but opposite in direction to the applied force (Fig. 2-8). This is a manifestation of Newton's third law of motion. Deformation, or failure of integrity, of the vertebral body may result.

COUPLES (PARALLEL-AXIS THEOREM FOR MOMENTS)

The physical principle of a *couple* (not to be confused with the phenomenon of coupling—see below) is used to understand this latter point. A couple is a pair of forces, applied to a structure, that are of equal magnitude and opposite direction, having lines of action that are *parallel* but that do not *coincide.* Figure 2-9A illustrates a couple consisting of two forces, each of magnitude F, acting upon a structure and separated by a perpendicular distance D. The resultant force is zero ($F - F = 0$).

The fact that the resultant force is zero means that the couple brings about no *translational* movement of the structure; that is, the structure does not move in a linear manner. The only effect of the couple is to produce *rotation.* By definition, the resultant torque (bending moment) about any arbitrary point (e.g., O) is:

$$\text{resultant torque} = x_1F - x_2F$$
$$= x_1F - (x_1 + D)F = -DF.$$

Since x_1 and x_2 do not appear in the result, the torque of the couple is the same about all points in the plane of the

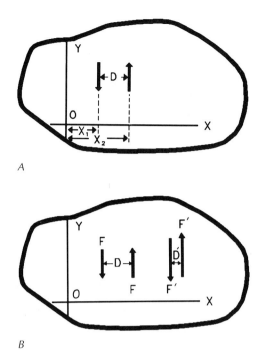

A

B

FIGURE 2-9 *A.* A couple acting upon a structure. In this case, translation will not occur, but rotation will occur if the couple is unopposed. *B.* Two couples of equal magnitude but opposite orientation result in the affected body's remaining in equilibrium. (See text.)

forces forming the couple and is equal to the product of the magnitude of either force and the perpendicular distance between their lines of action. A structure acted upon by a couple can be kept in equilibrium only by another couple of the same moment and the opposite direction. Figure 2-9*B* illustrates this point. The concept of the couple is important, particularly regarding the complex forces applied by instrumentation constructs.

SIMPLE CLINICAL PORTRAYALS OF FORCE PAIRS AND COUPLES

An axial load applied to a vertebral body at the point of the IAR results, by definition, in an equal (in magnitude) but opposite (in direction) reaction force (Fig. 2-8). This pair of forces may result in deformation or failure of the vertebral body, resulting in a burst fracture (Fig. 2-10*A*).

If, however, the load is applied in a plane at some distance from the IAR, a bending moment is created (Fig. 2-6). This bending moment is matched with an equal (in magnitude) but opposite (in direction) reaction bending moment. This pair of forces may similarly result in deformation or failure of the vertebral body, resulting in a wedge compression fracture (Fig. 2-10*B*). This type of deformation or failure may occur in any plane, depending on the point of application of the force vector (load). This is illustrated for

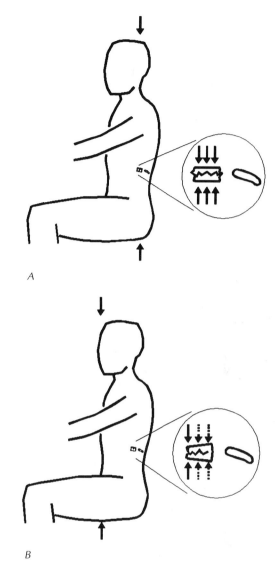

A

B

FIGURE 2-10 *A.* If the load, as applied in Fig. 2-8, is sufficient to result in vertebral body failure, the failure is of a burst-fracture nature. *B.* If, however, a load is applied in a plane ventral to the IAR, an asymmetrical bending moment force pair will be applied to the IAR, resulting in a wedge compression fracture.

a lateral bending component in Fig. 2-11*A* and for a combination anterior and lateral bending component in Fig. 2-11*B*.

HOOKE'S LAW

No solid is perfectly rigid. When several external forces act on a solid at rest and the resultant net force is zero, the solid remains at rest. Its size, or shape, or both, however, will be altered by the external forces; that is, the solid will be deformed. *Hooke's law* states that for small displacements, the size of the deformation is proportional to the deforming force. This law is important when one considers the forces

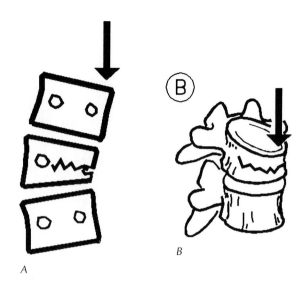

A

B

FIGURE 2-11 The force-pair-generated bending moment, as depicted in Fig. 2-10, may occur in any plane. *A.* Lateral bending. *B.* A combination of flexion and lateral bending.

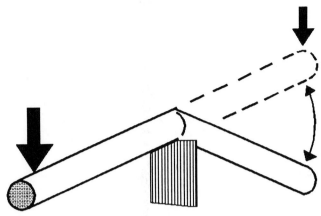

FIGURE 2-13 A rod, if bent over a fulcrum, may incur a permanent set if the stresses incurred were within the plastic zone *(solid lines)* or may return to its original shape *(dotted lines)* if the stresses incurred did not exceed the limits of the elastic zone.

applied to the spine by a spinal instrumentation construct (as well as the response of the construct to these forces).

For larger displacements, however, the *neutral zone* is exceeded and the *elastic limit* is reached. This is the point at which the force departs from the linear relationship between the size of deformation and the deforming force is lost (Fig. 2-12). Exceeding the elastic limit causes the solid to acquire a *permanent set,* so that if the external forces are removed the solid does not spring back to its undeformed configuration (Fig. 2-13). The solid will ultimately fail if further forces are applied. This point is the *point of failure.* For most materials, the elastic limit occurs close to the point where a permanent set is produced. Figure 2-12 depicts these points.

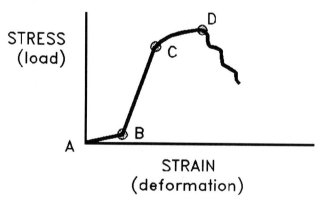

FIGURE 2-12 A typical stress/strain curve for a biological tissue, such as a ligament. *AB,* the neutral zone. *BC,* the elastic zone. When the elastic limit (*c*) is reached, permanent deformation can occur (permanent set). *CD,* the plastic zone where a permanent set occurs. Past *D,* failure occurs and the load diminishes.

ELASTIC MODULUS

For small deformations, Hooke's law applies, using the *elastic modulus:*

$$\text{elastic modulus} = \frac{\text{stress}}{\text{strain}}$$

where the elastic modulus is a constant that is characteristic of a given material. *Stress* is defined as the force applied to an object (load), while *strain* is defined as the response of the object to the force (deformation).

Three types of elastic moduli exist: *Young's modulus,* a measure of the elastic properties of a body that is stretched or compressed; *shear modulus,* a measure of the shear deformation experienced by a body that is subjected to transverse forces of equal and opposite direction, applied at opposite faces of the body; and *bulk modulus,* the elastic deformation of a solid when it is squeezed.

SECTION MODULUS AND THE MOMENT OF INERTIA

In order to understand the properties of spinal implants and instrumentation constructs, two additional concepts are needed: that of the *section modulus* (Z) and that of the *moment of inertia* (I). The section modulus is an indicator of the strength of an object, such as a rod or screw. The moment of inertia is an indicator of the object's stiffness and is a measure of an object's distribution about its centroid (e.g., the center of the rod). Considering a rod with a diameter *D*, the section modulus (*Z*) is defined by the equation:

$$Z = \frac{\pi \times D^3}{32}$$

The moment of inertia (*I*) is defined by the equation:

$$I = \frac{\pi \times D^4}{16}$$

It is quite obvious, therefore, that the diameter of a rod (or the core diameter of a screw) substantially affects strength (resistance to failure in flexion) and stiffness (to the third and the fourth power, respectively).

Stress (*θ*) is a measurement of the force per unit area applied to a structure and is defined by the equation:

$$\theta = \frac{\text{bending moment}}{Z}$$

Strain is the change in length or angle of a material subjected to a load. Strain may be either normal (linear) or shear (angular) in nature. Normal strain reflects tensile or compressive force-resisting abilities of a material; shear strain reflects angular deformation-resisting abilities of a material.

COUPLING

Coupling is the phenomenon whereby a movement of the spine obligates a separate movement about another axis. In the cervical region, for example, lateral bending results in rotation of the spinous processes away from the concave side of the direction of the bend. This is due, in part, to the orientation of the facet joints, as well as to the presence of the uncovertebral joints. In the lumbar region, however, the coupling movements associated with lateral bending are in the opposite direction, with the spinous processes rotating

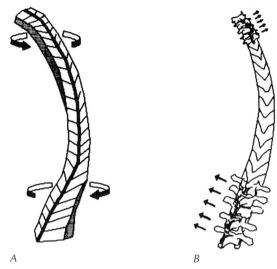

A   *B*

FIGURE 2-14 Perhaps the most important manifestation of the coupling phenomenon is the relationship between lateral bending and rotation in the cervical and lumbar regions. This is depicted diagramatically (*A*) and anatomically (*B*). Note that the coupling phenomenon results in rotation, in opposite directions, of these two regions. Also note that the thoracic spine does not exhibit significant coupling.

in the same direction as the concave side of the direction of the bend. The phenomenon of coupling also explains the association of the obligatory rotatory component associated with degenerative scoliosis of the lumbar spine (Fig. 2-14).

REFERENCES

1. White AA, Panjabi MM: *Clinical Biomechanics of the Spine*, 2d ed. Philadelphia: Lippincott, 1990: 1–125.
2. Smith TM, Fernie GR: Functional biomechanics of the spine. *Spine* 1991; 16:1197–1203.
3. Gertzbein SD, Holtby R, Tile M, et al: Determination of a locus of instantaneous centers of rotation of the lumbar disc by Moire fringes: A new technique. *Spine* 1984; 9:409–413.
4. Benzel EC, Hadden TA, Saulsbery CM: A comparison of the Minerva and halo jackets for stabilization of the cervical spine. *J Neurosurg* 1989; 70:411–414.

Chapter 3

Stability and Instability of the Spine

TRADITIONAL CONCEPTS

White and Panjabi define *clinical stability of the spine* as the ability of the spine under physiological loads to limit patterns of displacement so as not to damage or irritate the spinal cord or nerve roots and, in addition, to prevent incapacitating deformity or pain due to structural changes.[1] Spinal stability is a phenomenon of increments (shades of gray, so to speak); it is not absolutely present or absent. Depending on circumstances, the spine is expected to provide varying degrees of support (stability). Therefore, spinal stability should be defined according to circumstances.

The converse of stability, obviously, is *instability*. Whereas stability is difficult to define, instability is somewhat more easily quantitated and assessed. A consideration of instability is perhaps more appropriate clinically and is, therefore, undertaken here.

Instability should, perhaps, be defined more generally, with specific consideration given to the type of instability. *Instability* is the inability to limit excessive or abnormal spinal displacement. The use of the word "excessive" reflects the difficulty of quantitation in clinical spine medicine. An attempt to impart an understanding of, and a sense of how to deal with, the uncertainty associated with the quantitation of instability is undertaken below.

There are two fundamental categories of instability: acute and chronic. Acute instability may be broken down into two subcategories: overt and limited. Chronic instability can likewise be broken down into two subgroups: glacial instability and the instability associated with dysfunctional segmental motion (see below).

THE QUANTITATION OF ACUTE INSTABILITY

One has only to read the voluminous literature on acute spinal instability and the definitions thereof to appreciate the difficulties associated with this definition process.[2–24] Numerous authors have tried to quantitate the degree or extent of acute instability by a point-system approach. White and Panjabi described a region-specific point system in which an accumulation of 5 or more points indicated the presence of an unstable spine. Their regional point system emphasizes differences between the cervical, thoracic and thoracolumbar, and lumbar regions.[1] These are essentially assessments of overt and limited instability, as defined below.

Stability determination algorithms are ultimately intended to delineate the most appropriate management scheme in any given clinical situation. This does not rely significantly on regional differences within the spine. In this vein, the multiple schemes for the determination of the extent of acute instability of White and Panjabi[1] are combined here into a scheme that is not region-specific (Table 3-1). It must be recognized that the determination of the extent of acute instability is often difficult and, in addition, depends on the philosophy or orientation of the surgeon and on the limitations of the available diagnostic armamentarium.

In light of the foregoing, White and Panjabi recommended a stretch test for the assessment of acute cervical spine instability.[1] This involves progressive addition of cervical traction weight (to 33 percent of the patient's weight) with serial radiographic and clinical assessments. A positive test (indicating the presence of instability) is one that shows a disk interspace separation of more than 1.7 mm or a change in angle between vertebrae of more than 7.5 degrees between the prestretch and poststretch conditions. The merits of this test are uncertain. First, it is clearly not without risks, whether those risks be immediately obvious or occult. The risk of the tethering of the spinal cord over a ventral mass goes without saying. Perhaps the most significant and least immediately recognized risk of such a procedure is the risk of a false-negative test—that is, the seeming presence of stability in an unstable situation. This is in spite of the fact that the test has been used as a determinant of eligibility for participation in contact sports. One must remember that, particularly in athletes, the resistance to

TABLE 3-1 Quantitation of acute instability in subaxial cervical, thoracic, and lumbar injuries[a] (point system[b])

Condition	Points assigned
Loss of integrity of anterior (and middle) column[c]	2
Loss of integrity of posterior column(s)[c]	2
Acute resting translational deformity[d]	2
Acute resting angulation deformity[d]	2
Acute dynamic translation deformity exaggeration[e]	2
Acute dynamic angulation deformity exaggeration[e]	2
Neural element injury[f]	3
Acute disk narrowing at level of suspected pathology	1
Dangerous loading anticipated	1

[a]Modified from White and Panjabi,[1] with care taken to avoid duplication or overlapping of point criteria.

[b]A score of 5 points or more implies the presence of overt instability (see text). A score of 2 to 4 points implies the presence of limited instability (see text).

[c]By clinical examination, MRI, CT, or x-ray. A single point may be allotted if incomplete evidence exists; e.g., only MRI evidence of posterior ligamentous injury (i.e., evidence of only interspinous ligament injury on T2-weighted images). Columns are defined as per Bailey, Denis, and Louis.[25,26,28]

[d]From static resting anteroposterior and lateral spine x-rays. Must be the result of an acute clinical process. Tolerance for this criterion is variable with respect to surgeon and clinical circumstances. Guidelines as per White and Panjabi.[1]

[e]From dynamic (flexion and extension) spine x-rays. Recommended only after other mechanisms of instability assessment have been exhausted, and then only by an experienced clinician. Usually indicated only in cervical region. Must be the result of an acute clinical process. Tolerance for this criterion is variable with respect to surgeon's opinion and clinical circumstances. Guidelines as per White and Panjabi.[1]

[f]Three points for cauda equina, 2 points for spinal cord, or 1 point for isolated nerve root neurological deficit. *The presence of neural element injury indicates that a significant spinal deformation occurred at the time of impact, implying that structural integrity may well have been disturbed.*

stretching by muscle action (voluntary or involuntary) may easily conceal ligamentous deficiencies.

One must keep in mind that flexion and extension x-rays may not be helpful, and in fact may be misleading, following trauma. If pathology is observed and iatrogenic injury via the act of flexion and extension is not incurred, they are useful. However, they are not without risk if spinal instability is present. Perhaps their greatest risk is the fact that a "normal" flexion-extension x-ray, which implies a safe clinical situation, indeed may not reflect a normal situation. (That is, the test may be false-negative.) Incomplete patient cooperation and "guarding" against excessive spinal movement due to underlying acute pathology can disguise a pathological process that may lead to catastrophe if treated improperly.

Determination of the presence of more chronic forms of instability should be considered separately. These clinical situations are obviously different, as are the surgeon's expectations and the patient's risks.

"Column" Concepts of Spinal Integrity

Many instability definition schemes use point systems to quantitate the extent of spinal integrity (or loss thereof) and to ultimately determine the presence or absence of spinal stability (see Table 3-1). These schemes are usually based on a "column" concept of spinal structural integrity, such as those described by Louis; by Bailey, Holdsworth, and Kelly and Whitesides; and by Denis (Fig. 3-1).[13,25–28] The consideration of "columns" in defining the extent of instability is of some value, since it helps the physician to conceptualize and categorize case-specific phenomena. The three-column (one anterior and two lateral columns) theory of Louis[28] is based on the fact that the spine bears weight principally by the acceptance of axial loads along the three vertical bony and soft tissue columns—the vertebral body and intervertebral disks, and the two facet joint complexes—at each segmental level (Fig. 3-1). Although this is indeed true, the concept of Louis assists in the instability assessment process only when predominantly axial loads are considered. It assesses bony-component failure much more effectively than soft-tissue-component failure, because of its obvious association with the bony columns of the spine (vertebral body and facet joints). This aspect of stability is easily assessed by x-ray and CT. It can be quantitated by assessing the extent of collapse or fracture. However, except for the case of significant vertebral body failure, a correlation between the extent of bony injury and the presence of overt

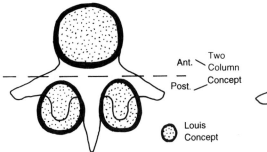
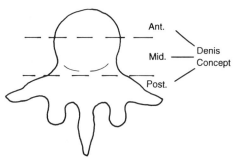

FIGURE 3-1 The ''column'' concepts of spinal instability. The concept described by Louis (*left*) assigns significance to the vertebral body and the facet joint complexes (lateral masses) on either side of the dorsal spine. Denis's three-column concept (*right*) assigns significance to the region of the neutral axis and the integrity of the posterior vertebral body wall (the middle column). The two-column construct (*left*) relies on anatomically defined structures, the vertebral body (anterior column) and the posterior elements (posterior column). Louis's three-column concept (*left*) similarly relies on anatomically defined structures. (*From White and Panjabi.*[1])

spinal instability may be tenuous. Furthermore, the three-column theory of Louis does not facilitate the assessment of the distraction, flexion, and extension components of the injury.

The two- and three-column concepts of Bailey, Holdsworth, and Kelly and Whitesides (two-column) and Denis (three-column)[13,25–27] are more applicable to this situation (Fig. 3-1). They not only assist in assessing the bony collapse associated with axial load-bearing, but also offer insight in the assessment of the distraction, flexion, and extension components of the injury (i.e., injury to the posterior elements) of the spinal column. Denis's three-column theory, which adds the concept of a middle column to the two-column theories, allows specific assessment of that component of the spinal column in the region of the *neutral axis*. The neutral axis is that longitudinal region of the spinal column that bears a significant portion of the axial load and about which spinal element distraction or compression does not excessively occur with flexion or extension (Fig. 3-2). Usually, the neutral axis is located in the region of the midpos-

terior aspect of the vertebral body; that is, the middle column of Denis. Usually it encompasses the instantaneous axis of rotation (IAR) in the sagittal plane (see Chap. 2).

The three columns of Denis[26] are conceptually useful for the determination of the presence or absence of acute instability. The point system used here employs his scheme.

CATEGORIZATION OF INSTABILITY

In order to facilitate the understanding and, hence, the clinical application of the terms *stability* and *instability*, a more simplistic approach is taken here for the subaxial cervical, thoracic, and lumbar spine. This is done because strict criteria for the universal definition of stability and instability are impossible to derive. Therefore, one must realize up front that the clinical decision-making process, as it pertains to the definition of instability, is somewhat tenuous, and that it relies heavily on clinical judgment and the surgeon's intuition.

FIGURE 3-2 The depiction of the neutral axis (*shaded areas*). The neutral axis is the longitudinal region of the spinal column that bears much of the axial load and about which spinal element distraction or compression does not significantly occur with the assumption of flexed (*A*), neutral (*B*), or extension (*C*) postures.

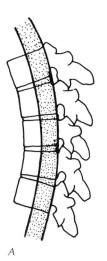
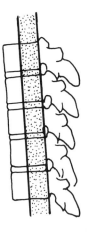
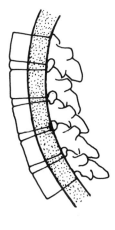

A   *B*   *C*

Instability is divided herein into two categories: acute and chronic. Each is unique. However, neither of these categories is clearly defined. Each uses, at least in part, the concepts of each of the column theories discussed.

Instability, being a phenomenon that is unique to a specific clinical circumstance, is most appropriately defined separately for each category, as opposed to the schemes of White and Panjabi, which define instability in a global sense but quantitate it on a region-specific basis.[1] The scheme used here for acute instability categorizes instability (overt and limited; see below) with regard to the potential for catastrophe. The scheme used here also differs from that of White and Panjabi by its deemphasis of region-specificity.

Four subcategories of instability are also defined here. These are referred to throughout the text. These categories are (1) overt instability, (2) limited instability, (3) glacial instability, and (4) the instability associated with dysfunctional segmental motion (Table 3-2). The first two are acute and the second two chronic. None are applicable to all clinical situations. Overt and limited instability are applicable to acute posttraumatic situations or cases of spinal involvement by tumor or infection. Thus the relatively acute disruption of spinal integrity is implied. Both of these categories of instability may have a chronic component as well. For example, if an overtly unstable spine is not surgically stabilized and does not acquire stability nonoperatively, the acute overt instability persists into a chronic phase. Similarly, if a spine with acute limited instability does not heal properly, excessive ligamentous laxity may persist and become chronic. The latter may be difficult to differentiate, at times, from glacial instability or dysfunctional segmental motion. Glacial instability and dysfunctional segmental motion are usually manifestations of a process more chronic than overt or limited instability. They are usually associated with degenerative disease or the long-term sequelae of trauma, tumor, or infection.

The point system presented here for overt and limited instability (acute instability, Table 3-1) is relatively independent of spinal level (excepting the occiput and upper cervical spine). It depends, instead, on the category of spinal instability considered. Therefore, Table 3-1 is appropriate for consideration only with regard to the delineation of the presence or absence of acute spinal instability.

In any given clinical situation one may ask if overt instability, limited instability, glacial instability, or dysfunctional segmental motion exists. If none of these are present, the spine is stable. If instability exists in one or more of these subcategories, the decision-making process is dictated by the clinical situation and the anticipated loads to be applied to the spine.

Ultimately, the need to define the subcategory of instability present in any given clinical situation is based on the need to attend to the patient's pathology. Obviously, there are numerous potential options for treatment. These include surgery for decompression and/or stabilization, bed rest, external splinting, and medications for pain and/or inflammation. Each subcategory of instability, therefore, is associated with a series of indications for treatment and for the type of treatment scheme to be used. These schemes may be complex. They should, however, be clearly established in the mind of the clinician. As long as the surgeon's scheme is individually "thought out" and based on sound principles, it should serve the surgeon (and the patient) well.

In order to optimize patient management, the spine surgeon should first determine the extent of instability present. Then must be considered the patient's symptoms (complaints), the category of instability, the extent of neurological compromise, the risks of further neurological injury, and the desires and concerns of the patient. For example, a patient with a spine injury that is moderately unstable (fractured facet joint with posterior interspinous ligament disruption identified clinically and by MRI; i.e., limited instability) is at moderate risk for deformity progression and delayed neurological injury. Therefore, the surgeon could recommend stabilization and fusion surgery. If the patient agrees, the surgery should be performed if it is not medically contraindicated. On the other hand, a patient who has significant laxity at the L4-L5 motion segment (dysfunctional segmental motion), but whose symptoms have responded to conservative management, should *not* have surgery—regardless of the patient's desires. In the former case, surgery is used as a management option to prevent further harm. In the latter case, in spite of the presence of an unstable spine (ligamentous laxity; dysfunctional segmental motion), the patient is without symptoms and should not have surgery. *Spinal instability has widely disparate implications in different clinical circumstances.* In the former case the ability of the spine to resist "excessive" displacement was thought to be deficient, requiring surgical stabilization. In the latter case it was not thought to be deficient, since the laxity was not progressive and did not cause refractory pain or neurological deficit.

The terms *overt instability* and *limited instability* are applicable to situations where there is a risk of acute loss of stability. The term *glacial instability* is applicable in more chronic situations. Glacial instability is confirmed by serial assessments or by incriminating evidence (e.g., a translational deformation of the spine in the presence of a pain syndrome consistent with the deformation). The term *dysfunctional segmental motion* is much less objectively defined. It

---

TABLE 3-2   Instability categorization scheme

Acute instability
    Overt instability
    Limited instability
Chronic instability
    Glacial instability
    Dysfunctional segmental motion

applies to situations where overt or limited clinical instability is not present, but where pain, combined with abnormal significant spinal motion, is present. Each is defined below.

ACUTE INSTABILITY

Overt Instability

Overt instability is defined as the inability of the spine to support the torso during normal activity. This situation occurs most commonly following trauma or surgical intervention, or in the face of neoplasia, advanced degenerative disease, or infection. With an overtly unstable spine, the integrity of the spine is insufficient to prevent the sudden development (or exaggeration) of spinal deformity. For overt instability to occur, a loss of integrity of the vertebral body and/or disk, such as occurs following a compression fracture (see below), must be associated with a loss of integrity of the posterior elements (posterior columns). This results in a circumferential loss of spinal integrity.[29] The patient illustrated in Fig. 3-3 has an overtly unstable spine. All three columns are disrupted. The usual treatment of choice is surgical stabilization and decompression, followed by bracing (Fig. 3-3).

Posterior ligamentous disruption (particularly of the interspinous ligament) is difficult to assess by CT. Plain x-rays are helpful only if the spinous processes are splayed. Clinical examination is often more useful than all non-MRI imaging modalities for the determination of the presence of posterior column disruption. The presence of pain to palpation over the fracture level, or a loss of midline soft tissue definition (loss of the midline crease over the spinous processes), implicates posterior soft tissue disruption (Fig. 3-4) and, therefore, posterior spinal instability.

MRI may be useful in the assessment of overt instability. MRI clearly delineates soft tissue changes consistent with trauma (Fig. 3-5). Table 3-1 presents a point system that can be used to assist the surgeon in the decision-making process. This system uses MRI when the delineation of soft tissue disruption may be useful for the establishment of the loss of spinal integrity (e.g., the demonstration of posterior column disruption). Often the MRI may not be necessary. However, when the determination of soft tissue injury is imperative, it is invaluable.

Limited Instability

Injuries such as the obvious overtly unstable injury illustrated in Fig. 3-3 are clear-cut. Lesser injuries, however, present more of a diagnostic and decision-making dilemma.[29] *Limited instability* is defined as the loss of *either* ventral or dorsal spinal integrity, with the preservation of the other—which is sufficient to support some normal activities. If both ventral and dorsal loss of integrity are

present, overt instability usually exists. The ventral type is often associated with an isolated endplate or vertebral body fracture. A true burst fracture resulting in a collapse of the vertebral body, without other focal injuries to the spinal elements at or near the affected spinal level(s), should be considered such an injury (Fig. 3-6*A* and *B*). The dorsal type is either ligamentous (a spinal strain, of sorts) and/or bony (the result of laminar or facet fracture) in nature. Acutely, MRI aids in the definition of this type of instability, as it does with overt instability (Fig. 3-6*C*).[30,31] Under most circumstances conservative nonoperative management, using bracing, is the treatment of choice if neural decompression is not a consideration. Surgery may be indicated if there is a significant risk of chronic instability.

Not uncommonly, overt instability is mistaken for limited instability. An underestimation of the extent of either ventral or dorsal spinal injury may lead to this misinterpretation—a misinterpretation less likely if MRI is liberally employed. Delayed deformity progression may result. In this situation, overt instability may evolve into a chronic state (glacial instability).

Chronic forms of both overt and limited instability exist. If either of these types of instability does not heal following the acute phase, the instability may persist and evolve into a chronic phase. In this phase MRI may be less useful in instability definition, because of its relative inability to depict ligamentous injury after soft tissues have healed.

A Point System

The differentiation between overt and limited instability can be difficult, if not impossible, in some cases. The extent of vertebral body height loss or the extent of posterior ligamentous injury often bears on the diagnosis. A point system, as depicted in Table 3-1, may be helpful in this process. With this system, regardless of where in the subaxial spine the injury is located, a score of 5 or more points indicates overt instability and a score of 2 to 4 points indicates limited instability. *However, the spine surgeon must rely on common sense combined with clinical astuteness. If this or any other scheme is used without these two faculties, errors will be common. There is no substitute for common sense.*

In most cases MRI, combined with plain spine x-ray, is more sensitive than other imaging modalities in the diagnosis of an unstable spine. MRI is particularly useful in determining the extent of instability. It allows the surgeon to accurately assess the integrity of the middle column of Denis and, thus, the extent of neural impingement. More important, however, it is the only imaging modality that provides direct information on the presence or absence, and the extent, of injury to ligamentous structures. T2 sagittal images are most useful in this regard.[30] T2 images provide the clearest definition of ligamentous and other soft tissue injury (Fig. 3-5). Axial images are relatively unhelpful.

An important consideration in the use of MRI for the

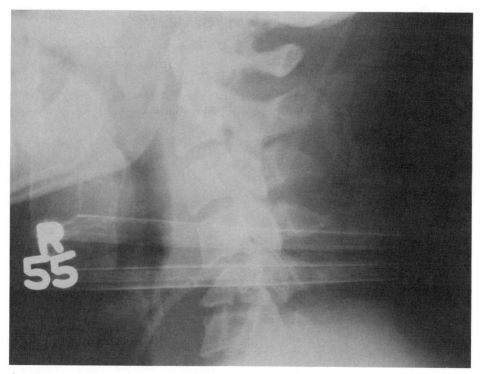

A

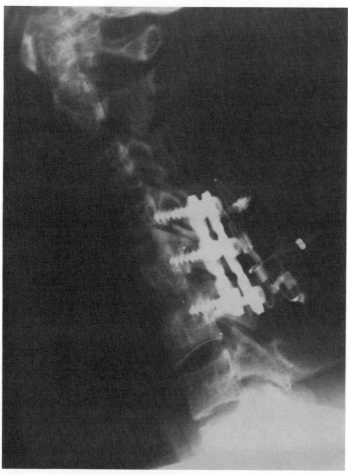

B

FIGURE 3-3 The lateral x-ray (*A*) of a patient who incurred a circumferential disruption of the spinal column. This overtly unstable spine demonstrates disruption of all columns of each of the column systems. Circumferential (anterior and posterior) stabilization may be necessary in this case (*B*).

determination of spinal integrity is the field strength of the scanner. High-field-strength scanners (1.0 to 1.5 T) give high resolution, but offer relatively poor differentiation between soft tissue types (contrast between tissues). On the other hand, low-field-strength scanners (0.064 to 0.5 T) provide less resolution but offer greater contrast between tissues. The greater ability of low-field-strength scanners to differentiate between noninjured and injured tissues, by visualizing blood or edema, is useful (Fig. 3-7A and B).[30,31]

CHRONIC INSTABILITY

Glacial Instability

Glacial instability is defined as spinal instability that is not overt and that does not pose a significant chance of the rapid development or progression of kyphotic, scoliotic, or translational deformities; but in which, as in the motion of a glacier, the deformity progresses gradually, and substantial external forces do not cause immediate movement or progression of deformity.[29] Glacial instability is chronic. It may or may not be associated with a potential for catastrophic spinal column disruption following the application of submaximal external loads. MRI does not demonstrate evidence of acute soft tissue injury. Serial spine x-rays, however, may demonstrate deformity progression over time (usually months or years). This type of instability may take the form of a progressive translational, rotational, or angulation deformity. Treatment may range from no treatment at all to surgical stabilization. The decision-making process must take into account the nature of the relationship of the neural elements to their bony and soft tissue confines, the possibility of impending or worsening neurological deficit, the possibility of unsightly deformity, and the subjective complaint of pain.

There are various etiologies of glacial instability: spondylosis, trauma, tumor, congenital defect, and infection. The most common glacial instability is the type associated with lumbar spondylolisthesis, either degenerative, iatrogenic, or isthmic. Excessive mobility and progressive slippage (deformity progression) may be present. This implies the presence, along with glacial instability, of dysfunctional segmental motion.

Following trauma or other spine-deforming pathological processes (degenerative disease, tumor, or infection), a biomechanically disadvantageous situation may exist wherein deformity progression is encouraged by an increased length of an applied moment arm. This may be compounded by the presence of posterior ligamentous laxity, which first may have been manifest as posterior ligamentous instability. The inability to limit flexion, combined with a tendency to flex, may cause a progressive flexion deformity.

Cancer or infection may destabilize the spine so that progressive deformation occurs, but overt instability is not yet present. Pain most often coexists, as it often does with other

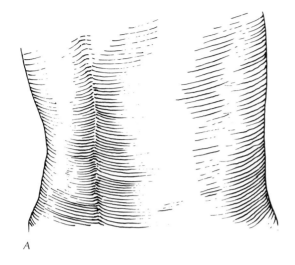
A

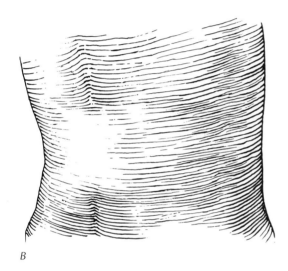
B

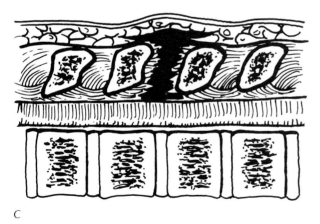
C

FIGURE 3-4 Posterior instability in the thoracic and lumbar region can be suggested, particularly in thin patients, by physical examination. The presence of tenderness over the spinous processes or the absence of the normal midline crease (*A*), on account of swelling or hematoma formation below the skin (*B*), suggests underlying soft tissue injury (*C*). This, in turn, suggests—but does not prove—the presence of posterior spinal instability.

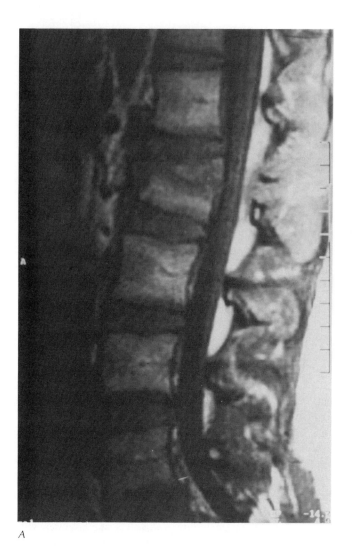

A

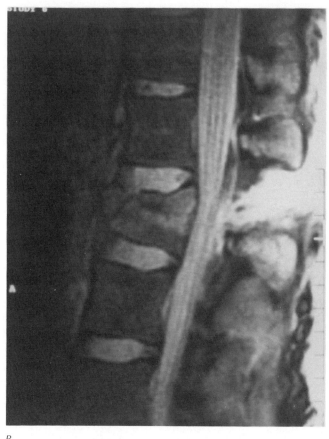

B

FIGURE 3-5 An MRI scan may confirm the presence of paraspinous (interspinous) soft tissue injury. In cases showing no other evidence of posterior injury, except perhaps cervical tenderness, MRI may be particularly helpful. Note the increased signal intensity in the interspinous regions, projecting ventrally to the level of the ligamentum flavum. The T1-weighted image (*A*) is less revealing in this regard than the T2-weighted image (*B*).

glacially unstable situations. This helps in establishing the diagnosis.

Dynamic x-rays (flexion and extension films) may be useful for the establishment of the diagnosis of associated dysfunctional motion segment (see below); for example, they may demonstrate excessive or inappropriate movement. As previously emphasized, if excessive movement is not present on dynamic imaging, the absence of instability cannot be assumed. Pain and guarding may result in a protection from movement that might have been demonstrated if the pain and guarding were not present. This is true for all subcategories of instability.

Dysfunctional Segmental Motion

A *dysfunctional motion segment* involves neither the overt disruption of spinal integrity nor deformity progression.

Most patients with glacial instability can also be considered to have a dysfunctional motion segment. However, all types of glacial instability have, as a component of their instability, deformity progression, with or without excessive motion. Dysfunctional segmental motion is defined as *a type of instability related to disk interspace or vertebral body degenerative changes, tumor, or infection that results in the potential for pain of spinal origin.* The mere concept of dysfunctional segmental motion is controversial; the diagnosis is most often conjectured and is infrequently clearly and objectively established. The associated instability has also been called *mechanical instability,* among other things. The term *dysfunctional segmental motion* is used here because of its less controversial nature and its more accurate reflection of the suspected pathological process involved.

A characteristic pain pattern (usually worsened by activity and improved by rest and the positioning of the torso in

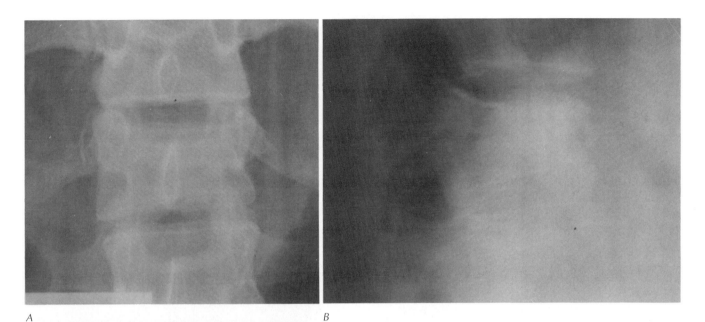

A   *B*

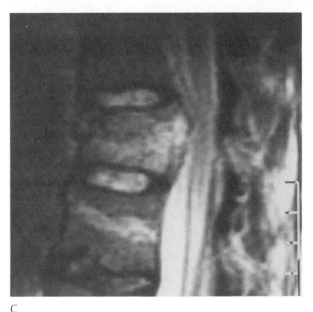

FIGURE 3-6 Anteroposterior (*A*) and lateral (*B*) x-rays of a thoracolumbar fracture. The x-rays suggest that posterior instability is not present, via the demonstration of normal posterior element relationships. *C*. An MRI scan confirms the absence of posterior element injury. This fracture, therefore, has a 2- or 3-point score (depending on the anticipated loading) by the scheme outlined in the text and in Table 3-1. Hence it is not overtly unstable (limited instability).

C

such a manner that spinal stresses are minimized) suggests the diagnosis. This pain pattern is similar to that associated with glacial instability. When this pain pattern is combined with degenerative disk interspace changes or tumor or infection involving either the disk interspace, the vertebral body, or some other vertebral component, the diagnosis of dysfunctional segmental motion is suggested. The pain pattern implicates an exaggeration of reflex muscle activity that is enlisted in order to maintain an acceptable amount of spinal stability (implying that adequate intrinsic stability is not provided by the spine proper). Plain x-rays, MRI, and diskography have been touted as useful for the diagnosis of a spinal pain generator (harbinger of the symptoms associated with dysfunctional segmental motion). A lack of objective data, however, impugns these techniques. Plain x-rays

offer the greatest advantage for clearly assessing potentially dysfunctional motion segments (Fig. 3-8). MRI demonstrates changes in the bone and in the disk interspace. Although MRI is extremely useful for the diagnosis of overt and limited instability, its sensitivity for detecting degenerative and inflammatory changes in the spine minimizes its utility in the diagnosis of dysfunctional segmental motion. Hence it is more useful for determining instability in acute situations than in chronic ones.

Although diskography demonstrates degenerative changes in the disk interspace, with provocative tests used to select painful joints, it, like MRI, is not discerning as a diagnostic tool for the determination of the cause of disk-related pain. As with MRI, convincing correlations with surgical outcome are lacking. Bone scanning has also been used

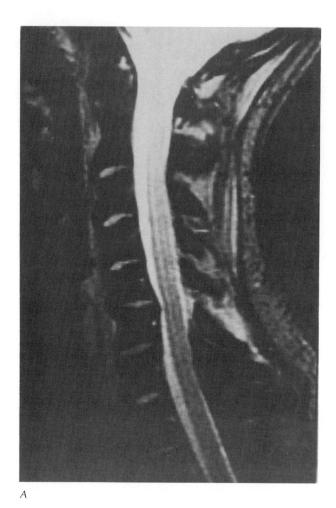

A

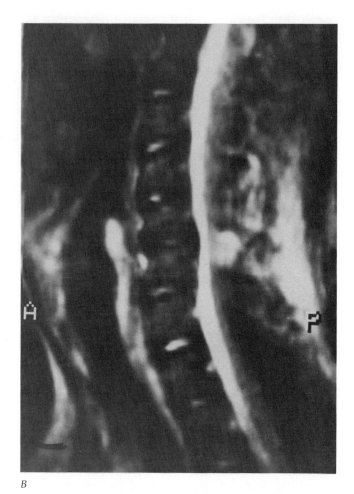

B

FIGURE 3-7 The field strength of an MRI scanner is a factor in both anatomic resolution definition and soft tissue injury definition. A high-field-strength scanner (1.5 T) has better anatomic resolution but worse soft tissue injury definition sensitivity than a low-field-strength scanner (0.064 T). This is illustrated by images from one patient who underwent MRI scans by both techniques within a short period. *A.* High-field-strength scan. *B.* Low-field-strength scan.

to define unstable spinal segments (or, at least, the spinal segments contributing to pain). It, likewise, has not been proven to be clinically useful.

The presence of dysfunctional segmental motion, as ascertained by abnormal segmental movement demonstrated radiographically or by determination of the IAR or of the center of rotation (COR),[32-40] may aid in this aspect of diagnosis. These types of movement may not be obvious on flexion and extension x-rays. Exaggerated examples are depicted in Fig. 3-9. In fact, the case presented in Fig. 3-8 may represent not only translational movement but also a pivoting movement. Techniques for discerning pathological motion are important for the accurate determination of the "appropriate" level(s) for fusion.

Dysfunctional segmental motion may be implied by the observation of excessive degenerative changes at a given segmental level. For this degeneration to have occurred, excessive stresses or motion must have been predisposing factors in the disk interspace changes.

Variations in the method of calculation of the IAR or COR may lead to differing results. For example, the use of different vertebral bodies as the "standard" can result in misleading determinations. Hence one must be careful in this regard if the precise location of the IAR is used to determine a clinical management scheme. This underscores the artificial nature of IAR and COR calculations. The IAR and COR are relative. Similarly calculated IARs can be compared with each other, but not with IARs determined by other techniques.

It cannot be overemphasized that the lack of objectivity makes the diagnosis of dysfunctional segmental motion often controversial and, simultaneously, subject to abuse. Fusion and instrumentation operations are lucrative to the surgeon. Likewise, the diagnostic algorithm used is often lucrative to the diagnostician. These factors, combined with the inability to objectively assess either operative indications or surgical results, enhance the potential for abuse in the establishment of this diagnosis.

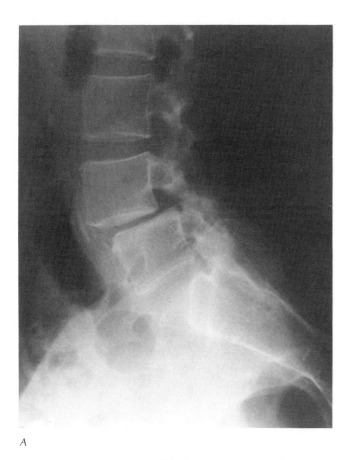

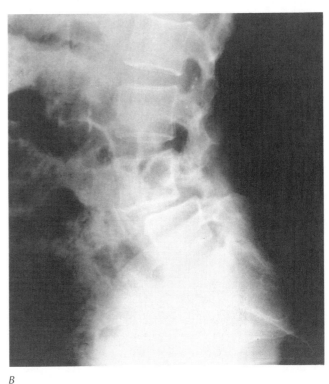

A

B

FIGURE 3-8 The presence of dysfunctional segmental motion is suggested on plain x-ray by disk interspace degeneration or excessive segmental spinal movement. Flexion (*A*) and extension (*B*) lumbar spine x-rays demonstrate these points.

THE CONTRIBUTION OF THE RIB CAGE AND MUSCLES TO STABILITY

The Rib Cage

The ribs and sternum make an important contribution to stability in the mid- and upper thoracic spine. The two entities function together to enhance stability. The costovertebral joints play a pivotal role in this process[1,41]; the role of the costosternal joints may be even more significant. The

bony cylindrical shell about the chest provides an added degree of stiffness to the spine.

The stiffness of the spine is greatly increased if all parts of the rib cage are intact. The intact rib cage augments the axial load-resisting ability of the spine fourfold. The removal or loss of either the ribs themselves or their attachment to an intact sternum nearly completely negates this advantage (Fig. 3-10).[1]

FIGURE 3-9 Dysfunctional segmental motion is present if a smooth flexion or extension does not occur at the motion segment in question. This can be assessed by determination of the location of the IAR (Chap. 2). Several types of dysfunctional segmental motion can occur: true translation (*A*), excessive angulation (with flexion or extension) without translation (*B*), translation with angulation (*C*), and pivotal movement about a pathological axis (*D*). The case presented in Fig. 3-8 suggests a combination of the types of dysfunctional segmental motion demonstrated in *A* and *D*.

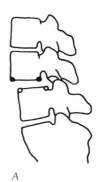 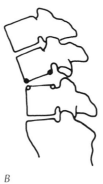 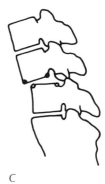 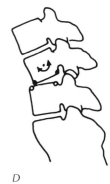

A   *B*   *C*   *D*

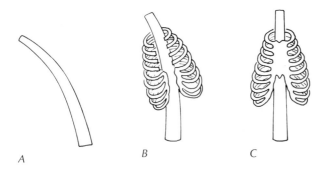

FIGURE 3-10 An illustration of the stability provided to the spine by the rib cage. *A.* The spine without a rib cage can bend excessively. *B.* The addition of the rib cage moderately increases stability. *C.* Sternal attachments are required for achievement of the full stabilization potential of the rib cage. Removal of the effects of either the sternum or the ribs causes a significant diminution of stability.

The Muscles

Muscles, by virtue of their attachments to the spinal elements at every segmental level, provide significant stability. The obvious absence of their effect in the biomechanics laboratory is a significant problem for researchers attempting to study the biomechanics of stability.

In general, any imbalance of muscular forces causes movement about a motion segment. Conversely, a balanc-

ing of muscle and other intrinsic forces about a motion segment results in no net movement. In both of these situations it is assumed that no other forces are applied to the spine.

Muscular activity at a distance from the spine effects spinal movement and can augment spinal stability. The most important example of this is the rectus abdominis and associated anterior abdominal wall muscles. These muscles provide substantial spinal stability by virtue of their attachments to structures ventral to the spinal column (e.g., the sternum, ventral rib cage, and ventral pelvis). This, in turn, results in spinal flexion or lateral bending if contraction occurs. Simultaneous contraction of the erector spinae and rectus abdominis muscles results in no motion if each counterbalances the other. This gives a stabilizing effect (Fig. 3-11). This is a good example of balanced forces applied to the spine by opposing muscles, resulting in augmented stability.

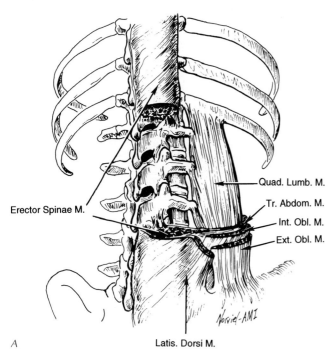

Erector Spinae M.

Quad. Lumb. M.
Tr. Abdom. M.
Int. Obl. M.
Ext. Obl. M.

Latis. Dorsi M.

A

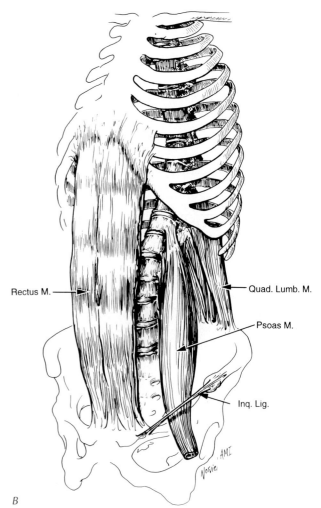

Rectus M.

Quad. Lumb. M.
Psoas M.
Inq. Lig.

B

FIGURE 3-11 The effects of muscles on stability. Muscles provide stability by virtue of the orientation of their attachments to the spine (*A*). In some situations, as with the rectus abdominis muscle, the muscle may influence spinal movement indirectly (i.e., without direct attachment to the spine) (*B*). Similarly, this muscle (as well as all others) may stabilize the spine by balancing opposing muscle function, thus resulting in no movement. A

significant degree of stability is thus provided. Lateral bending is achieved via the contraction of muscles attached to the lateral aspect of the spine—for example, the quadratus lumborum, attached to the transverse processes (*A* and *B*). The balancing of the right and the left muscle actions likewise results in no movement.

THE CONTRIBUTION OF SPINAL DEFORMATION TO INSTABILITY

The contribution of a spinal deformation to instability may be significant. Deformation plays a major role in acute instability (Table 3-1).[1] The quantitation of an angular deformity can be accomplished by defining Cobb's angle (Fig. 3-12).[42] As Cobb's angle increases, an increased moment-arm length is applied to the spine. In the case of a kyphotic deformation the posterior ligamentous structures are stressed excessively, since their main function is to resist tensile loads. Simultaneously, the ventral structures (vertebral body, etc.)

are also stressed—but in compression (axial loading). These concepts apply to angular deformations in any plane.

Voutsinas and MacEwen pointed out the deceptive nature of Cobb's angle. Similar Cobb's angles may be indicative of widely disparate radii of curvature at the segmental level (Fig. 3-12*A* and *B*).[43]

UPPER CERVICAL SPINE INSTABILITY

The assessment of the stability of the upper cervical spine is complicated by the complex anatomy of this region. This is compounded by the relative success of nonsurgical management of injuries in this region. Thus, the definition of an unstable spine is even more uncertain in this region than in the subaxial regions.

White and Panjabi presented criteria for the determination of instability (overt) of the upper cervical spine.[1] These criteria have been modified slightly for presentation here (Table 3-3). This may oversimplify the clinical determination of the unstable spine, but it does provide a foundation from which to begin to understand stability assessment in this region.

Ligamentous or bony disruption with a resultant loss of translation-resisting integrity constitutes an overtly unstable spine (Table 3-3). Ligamentous or bony disruption that does *not* result in overt loss of translation-resisting integrity constitutes limited instability. This interpretation of the unstable upper cervical spine, although vague, should suffice if the clinician uses the principles presented above as well as common sense. The stability of the upper cervical spine is further addressed in Chaps. 5 and 25.

Glacial instability and the instability associated with dysfunctional segmental motion are less commonly considered in the upper cervical spine than in the subaxial regions. Their definitions in the upper cervical spine are the same as in the subaxial regions.

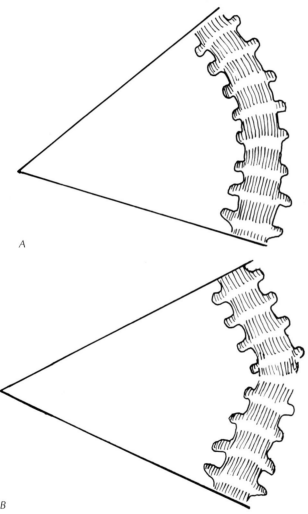

A

B

FIGURE 3-12 The determination of Cobb's angle in a spine with a moderate scoliotic deformity (*A*). If a spinal deformity with a greater Cobb's angle has an axial load applied, the bending moment applied to the region of the deformity is exaggerated. This illustrates the importance of spinal deformity in the determination of acute spinal instability (Table 3-1). The radii of curvature of two spinal deformities may be widely disparate despite their having the same Cobb's angle. A lesser radius of curvature is observed at the injured segment in a situation where an acute segmental angulation occurs (*B*), compared to less acute multisegmental angulations (*A*). Note that each has the same Cobb's angle.

TABLE 3-3 Criteria for C0-C1-C2 instability

Extent of motion	Site/nature of motion
>8 degrees	Axial rotation C0-C1 to one side
>1 mm	C0-C1 translation in the sagittal plane
>7 mm	Overhang C1-C2 (total right and left)
>45 degrees	Axial rotation C1-C2 to one side
>4 mm	C1-C2 translation in the sagittal plane
<13 mm	Posterior body C2-posterior ring C1 in the sagittal plane
	Avulsed transverse ligament of the atlas

SOURCE: After White and Panjabi.[1]

SPINAL INSTRUMENTATION AND INSTABILITY

Spinal instrumentation augments the stability of the spine. It does so by various mechanisms and by the application of various biomechanical principles. Obviously, the type of instability encountered dictates the type of instrumentation construct used, as well as its mode of application. Phenomena such as instrumentation construct load-sharing and load-bearing play important roles in the decision-making process. The loss of anterior axial load-bearing ability generally shifts the IAR in a dorsal direction. Conversely, the loss of posterior axial load-bearing ability generally shifts the IAR in a ventral direction. The IAR is shifted in a predictable manner by the loss of integrity of ventral and posterior spinal integrity. The placement of spinal implants also shifts the IAR in a predictable manner, usually toward the region of the nonpathological neutral axis.[15] These factors are discussed in detail in the chapters that follow.

REFERENCES

1. White AA, Panjabi MM: *Clinical Biomechanics of the Spine,* 2d ed. Philadelphia: Lippincott, 1990:30–342.
2. Bucholz RW, Gill K: Classification of injuries to the thoracolumbar spine. *Orthop Clin North Am* 1986; 17:67–83.
3. Clark WM, Gehweiler JA, Laib R: Twelve significant signs of cervical spine trauma. *Skeletal Radiol* 1979; 3:201.
4. Cope R, Kilcoyne RF, Gaines RW: The thoracolumbar burst fracture with intact posterior elements. Implications for neurologic deficit and stability. *Neuro-Orthopedics* 1989; 7:83–87.
5. Cyron BM, Hutton WC: Variation in the amount and distribution of cortical bone across the pars interarticularis of L5: A predisposing factor in spondylolysis? *Spine* 1979; 4:163–167.
6. DuPuis PR, Yong-Hing K, Cassidy JD, et al: Radiologic diagnosis of degenerative lumbar spinal instability. *Spine* 1985; 10:262–276.
7. Dvorak J, Fohlich D, Penning L, et al: Functional radiographic diagnosis of the cervical spine: Flexion/extension. *Spine* 1988; 13:748–755.
8. Dvorak J, Panjabi MM, Chang DG, et al: Functional radiographic diagnosis of the lumbar spine: Flexion-extension and lateral bending. *Spine* 1991; 16:562–571.
9. Dvorak J, Panjabi MM, Novotny JE, et al: Clinical validation of functional flexion-extension roentgenograms of the lumbar spine. *Spine* 1991; 16:943–950.
10. Friberg O: Lumbar instability: A dynamic approach by traction-compression radiography. *Spine* 1987; 12:119–129.
11. Froning EC, Frohman B: Motion of the lumbosacral spine after laminectomy and spine fusion. *J Bone Joint Surg* 1968; 50A:897–918.
12. Henley EN, Matteri RE, Frymoyer JW: Accurate roentgenographic determination of lumbar flexion-extension. *Clin Orthop* 1976; 115:145–148.
13. Holdsworth FW: Fractures, dislocations and fracture dislocations of the spine. *J Bone Joint Surg* 1963; 45B:6–20.
14. Holdsworth FW: Fractures, dislocations and fracture dislocations of the spine. *J Bone Joint Surg* 1970; 52A:1534–1551.
15. Jelsma RK, Kirsch PT, Rice JF, et al: The radiographic description of thoracolumbar fractures. *Surg Neurol* 1982; 18:230–236.
16. Kaneda K, Kuniyoshi A, Fujiya M: Burst fractures with neurologic deficits of the thoracolumbar-lumbar spine. *Spine* 1984; 9:788–795.
17. Keene JS: Radiographic evaluation of thoracolumbar fractures. *Clin Orthop* 1984; 189:58–64.
18. McAfee PC, Yuan HA, Frederickson BE, et al: The value of computed tomography in thoracolumbar fractures. *J Bone Joint Surg* 1983; 65A:461–473.
19. Pearcy M, Shepherd J: Is there instability in spondylolisthesis? *Spine* 1985; 10:175–177.
20. Penning L, Blickman JR: Instability in lumbar spondylolisthesis: A radiologic study of several concepts. *AJR* 1980; 134:293–301.
21. Penning L, Wilmink JT, van Woerden HH: Inability to prove instability. A critical appraisal of clinical-radiological flexion-extension studies in lumbar disc degeneration. *Diagn Imaging Clin Med* 1984; 53:186–192.
22. Riggins RS, Kraus JF: The risk of neurological damage with fractures of the vertebrae. *J Trauma* 1977; 17:126–133.
23. Smith WS, Kaufer H: Patterns and mechanisms of lumbar injuries associated with lap seat belts. *J Bone Joint Surg* 1969; 51A:239–254.
24. Whitesides TE Jr: Traumatic kyphosis of the thoracolumbar spine. *Clin Orthop* 1977; 128:78–92.
25. Bailey RW: Fractures and dislocations of the cervical spine: Orthopedic and neurosurgical aspects. *Postgrad Med* 1964; 35:588–599.
26. Denis F: The three-column spine and its significance in the classification of acute thoracolumbar spine injuries. *Spine* 1983; 8:817–831.
27. Kelly RP, Whitesides TE: Treatment of lumbodorsal fracture-dislocations. *Ann Surg* 1968; 167:705–717.
28. Louis R: Spinal stability as defined by the three-column spine concept. *Anat Clin* 1985; 7:33–42.
29. Benzel EC: Biomechanics of lumbar and lumbosacral spine fracture, in Rea GL, Miller CA (eds). *Spinal Trauma: Current Evaluation and Management.* American Association of Neurological Surgeons 1993: 165–195.
30. Benzel EC, Hart BL, Ball PA, et al: MRI for the evaluation of patients with non-obvious cervical spine injury. (submitted)
31. Orrison WW, Hart BL, Benzel EC, et al: MRI, CT and plain film comparison in acute cervical spine trauma. (Submitted.)
32. Gertzbein SD, Holtby R, Tile M, et al: Determination of a locus of instantaneous centers of rotation of the lumbar disc by moire fringes. A new technique. *Spine* 1984; 9:409–413.
33. Haher TR, Bergman M, O'Brien M, et al: The effect of the three columns of the spine on the instantaneous axis of rotation in flexion and extension. *Spine* 1991; 16:s312–s318.
34. Mensor M, DuVall G: Absence of motion at the fourth and fifth lumbar interspaces in patients with and without low back pain. *J Bone Joint Surg* 1959; 39B:6–22.
35. Moll JMH, Wright V: Normal range of spinal mobility. *Ann Rheum Dis* 1971; 30:381–386.
36. Panjabi MM, Goel VK, Walter SD, et al: Errors in the center and angle of rotation of a joint: An experimental study. *J Biomech Eng* 1982; 104:232–237.
37. Pennal G, Conn G, McDonald G, et al: Motion studies of the lumbar spine: A preliminary report. *J Bone Joint Surg* 1972; 54B:442–452.
38. Stokes IA, Wilder DG, Frymoyer JW, et al: Assessment of patients with low back pain by biplanar radiographic measurement of intervertebral motion. *Spine* 1981; 6:233–240.
39. Tanz S: Motion of the lumbar spine: A roentgenologic study. *AJR* 1953; 69:399–412.
40. Webb JK, Broughton RBK, McSweeney T, et al: Hidden flexion injury of the cervical spine. *J Bone Joint Surg* 1976; 58B:322–327.
41. Andriacchi TP, Schultz AB, Belytschko TB, et al: A model for studies of mechanical interactions between the human spine and rib cage. *J Biomech* 1974; 7:497–507.
42. Cobb JR: Spine arthrodesis in the treatment of scoliosis. *Bull Hosp Joint Dis* 1958; 19:187–209.
43. Voutsinas SA, MacEwen GD: Sagittal profiles of the spine. *Clin Orthop* 1986; 210:235–242.

Part II

Spine and Neural Element Pathology

Chapter 4

Degenerative and Inflammatory Diseases of the Spine

INTRODUCTION

The management of degenerative and inflammatory spine diseases is complex. Degenerative alterations of the bony spine and ligamentous instability predominate as complicating factors. Degenerative and inflammatory spine diseases, as presented here, include primary degenerative diseases of the spine (e.g., spondylosis and Scheuermann's disease), as well as inflammatory diseases of the spine [e.g., rheumatoid arthritis, ankylosing spondylitis, ossification of the posterior longitudinal ligament (OPLL), ankylosing hyperostosis, and related processes].

This chapter will focus on the biomechanics of the cervical, thoracic, and lumbar regions as they are affected by these various disease entities. Because of the high incidence of spondylosis, it will focus predominantly on the spondylotic degenerative process.

PATHOGENESIS

The degenerative process involves the disk interspace, facet joints, and intra- and paraspinal tissues. Degenerative changes of the intervertebral disk typically involve one, or a combination, of four processes: (1) loss of disk interspace height, (2) irregularities in the disk endplate, (3) sclerosis of the disk interspace, and (4) osteophyte formation. Soft tissue proliferation may accompany this process as an associated phenomenon or may be a primary process (Fig. 4-1). *Degenerative disk disease* is defined by Kramer as biomechanical and pathological conditions of the intervertebral segment caused by degeneration, inflammation, or infection.[1] Like the changes associated with disk interspace degeneration, facet joint degenerative changes are often associated with increased laxity of movement. As the degenerative process proceeds, however, an element of stability is often conferred.

Intra- and paraspinal tissue inflammation, calcification, and hypertrophy are commonly associated with spondylosis (e.g., hypertrophy of the ligamentum flavum), rheumatoid arthritis (e.g., bursa inflammation, pannus formation), and OPLL (calcification and hypertrophy of the posterior longitudinal ligament). Ankylosing spondylitis is the only inflammatory or degenerative disease not associated specifically with soft tissue changes; however, it is associated with increased stability via decreased allowed motion.

The pathogenesis of degenerative disk disease varies according to the underlying disease process. Fundamentally, aberrant physiological responses to stresses placed on the spine and accelerated deterioration of the integrity of spinal elements underlie the pathological process, regardless of the disease entity or region of the spine involved. Before one can appreciate the degenerative process and accompanying pathology, one must appreciate the normal physiological processes associated with the disk interspace and related structures.

Anatomy and Physiology of the Disk Interspace[1,2]

The disk interspaces account for approximately 20 percent of the height of the spine. The disk consists of an outer annulus fibrosus and an inner nucleus pulposus. It is bordered rostrally and caudally by a cartilaginous plate. The latter is part of the vertebral body and is composed of hyaline cartilage. The medullary bone of the vertebral body is connected to the cartilaginous plate and provides it, as well as the disk proper, with nutrients via diffusion through fine pores (laminae cribosae).

The annulus fibrosus is composed of laminated bands of fibrous tissue (predominantly collagen) oriented in opposite directions, with consecutive layers situated in an alternating manner, at about a 30-degree angle from the disk interspace. The inner bands of the annulus are attached to the cartilag-

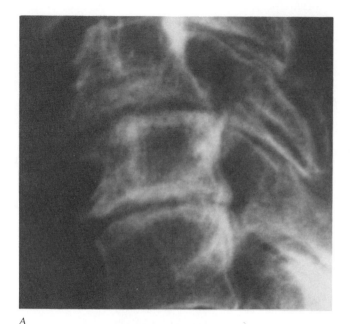

A

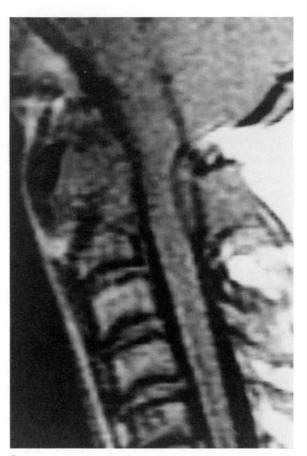

B

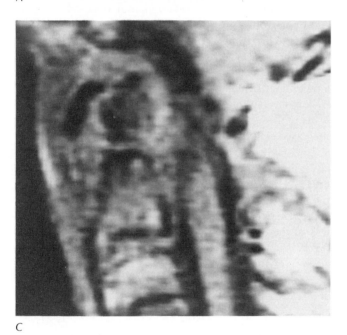

C

FIGURE 4-1 The radiographic appearance of the spondylotic degenerative process. *A.* Disk interspace height loss, osteophyte formation, sclerosis of the endplate, and irregularities of the endplate are demonstrated by a lateral cervical spine x-ray of a patient with spondylotic myelopathy. *B.* Soft tissue proliferation is demonstrated by pannus formation in a patient with rheumatoid arthritis. *C.* An asymmetric collapse of the articular pillars has resulted in the positioning of the dens lateral to the midline. The dens is visualized with surrounding soft tissue pannus formation.

inous plate, while the marginal zone is attached to the ring epiphysis of the vertebral body and the osseous tissue of the vertebral body. These latter attachments (Sharpey's fibers) are stronger than the more medial attachments to the cartilaginous plate. The annulus fibrosus is stronger and more abundant anteriorly and laterally than posteriorly. In fact, in youth the anterior annulus fibrosus merges into the nucleus fibrosus. The fact that the posterior fibers of the annulus fibrosus are weaker contributes to the manifestations of the disk degeneration process (see below).

The nucleus pulposus, a remnant of the notochord, is located in the posterior portion of the intervertebral disk. It consists of reticular bands of closely packed nuclei surrounded by a liquid mucoid ground substance. The water content of the nucleus pulposus decreases from about 90 percent at birth to about 70 percent by age 70. The water, however, is not free. It is reversibly bound to macromolecules via their intense hydroscopic properties. In fact, the water content changes from morning to afternoon, which implies changes in response to weight-bearing (see below). In fact, pressure-dependent fluid movement in and out of the intervertebral disk leads to measurable changes in a person's height from the awakening supine position to the late afternoon erect position. Multiple authors have observed this fact which is summarized nicely by Kramer.[1]

The latter point implies that water escapes and enters the disk through a semipermeable membrane. Other small molecules, such as waste products and nutrients, must also pass through this membrane. The changes in the water content of the disk in response to weight-bearing imply a hydrostatic pressure effect on disk interspace physiology. The hydrostatic pressure within the intervertebral disk in the erect position is many times greater than that within surrounding tissue. In order for the disk to retain water, fluid movement must occur against this very steep pressure gradient. The mechanism through which this occurs is an osmotic pressure–driven counterforce to the hydrostatic pressure. The macromolecules in the interior of the disk take up fluid on account of their hydroscopic capacity. In equilibrium, the following equation is manifest:

Extradiskal hydrostatic pressure	+	intradiskal oncotic pressure	=	intradiskal hydrostatic pressure	+	extradiskal oncotic pressure

Whenever one side comes to outweigh the other (e.g., because of weight-bearing), equilibrium is disrupted and fluid moves across the semipermeable membrane. Increased weight-bearing causes intradiskal fluid to escape via hydrostatic forces. This increases the concentration of the macromolecules within the disk interspace and results in an increase in intradiskal oncotic pressure. This, in turn, increases the absorption capacity of the disk. In addition to the biomechanical effects, this fluid movement allows the passage of nutrients and waste products across the membrane. Therefore, the greater the activity of the subject, the more active this form of transport. Traction is an obvious mechanism by which the intradiskal pressure can be reduced, thus causing an increase in intradiskal water content and an increase in disk height. These points are summarized in Fig. 4-2.

The facet joint, being a synovium-lined diarthrodial joint, is subject to the ravages of inflammatory disease processes (see below). In the strictest sense, the disk interspace is not subject to this type of pathological insult.

Biomechanics of the Intervertebral Motion Segment

During axial loading of a disk interspace, the intradiskal pressures are symmetrically distributed. Eccentrically placed loads, however, result in the asymmetric distribution of pressures within the disk. This, in turn, causes the nucleus pulposus to move within the disk from a region of high pressure (high load) to a region of low pressure (low load); for example, forward flexion results in the posterior

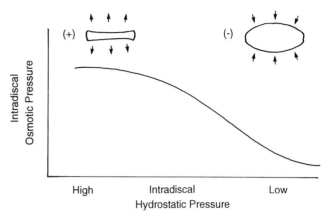

FIGURE 4-2 Osmotic and hydrostatic factors affecting the disk interspace (after Kramer[1]). Note that an increased intradiskal pressure, resulting from an increase in weight-bearing, causes fluid to migrate out of the intradiskal space *(arrows)*. This, in turn, increases the concentration of macromolecules and the oncotic pressure within the disk space (+). Hence the absorption capacity of the disk is increased. Decreasing intradiskal pressure has the opposite effect. *(Adapted from J. Kramer.[1])*

migration of the nucleus pulposus. Conversely, the annulus fibrosus responds to asymmetric force application to the disk interspace by bulging on the side of the disk with the greatest stress applied; that is, the annulus bulges on the side opposite the direction of migration of the nucleus pulposus (Fig. 4-3).

PATHOPHYSIOLOGY OF DISK DEGENERATION AND THE SPONDYLOTIC PROCESS[1-3]

Spondylosis is defined as "vertebral osteophytosis secondary to degenerative disc disease."[3] Spondylosis is not to be confused with inflammatory processes that are associated with osteophyte formation. The latter disease entities are grouped together as arthritides. The osteophytes of spondylosis are associated with degeneration of the intervertebral disk, which is an *amphiarthrodial joint* (i.e., one where there is no synovial membrane). Arthritis, on the other hand, classically involves the synovial membranes of *diarthrodial joints* (joints lined with synovium—e.g., the facet joints). The presence of spondylosis is defined, therefore, by the presence of noninflammatory disk degeneration. The process of disk degeneration is complex and involves many alterations of normal physiology.

Intradiskal Hydrostatic and Oncotic Pressure

Persistent elevation of intradiskal pressures causes narrowing of the disk interspace. This results in annulus fibrosus and facet joint capsule distortion and stretching, with acceleration of the degeneration process. The degeneration pro-

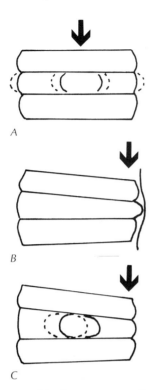

FIGURE 4-3 *A.* An axial load causes an equally distributed force application to the disk. *B.* An eccentric force application results in annulus fibrosus bulging on the side of the greatest force application—i.e., the concave side of the bend. *C.* The nucleus pulposus moves in the opposite direction. Dashed lines indicate the positions of structures during force application.

cess itself should be considered simply a manifestation of the normal aging process; but its pathological acceleration, or the deterrence of same, is of obvious clinical significance.

The water content of the disk interspace, as previously mentioned, decreases gradually throughout life. In addition, the vascularity of the disk also decreases, ranging from a well-vascularized disk at birth to essentially no vascular supply by age 30. These and other factors contribute to changes in the chemical and anatomic makeup of the disk Fibroblasts produce inferior-quality fibers and ground substance. The disk becomes dessicated and less able to function as a cushion. Fissures occur in the cartilaginous plates with defects resulting in internal herniations (Schmorl's nodes).[4] Gas accumulates in the disk (vacuum phenomenon). Mucoid degeneration, an ingrowth of fibrocartilage, and obliteration of the nucleus fibrosus ensue. Generalized disk deterioration results in instability. This, in turn, results in annulus tension and bulging, both of which result in pathological deformations.

Disk Deformation

The bulging of the annulus fibrosus causes the periosteum of the adjacent vertebral bodies to be elevated at the attach-

ment site of Sharpey's fibers. Bony reactions (subperiosteal bone formation) occur, resulting in spondylotic ridge (osteophyte) formation (Fig. 4-4*A*, *B*, and *C*). This process most commonly results in spinal canal encroachment in the cervical and lumbar regions, relatively sparing the thoracic region (Fig. 4-4*D*). This is due to the fact that the natural lordosis in these spinal regions results in concavity of the spinal curvature and, hence, the tendency toward annular bulging in the direction of the spinal canal. The spondylotic process is lessened by fusion or immobilization.[5]

Regarding a lateral bending deformity (scoliotic curvature), osteophyte formation occurs predominantly *on the concave side of a curve,* where annulus fibrosus bulging is similarly most pronounced (Fig. 4-5). But the concave side of the spinal curvature is not the side of the spine that harbors the predisposition for disk herniation. This discrepancy warrants further attention.

The posterior migration of the disk into the spinal canal (disk herniation) occurs predominantly in a dorsal direction, whereas osteophytic spur formation commonly occurs in an anterior or lateral direction. Flexion and lateral bending cause annulus fibrosus bulging and encourage osteophyte formation along the concave side of the curve. Conversely, the thin posterior annulus fibrosus and relatively weak posterior longitudinal ligament (particularly laterally) combine with the migratory tendencies of the nucleus pulposus to encourage posterolateral disk herniation (Fig. 4-6).

Many factors play roles in inducing posterior and lateral location of disk herniation. These include the migratory tendencies of the nucleus pulposus, the relatively weak lateral portion of the posterior longitudinal ligament, and the thin posterior portion of the annulus fibrosus. Most disk herniations do not occur (or, to put it more correctly, do not become manifest) immediately following trauma. Labora-

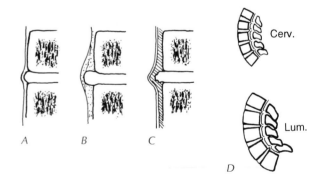

FIGURE 4-4 Osteophyte formation results from subperiosteal bone formation, which results from elevation of the periosteum by disk bulging (*A*). A spondylotic ridge then develops (*B* and *C*). This commonly encroaches on the spinal column in the cervical and lumbar regions, because the lordotic spinal curvature causes the disk bulging and osteophyte formation to occur toward the spinal canal (*D*). This is less common in the thoracic region, because the concavity is oriented away from the spinal canal. See also Fig. 4-5.

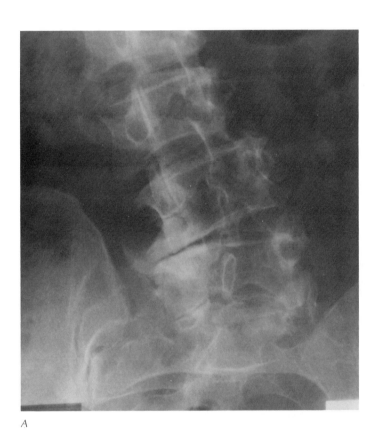

A

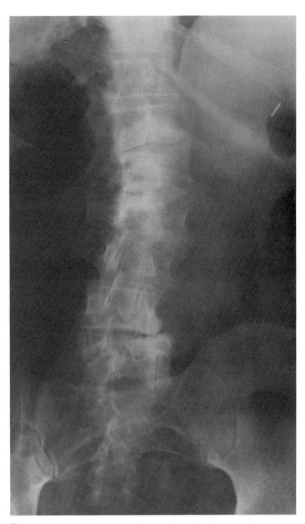

B

FIGURE 4-5 Spondylotic ridges (osteophyte formation), associated with scoliosis, predominantly occur on the concave side of a curve—i.e., on the side of chronic or long-term annulus fibrosus bulging (*A*). This is demonstrated at two separate levels, on opposite sides of the spine, in a patient with a bi-concave curve (*B*).

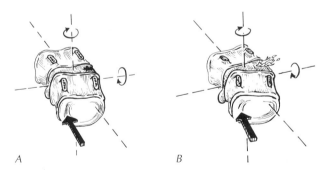

A   *B*

FIGURE 4-6 The application of an axial load, lateral bending, and flexion causes the nucleus pulposus to migrate in the direction of the region of the annulus fibrosus that is under tension and prone to tearing (*A*). This may result in disk herniation in the posterior paramedian location if the disk is degenerated (and thus predisposed to pathological migration) (*B*).[2,6]

tory investigations that attempt to determine the mechanism of disk herniation are lacking; that lack has hampered investigations in this area for years. Adams and Hutton, however, determined that a high percentage of lumbar disks in the laboratory could be encouraged to herniate if (1) the disk was degenerated and (2) a specific force pattern was delivered acutely to the motion segment. This force pattern includes (1) flexion (causing posterior nucleus pulposus migration), (2) lateral bending away from the side of disk herniation (causing lateral nucleus pulposus migration), and (3) application of an axial load (causing an increase in intradiskal pressure).[6] As shown in Fig. 4-6, this complex loading pattern causes (1) the application of tension to the weakest portion of the annulus fibrosus (posterolateral position—the location of the herniation), (2) migration of the nucleus pulposus toward this position, and (3) an asymmetric increase in intradiskal pressure. A degenerated disk is requisite for the occurrence of this process. These factors, plus the increasing frequency of annulus fibrosus tears with age and the observation of peak nucleus fibrosus pressures in the 35- to 55-year age group, are among the factors giving rise to an increased incidence of disk herniation in this age group (Fig. 4-7).

There is controversy about the necessity of the routine pathological examination of the operatively resected degenerated disk. One must weigh carefully the cost and advantage, to the patient, of submitting disk specimens for pathological examination. It appears that, unless the surgeon suspects an atypical process on the basis of clinical history or examination, or of gross inspection at the time of surgery, the routine examination of surgically resected intervertebral disk specimens is not warranted.[7]

Extradiskal Soft Tissue Involvement

The spondylotic process includes soft tissue pathological processes, in addition to disk and facet joint degeneration. In this regard, the hypertrophy and buckling of the ligamentum flavum is a major contributor to the development of myelopathy in the patient population afflicted with cervical spondylotic myelopathy.[8]

Osteoporosis

With aging, a decrease of bone formation with associated continued bone resorption leads to a decrease in bony integrity. This may lead, in turn, to the collapse of the vertebral body. Unlike the Schmorl's node, this collapse is not circumscribed. The thoracic kyphosis predisposes the spine to ventral vertebral body collapse in this region (Fig. 4-8). This applies to trauma, in general (see Chap. 5).

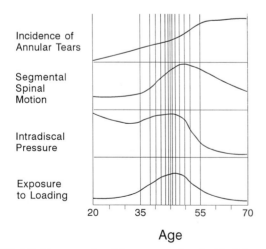

FIGURE 4-7 The age-related factors associated with disk herniation. The densities of the vertical lines correlate with the incidence of disk herniation. (*Adapted from J. Kramer.*[1])

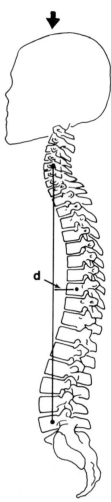

FIGURE 4-8 Osteoporosis can result in pathological fractures whose characteristics depend on the local configuration of the spine. In a region with a kyphotic posture, a ventral wedge compression fracture might be expected, because of the moment arm (*d*) applied to the spine at the apex of the kyphosis. In a region without significant kyphosis (e.g., the mid- and low lumbar region), a pancaking of the vertebral body (burst fracture) might be expected, because of the decreased length of the applied moment arm (*d* = 0).

Scheuermann's Disease

In the developing spine the intradiskal oncotic pressure is normally relatively high. This can result in focal sites of penetration of the endplate (Schmorl's nodes) with resulting destruction of the growth plate. The preexisting thoracic kyphosis, which is associated with asymmetrically high ventral intradiskal pressures, may lead to the exaggeration of focal endplate penetration in this circumstance. This phenomenon is known as *Scheuermann's disease* (osteochondrosis) and is associated with a disproportionate loss of ventral vertebral body height, Schmorl's nodes (predominantly ventrally located), irregularities of the vertebral endplates, and narrowing of the disk interspaces (predominantly ventrally).[9] As stated by Kramer, "The developmental disorders of Scheuermann's disease are secondary changes and are caused by increased pressure of the developing disc tissue on the anterior parts of the intervertebral segments in the kyphotic area of the spine."[1]

Because of the increased focal pressures exerted, degeneration of the disk is accelerated. Fibrous, and ultimately bony, fusion occurs.

NONSPONDYLOTIC, NONINFECTIOUS INFLAMMATION OF THE SPINE

Rheumatoid Arthritis

Rheumatoid arthritis affects spinal ligaments and the calcium content of bones, including the spine. It is associated with two separate processes that result in spinal deformity in the cervical region. The transverse ligament of the atlas weakens and stretches. This allows excessive flexion of the atlas on the axis (Fig. 4-9A).

In addition, rheumatoid arthritis often involves an inflammation of the disk interspace with narrowing of the disk height and defective vertebral endplates with reactive sclerosis (spondylodiskitis).[1,10] This, combined with facet joint weakening, may allow exaggeration of a flexion deformity by the "stair-stepping" of the vertebrae encouraged by the ligamentous and capsular (facet) joint laxity (Fig. 4-9B). Stair-stepping is much more commonly manifested in the cervical region than in the thoracic and lumbar regions.

Exaggerated upper cervical degenerative changes can lead to deformation and instability at the occiput-C1 level. This, in turn, may lead to migration of the dens upward through the ring of C1 (vertical subluxation) (Fig. 4-9C).

The etiopathogenesis of rheumatoid arthritis is not without controversy. The disk interspace destruction and instability in rheumatoid arthritis may be consequences of cervical instability caused by facet joint arthropathy and capsular and other posterior ligament laxity. This in turn, may lead to diskovertebral destruction.[11]

Catastrophic complications of rheumatoid arthritis are not uncommon.[12–14] These are often related to the sudden onset of quadriplegia following minimal trauma. This phenomenon is the foundation on which much of the spine-stabilization surgery for rheumatoid arthritis patients is based.

Ankylosing Spondylitis

Ankylosing spondylitis (Bekhterev's, or Marie-Strümpell, disease) causes a gradual ankylosis of the spine, combined with a progressive osteoporosis. The ankylosing process essentially involves the ossification of the ligamentous insertion sites on bone (entheses). It involves the intervertebral disk margin, the facet joint capsules, the anterior and posterior longitudinal ligaments, and the interspinous ligaments, resulting in a circumferential ankylosis (Fig. 4-10A and B). The ankylosing process begins with a spondylodiskitis. It is observed as a secondary process in rheumatoid arthritis. Characteristic spinal deformities develop and progress. The combination of these deformities, the spinal ankylosis, and the associated osteoporosis results in a substantial propensity toward spinal fracture. Fracture may occur through the region of the intervertebral disk or the vertebral body (Fig. 4-10B). The management of such fractures is fraught with difficulty and complications.[15]

Spinal deformities associated with ankylosing spondylitis may become remarkably debilitating. Their prevention with appropriate education regarding postural management (e.g., sleeping without a pillow during the early phases of the disease while the permanent postural configuration is being defined) is emphasized. Radical surgical management has been used successfully in severe cases.[16]

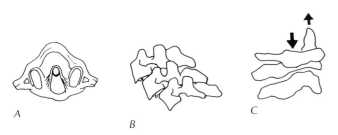
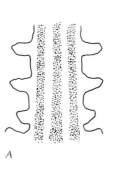
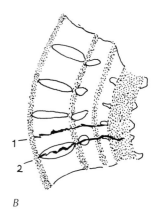

FIGURE 4-9 The pathogenesis of rheumatoid arthritic spinal involvement. *A.* Laxity of the transverse ligament of the axis leads to instability and an increase in the size of the predental space. *B.* Stair-stepping of the cervical vertebral bodies in response to ligamentous laxity, disk degeneration, and facet joint arthropathy. *C.* Vertical subluxation may also occur secondarily to cartilage loss, bony erosion, and collapse of the occiput-C1 and C1-C2 facet joints.

FIGURE 4-10 Ankylosing spondylitis. Ankylosis of the vertebral bodies, facet joints, and interspinous ligaments occurs. This may result in the radiographic appearance of longitudinal fusion masses along these structures. This is visible on both the anteroposterior (*A*) and lateral (*B*) views. Fracture formation in the region of the vertebral body (*1*) and disk interspace (*2*) is illustrated in *B*.

Ossification of the Posterior Longitudinal Ligament (OPLL)

OPLL predominantly affects the cervical spine. It most commonly affects Mongolians, but also occurs in Caucasians.[17] The ossification process results in a calcification (i.e., conversion into hydroxyapatite) of the posterior longitudinal ligament, as well as its thickening.[18] This, in turn, results in encroachment on the spinal canal. This process increases the rigidity of the spine.[19]

Surgical management of this disorder can be undertaken by either an anterior or a posterior approach. Anterior approaches appear to be the more popular.[20,21] Regardless of the surgical approach, the maintenance of normal spinal curvatures and spinal column integrity optimizes the outcome.[22]

Ankylosing Hyperostosis

Ankylosing hyperostosis (Forestier disease) involves the presence of focal spinal ankylosis, intact vertebral endplates, normal intervertebral disk height, and ossification of the anterior longitudinal ligament.[23] It occurs in the thoracic, lumbar, and cervical spines, in order of decreasing frequency. Clinical symptoms are uncommon. This disorder is the anterior longitudinal ligament counterpart of OPLL. It is differentiated from OPLL by its involvement of the ventral vertebral body region and from ankylosing spondylitis by the lack of posterior (facet joint region) involvement.

The ossification bridges out into the ventral paravertebral soft tissues, forming bony bridges.[24,25] Fractures of the spine afflicted by ankylosing hyperostosis present challenging management problems.[26]

Other Nondegenerative Disorders

Compressive myelopathy from calcification of the ligamentum flavum is a rare cause of degenerative compression of the spinal cord. It occurs predominantly in the cervical spine,[27-29] but has been observed in the thoracic spine.[30]

Tophaceous gout has also been reported as a cause of spinal cord compression.[31] This is related to hyperuricemia. Gout, in some cases, may be implicated in chronic back pain.

Regional Variations

Degenerative diseases of the spine that involve the cervical spine include spondylosis, rheumatoid arthritis, ankylosing spondylitis, and OPLL. Because of the relative ease of access to the cervical spinal cord from both the ventral and dorsal directions, surgical management of cervical spine degenerative diseases is common.

Degenerative diseases of the thoracic spine, although uncommon, deserve serious attention. They include many of the processes affecting the cervical spine, ankylosing hyperostosis, and Scheuermann's disease. The surgical approach to these problems is often complicated by the need for decompression of the ventral aspect of the thoracic spine. Surgical considerations differ from those in the cervical region, on account of the opposite curvatures of the thoracic and the cervical spine (cervical lordosis and thoracic kyphosis).

Surgical considerations in the lumbar spine, too, differ substantially from those in the cervical and thoracic regions. Although the intrinsic curvature of the lumbar spine is lordotic, the massive size of the vertebral bodies and the forces they resist make the lumbar spine unique.[32] The often-near-vertical orientation of the lumbosacral joint space is an additional confounding factor. The sagittal orientation of the facet joints and the usual manner of progression of facet joint degenerative changes also differentiate lumbar degenerative processes from thoracic and cervical ones.

SPINAL CONFIGURATION

The surgical approaches for both decompression and stabilization of degenerative diseases of the spine often include a combination of decompression, fusion, and instrumentation, performed from either a ventral or a dorsal exposure, or from both. The surgical approach to be used for any given spinal disorder, including the application of an instrumentation construct, should be determined, at least in part, by the intrinsic curvature of the spine.

The Cervical Spine

The spondylotic degenerative process results in a loss of height, predominantly at the disk interspace. Initially, this loss of height occurs in the ventral aspect of the disk.

The disk space is thicker ventrally than dorsally. This contributes to the normal cervical lordosis. As the ventral aspect of the disk interspace decreases, the lordotic posture is diminished and eventually is lost. This straightening of the spine then increases the forces placed on the ventral aspects of the vertebral bodies by increasing the length of the moment arm, thus exposing the ventral aspects of the vertebral bodies to increased stresses and a tendency toward compression. As the loss of lordosis progresses and the kyphosis-producing forces on the spine increase, the vertebral bodies begin to lose height ventrally more than dorsally (Fig. 4-11). This is encouraged by the gradual loss of calcium. The process of collapse of the disk interspace and the vertebral body results in the development of a forward bending of the dural sac and spinal cord. This contributes to the overall pathological relationship between the neural elements and the surrounding bony and soft tissues.

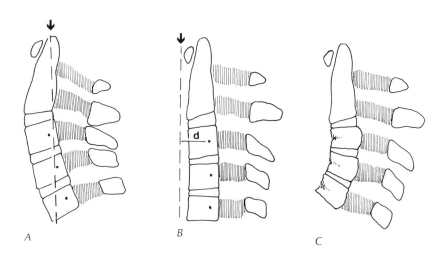

FIGURE 4-11 The nonpathological situation where the posterior vertebral body height is less than the ventral height. This results in the normal lordotic curvature in the cervical spine (*A*). Ventral disk interspace height loss (via the typical degeneration process) results in the loss of the nonpathological lordotic posture (*B*). This causes the creation and elongation of the moment arm applied to the spine, *d*, leading to ventral vertebral body compression. A further exaggeration of a pathological kyphotic posture may then ensue (*C*).

Since the assessment of the curvature of the spine is imperative to sound decision-making, a relatively precise definition of curvature types is necessary. An *"effective" cervical kyphosis* is a configuration of the cervical spine in which any part of the dorsal aspect of any of the vertebral bodies C3 through C7 crosses a line drawn in the midsagittal plane (on a lateral cervical spine tomogram, myelogram, or MRI scan) from the dorsocaudal aspect of the vertebral body of C2 to the dorsocaudal aspect of the vertebral body of C7. Conversely, an *"effective" cervical lordosis* is a configuration of the cervical spine in which no part of the dorsal aspect of any of the vertebral bodies C3 through C7 crosses this line. The definition of this imaginary line is associated with a zone of uncertainty ("gray zone"), within which the surgeon's bias and clinical judgment together determine whether lordosis or kyphosis is the predominant spinal configuration in the midsagittal section (Fig. 4-12). If, in the opinion of the surgeon, there is no "gray zone" (i.e., if only an "effective" kyphosis or an "effective" lordosis is possible), then surgical decision-making is simpler. On the other hand, if the surgeon discerns a "gray zone," the decision-making process is more complex. Perhaps patients whose spinal configuration falls in the "gray zone" should be defined as having a "straightened" spine.[33]

The surgical indications for myelopathy associated with degenerative diseases vary.[34-36] Both ventral and dorsal decompressive approaches are potentially useful for degenerative and inflammatory diseases of the spine; the choice should be for the approach that, in a given case, seems to carry the higher probability of success.[33,35,37-39] Spinal geometry is emphasized as an important determinant of the appropriateness of either the ventral or the dorsal approach in individual situations.[33,37] An "effective" lordosis may be a relative indication for a dorsal approach, whereas an "effective" kyphosis may be a relative indication for a ventral approach.

The Thoracic Spine

In the thoracic spine, disk height loss (predominantly ventral disk height loss) results in progression of the kyphotic deformity. This, however, is superimposed on a preexisting kyphotic deformity, thus exaggerating the deformity's progression. This tends to occur in Scheuermann's disease.

The rib cage, however, substantially adds to the stability of the thoracic spine. This stability is predominantly related to the rib's attachment to the vertebral and costovertebral

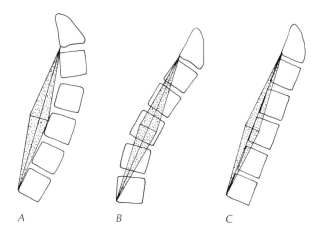

FIGURE 4-12 *A.* A midsagittal section of a cervical spine (as observed by MRI or myelography) configured in lordotic posture ("effective" cervical lordosis). A line has been drawn from the dorsocaudal aspect of the vertebral body of C2 to the dorsocaudal aspect of the vertebral body of C7 (*solid line*). The "gray zone" is outlined by the other lines. *B.* A midsagittal section of a cervical spine configured in kyphosis ("effective" cervical kyphosis). Note that portions of the vertebral bodies are located dorsal to the "gray zone." *C.* A midsagittal section of a "straightened" cervical spine. Note that the most dorsal aspect of a cervical vertebral body is located within, but not dorsal to, the "gray zone."[33]

joints and the sternum. The attachment of the rib to the sternum is crucial to the rib's contribution to stability (see Chap. 3).[1,2] The stability conferred by the rib cage minimizes progression of the thoracic kyphosis due to degenerative changes.

The Lumbar Spine

The lumbar spine is not protected by the rib cage. Furthermore, the coupling response to movements is different from that observed in the cervical region. This is attributed to the absence of the uncovertebral joints and the different orientation of the facet joints (see Chap. 1). These factors contribute to the progression of lateral bending deformities in the lumbar spine, rather than to kyphotic deformities as observed in the cervical and thoracic spine. An asymmetric loss of height of the lumbar intervertebral disk may progress

to an asymmetric collapse of the vertebral body. If this lateral bending (scoliotic deformity) occurs and progresses, it is associated with an obligatory rotation of the spine that is caused by the coupling characteristics of the lumbar spine. The osteophytes occur, as previously depicted, on the concave side of the curvature (see Chap. 1).

This obligatory association of a rotatory deformity with a lateral bending deformity (coupling) makes lumbar spinal instrumentation surgery in these patients more difficult and dangerous. Lateral transverse process dissection can result in injury to the nerve roots, because of their relatively dorsal location with respect to the transverse processes; deformity correction by the distraction of the concave side of the spine may result in stretching of shortened and tethered nerve roots (Fig. 4-13). Proximal (intradural) nerve roots are much less tolerant of stretching than their more peripheral nerve counterparts, on account of their lack of perineurium.

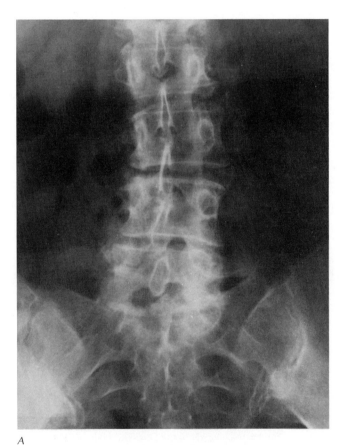

A

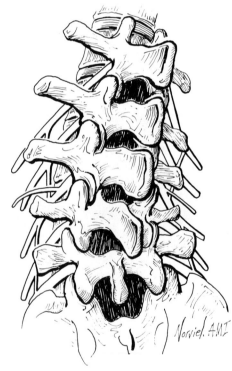

B

FIGURE 4-13 The obligatory rotation of the spine (rotatory component of scoliosis resulting from the coupling phenomenon), as illustrated on an anteroposterior x-ray (*A*), is associated with a propensity for nerve root injury during dissection along the transverse process on the concave side of the curvature. This is because of the juxtaposition of the exiting nerve root to the overlying transverse process created by spinal rotation (*B*). The nerve roots exiting on the concave side of the curve can be injured by stretching associated with surgical deformity correction. *The proximal (intradural) nerve roots are much less tolerant of stretching than their more distal peripheral nerve counterparts, because of their deficient perineurium.*

Spinal Configuration Definition

Except at its termini, the thoracic spine is in a kyphotic posture. The cervicothoracic and thoracolumbar junctions are transition zones between kyphotic and lordotic postures. The lumbar spine again assumes a lordotic posture much like that of the cervical spine. The clinical impact of degenerative changes on spinal curvature is not so evident in the thoracic and lumbar spine as in the cervical spine. The normal thoracic kyphosis can be exaggerated in the degenerated spine. This occasionally causes, or contributes to, spinal cord compressive processes, and predisposes the spine to further deformation (Fig. 4-8). The lumbar lordosis can precipitate or exaggerate sagittal plane translation deformities (Fig. 4-14).

SPINAL STABILITY

The intrinsic stability of the spine[40] plays a role in surgical decision-making. The surgeon may choose an anterior approach (which includes fusion) if the patient's spine is thought to be intrinsically unstable. This approach allows decompression and stabilization to be performed simultaneously. Alternatively, a posterior approach, with an accompanying posterior fusion, may be chosen.

Although posterior decompressive operations most certainly diminish intrinsic spinal stability, the extent of their effect on stability is often exaggerated.[35] An appropriately performed laminectomy should not significantly diminish intrinsic spinal stability. Raynor and coworkers[41] have demonstrated clearly that cervical laminectomy width is related to stability. In cases where laminectomy is laterally extended only to the lateral-most aspect of the dural sac, postoperative instability is rare.[35] Therefore, wide laminectomies that are extended past the medial one-quarter to one-third of the width of the facet and foraminotomies that disrupt facet integrity should be avoided—or, perhaps, should be accompanied by a fusion procedure (Fig. 4-15). Other authors have similarly described postlaminectomy spinal

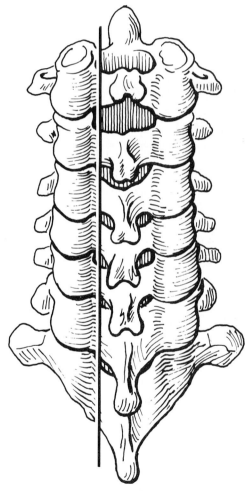

FIGURE 4-15 Surgical decompression via laminectomy should preserve the functional integrity of the facet joint. In the cervical region, this involves the preservation of at least two-thirds to three-quarters of the facet joint diameter. The valley between the facet joint and the lamina, located just lateral to the vertical line, corresponds to the medial aspect of the facet joint. Laminectomies rarely require extension laterally past this valley. In general, a laminectomy should not be taken lateral to this line.

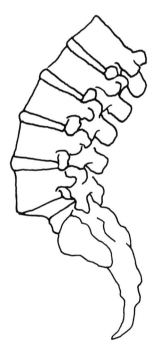

FIGURE 4-14 An exaggeration of the normal lumbar lordosis places excessive translational stresses on the lumbosacral junction when the patient is upright. This may result in a parallelogram-like translational deformation at the lumbosacral junction.

deformity complications[42] and have quantitated their presence in vitro.[40]

Osteophyte formation may contribute to spinal stability. The bridging of spinal segments by osteophytes may minimize or eliminate spinal segmental movement. The acquisition of stability via the spondylotic process becomes progressively more evident beyond the sixth decade of life. This process, taken to the extreme, is observed in ankylosing spondylitis. This increase in stability affords extra assurance as to the safety of an appropriately performed laminectomy. Stability augmentation, however, is not always present, particularly in patients with a kyphotic spinal configuration.

Accelerated degenerative changes and/or flexible kyphosis occur following fusion (whether surgical or secondary to the degenerative process). The longer moment arm associated with this process places significant stresses on the joints above and below the moment arm (fused segment). This, in turn, results in the acceleration of degenerative changes.[43,44]

CLINICAL APPLICATIONS

In general, ventral compressive lesions should be decompressed via a ventral surgical approach and dorsal lesions via a dorsal surgical approach. Patients with an "effective" kyphosis have a decreased probability of adequate ventral dural sac decompression following a dorsal decompressive operation. These patients should, perhaps, be approached by an anterior surgical decompression. In the presence of an "effective" kyphosis, a laminectomy cannot be expected to relieve ventral compression, because of a "sagittal bowstring" effect (see Chap. 7) whereby the dural sac and its contents are tethered over ventral osteophytes in a sagittal plane.

If an "effective" lordosis is present, a dorsal decompressive operation may be most appropriate, while an anterior operation may be less effective. If a "straightened" spine is present (bear in mind that the surgeon's bias and clinical judgment play a major role in determining the size of the "gray zone"), the patient can be treated with either an anterior or a posterior decompressive procedure.

REFERENCES

1. Kramer J: *Intervertebral Disc Disease: Causes, Diagnosis, Treatment, and Prophylaxis,* 2d ed. Stuttgart and New York: George Thieme Verlag, 1990: 14–47.
2. White AA, Panjabi MM (eds): *Clinical Biomechanics of the Spine,* 2d ed. Philadelphia: Lippincott, 1990: 1–125.
3. Weinstein PR, Ehni G, Wilson CB: *Lumbar Spondylosis: Diagnosis, Management and Surgical Treatment.* Chicago and London: Year Book, 1977: 13–87.
4. Resnick D, Niwayama G: Intravertebral disk herniations: Cartilaginous (Schmorl's) nodes. *Radiology* 1978; 126:57–65.
5. Baker WC, Thomas TG, Kirkaldy-Willis WH: Changes in the cartilage of the posterior intervertebral joints after anterior fusion. *J Bone Joint Surg* 1969; 51B:736–746.
6. Adams MA, Hutton WC: Prolapsed intervertebral disc. A hyperflexion injury. *Spine* 1982; 7:184–191.
7. Boutin P, Hogshead H: Surgical pathology of the intervertebral disc. Is routine examination necessary? *Spine* 1992; 17:1236–1238.
8. Stoltman HF, Blackwood W: The role of the ligamenta flava in the pathogenesis of myelopathy in cervical spondylosis. *Brain* 1964; 87:45–50.
9. Stoddard A, Osborn JF: Scheuermann's disease of spinal osteochondrosis. Its frequency and relationship with spondylosis. *J Bone Joint Surg* 1979; 61b:56–58.
10. Detenbeck LC: Rheumatoid arthritis of the spinal column. Pathologic aspects and treatment. *Orthop Clin North Am* 1971; 2:679–686.
11. Martel W: Pathogenesis of cervical discovertebral destruction in rheumatoid arthritis. *Arth Rheum* 1977; 20:1217–1225.
12. Mikulowski P, Wollheim FA, Rotmil P, et al: Sudden death in rheumatoid arthritis with atlanto-axial dislocation. *Acta Med Scand* 1975; 198:445–451.
13. Rana N: Natural history of atlanto-axial subluxation in rheumatoid arthritis. *Spine* 1989; 14:1054–1056.
14. Sharp J, Purser DW: Spontaneous atlanto-axial dislocation in ankylosing spondylitis and rheumatoid arthritis. *Ann Rheum Dis* 1961; 20:47–77.
15. Hunter T, Dubo H: Spinal fractures complicating ankylosing spondylitis. *Ann Intern Med* 1978; 88:546–549.
16. Simmons EH: Kyphotic deformity of the spine in ankylosing spondylitis. *Clin Orthop Rel Res* 1977; 128:65–77.
17. Klara PM, McDonnell DE: Ossification of the posterior longitudinal ligament in Caucasians: Diagnosis and surgical intervention. *Neurosurgery* 1986; 19:212–217.
18. Kubota T, Sato K, Kawano H, et al: Ultrastructure of early calcification in cervical ossification of the posterior longitudinal ligament. *J Neurosurg* 1984; 61:131–135.
19. Murakami N, Muroga T, Sobue I: Cervical myelopathy due to ossification of the posterior longitudinal ligament. *Arch Neurol* 1978; 35:33–36.
20. Abe H, Tsuru M, Ito T, et al: Anterior decompression for ossification of the posterior longitudinal ligament of the cervical spine. *J Neurosurg* 1981; 55:108–116.
21. Cloward RB: Removal of cervical ossified posterior longitudinal ligament at single and multiple levels. in Rengechary SS, Wilkins RH (eds): *Neurosurgical Operative Atlas.* Park Ridge, IL: American Association of Neurological Surgeons, 1991; 1:175–181.
22. Kamioka Y, Yamamoto H, Tani T, et al: Postoperative instability of cervical OPLL and cervical radiculomyelopathy. *Spine* 1989; 14:1177–1183.
23. Boachie-Adjei O, Bullough PG: Incidence of ankylosing hyperostosis of the spine (Forestier's disease) at autopsy. *Spine* 1987; 12:739–743.
24. Huang PS, Laha RK: Ankylosing hyperostosis of the cervical spine. *Surg Neurol* 1978; 9:273–274.
25. Stringer WL, Kelly DL, Johnston FR, et al: Hyperextension injury of the cervical spine with esophageal perforation. *J Neurosurg* 1980; 53:541–543.
26. Fardon DF: Odontoid fracture complicating ankylosing anterior hyperostosis of the spine. *Spine* 1978; 3:108–112.
27. Iwasaki Y, Akino M, Abe H, et al: Calcification of the ligamentum flavum of the cervical spine. *J Neurosurg* 1983; 59:531–534.
28. Kawano N, Matsuno T, Miyazawa S, et al: Calcium pyrophosphate dihydrate crystal deposition disease in the cervical ligamentum flavum. *J Neurosurg* 1988; 68:613–620.

29. Nakajima K, Miyaoka M, Sumie H, et al: Cervical radiculomyelopathy due to calcification of the ligamenta flava. *Surg Neurol* 1984; 21:479–488.

30. Omojola MF, Cardoso ER, Fox AJ, et al: Thoracic myelopathy secondary to ossified ligamentum flavum. *J Neurosurg* 1982; 56:448–450.

31. Leaney BJ, Calvert JM: Tophaceous gout producing spinal cord compression. *J Neurosurg* 1983; 58:580–582.

32. Benzel EC: Biomechanics of lumbar and lumbosacral spine fractures, in Rea GL, Miller CA (eds): *Spinal Trauma: Current Evaluation and Management*. Park Ridge, IL: American Association of Neurological Surgeons, 1993: 65–95.

33. Benzel EC: Cervical spondylotic myelopathy: Posterior surgical approaches, in Cooper PR (ed): *Degenerative Disease of the Cervical Spine*. Park Ridge, IL: American Association of Neurological Surgeons, 1993.

34. Ball PA, Saunders RL: The subjective myelopathy, in Saunders RL, Bernini PM (eds): *Cervical Spondylotic Myelopathy*. Boston: Blackwell, 1992:48–55.

35. Carol MP, Ducker TB: Cervical spondylitic myelopathies: Surgical treatment. *J Spinal Disord* 1988; 1:59–65.

36. Crandall PH, Batzdorf U: Cervical spondylotic myelopathy. *J Neurosurg* 1966; 25:57–66.

37. Batzdorf U, Batzdorff A: Analysis of cervical spine curvature in patients with cervical spondylosis. *Neurosurgery* 1988; 22:827–836.

38. Mann KS, Khosla VK, Gulati DR: Cervical spondylotic myelopathy treated by single-stage multilevel anterior decompression. *J Neurosurg* 1984; 60:80–87.

39. Mayfield FH: Cervical spondylosis: A comparison of the anterior and posterior approaches. *Clin Neurosurg* 1965; 13:181–188.

40. White AA, Johnson RM, Panjabi MM, et al: Biomechanical analysis of clinical stability in the cervical spine. *Clin Orthop Rel Res* 1975; 109:85–96.

41. Raynor RB, Pugh J, Shapiro I: Cervical facetectomy and its effect on spine strength. *J Neurosurg* 1985; 63:278–282.

42. Lonstein JE: Post-laminectomy kyphosis. *Clin Orthop Rel Res* 1977; 128:93–100.

43. Hunter LY, Braunstein EM, Bailey RW: Radiographic changes following anterior cervical fusion. *Spine* 1980; 5:399–401.

44. Whitehill R, Schmidt R: The posterior interspinous fusion in the treatment of quadriplegia. *Spine* 1983; 8:733–740.

Chapter *5*

Trauma, Tumor, and Infection

INTRODUCTION

This chapter focuses predominantly on trauma. Tumor and infection, however, often have biomechanical effects on the spine that are similar to those of trauma. Tumor- and infection-related fractures, dislocations (translocational deformities), and rotational injuries can occur, particularly when tumor or infection is associated with superimposed trauma, however slight or seemingly insignificant. For this reason, tumor, infection, and trauma will be discussed together as one entity.

The most common and illustrative types of spine injury are presented in order to portray the associated mechanisms of injury and pathological anatomy. Radiographic diagnosis of instability and pathological anatomy relies heavily on plain films (anteroposterior and lateral x-rays). CT, however, plays a significant role, particularly when posterior bony element disruption is in question.[1] MRI may be particularly useful in identifying soft tissue injury and neural element compromise (see Chap. 3).

LOSS OF STRUCTURAL INTEGRITY OF THE UPPER CERVICAL SPINE

The upper cervical spine is prone to traumatically induced injuries because of (1) the unique anatomy of that region, (2) the substantial spinal movements allowed there, and (3) the high incidence of exposure of that region to significant pathological stresses from trauma (usually in association with head trauma). The unique anatomy and spinal mobility of the region have been addressed in Chap. 1. The importance of the third factor, the high incidence of exposure to significant pathological stresses, is enhanced by the substantial forces often applied in head trauma.

Previously reported observations indicate that most upper cervical spine injuries result from blows to the head.[2-9] Another noteworthy cause of such injuries is sudden deceleration of the torso combined with restriction of movement of the cervical spine, which creates a flexion-dis-

traction force that can result in an applied bending moment (see below).[2] Spinal involvement with tumor or infection obviously lowers the tolerance for such injuries.

Very violent movements of the head can disrupt the usually stable and protective ligaments of the upper cervical spine. The kinetic energy absorbed by the calvarium in these cases may be sufficient to cause death by head injury. The spine injury incurred, however, may also be fatal.[3]

Relevant Anatomy

The C1 vertebra is essentially a ring with an interconnecting and transsecting transverse ligament (transverse ligament of the atlas) and articulating facets (both rostrally to the occiput and caudally to the axis) on both sides. A multitude of ligaments secure fixation to surrounding vertebral and cranial bony elements. These ligaments may fail under an excessive load. The orientations of the articulating facets make the ring of C1 prone to injury from axial loading, and the location of the posterior arch of C1 makes it prone to hyperextension and hyperflexion loading injuries (Fig. 5-1).

The pedicles of C2 are located more ventrally and medially than those at other spinal levels. They essentially form a posterolateral extension of the vertebral body, connecting the vertebral body proper with its superior articulating process (lateral mass). The pars interarticularis of C2 has a more rostrocaudal orientation. This affects the way in which loads are transmitted through the occiput-C1-C2 complex and the type of injuries sustained when loading to failure occurs; when an axial load is borne, the lateral masses accept the load (Fig. 5-2).

Factors Determining Type of Injury

The orientation of the force vector applied to the cervical spine is the predominant factor dictating the type of injury that results. The applied-force vector most commonly arises from a blow to the head, but may also result from a deceleration of the torso. The relative intrinsic strengths of C1

55

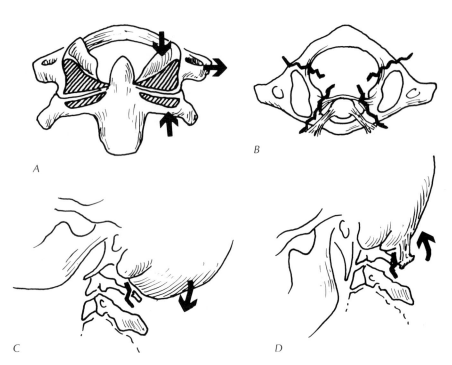

FIGURE 5-1 *A.* A coronal section of the C1-C2 articulations with surrounding elements. *B.* An axial load *(vertical arrows)* causes a laterally oriented resultant force vector *(horizontal arrow)* that, if substantial, causes a bursting of the ring of C1 via fracture of the ring in four locations (Jefferson fracture). *C.* Hyperextension of the calvarium can cause a fracture of the posterior arch of C1 by impingement on the posterior arch of C1 via the occiput or the lamina of C2. *D.* Hyperflexion can cause a similar injury, via ligamentous attachments. The latter two injuries do not usually degrade spinal stability, as can the C1 burst fracture.

and C2, as well as the surrounding spinal elements (including the adjacent vertebrae, calvarium, and supporting ligaments), secondarily dictate the type of injury by "setting the stage" for dissipating the energy of the applied-force vector.[10] The kinetic energy imparted predominantly dictates the magnitude of the injury.

The "stage-setting" aspect of the relative intrinsic strengths of the spinal elements is particularly obvious

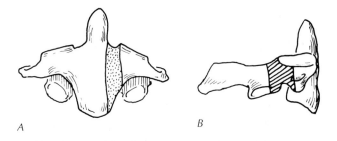

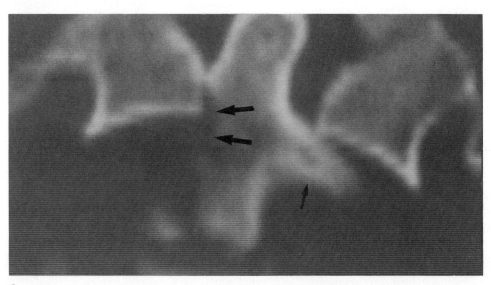

FIGURE 5-2 C2 and its articulations with surrounding elements. *A.* Coronal view. The shaded area *(dots)* marks the region of the C2 pedicle. *B.* Sagittal view. The diagonal bars mark the region of the pars interarticularis. *C.* Coronally reconstructed CT section through the mid-body of C2, illustrating the lack of support below the superior articulating facet of C2.

when more than one injury could theoretically result from the application of a single-force vector. For example, an axially applied load can result in a burst fracture of the atlas, a C2 burst-pedicle fracture, or a subaxial cervical spine burst fracture. The relative intrinsic strengths of the ring of C1, the body and pedicles of C2, and the subaxial cervical spine vertebral bodies dictate the type of injury incurred if a failure-producing force is, indeed, applied. Usually the ring of C1 or the subaxial cervical spine vertebral body is the weakest link, and a C1 burst fracture (Jefferson fracture—Fig. 5-1) or a subaxial cervical spine fracture is incurred. Occasionally, however, C2 is the weakest link (see below).

Applied-Force Vectors

In most cases the kinetic energy imparted to the upper cervical spine is directed to this region through the odontoid process via the anterior arch of C1 or the transverse ligament of the atlas, unless a true axial load is applied (Fig. 5-3). The direction (orientation) of the applied-force vector largely dictates the location of the fault line (location of fracture site or ligamentous disruption) (Fig. 5-4).[10] The location of the fault line is also influenced by the intrinsic strengths

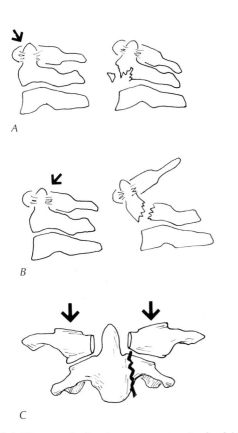

A

B

C

FIGURE 5-3 Blows to the head cause an extension load (*A*) or a flexion load (*B*) to be applied to the odontoid process, unless a pure axial load is applied. If a pure axial load is applied, the lateral masses bear this load. A fracture may result (*C*).

and weaknesses of C1 and C2 and the surrounding bony and soft tissue elements.

Although most failure-producing forces applied to the upper cervical spine are applied via the odontoid process, a true axial load injury, where the superior articulating processes (lateral masses) of C1 and C2 accept all of the load applied to the upper cervical spine, is an exception (see below). If structural failure of the upper cervical spine occurs, a bursting of C1—or, less frequently, a bursting of C2, or an occipital condyle fracture—may occur.[10,11]

Types and Mechanisms of Injury

The definition of mechanisms of injury in upper cervical spine fractures and dislocations has been complicated by the assumption that the injury types must be relatively few. The variety of *observed* mechanisms of injury confuses the situation. A variety of injury types do, indeed, exist. Figure 5-5 illustrates the force vectors that cause the various C1 and C2 fractures and dislocations. Several of the injury types that result from these force vectors have been under-recognized. Their structural natures, and what is known about their respective mechanisms of injury, will be discussed individually.

The injury types are discussed in the order of force vector application, starting with the judicial hangman's fracture and proceeding in a clockwise manner (Fig. 5-5*A*). Then lateral (coronal) injuries (Fig. 5-5*B*) and, finally, rotatory injuries are discussed.

The schema presented here is subject to change with the advent of new clinical and biomechanical data.

JUDICIAL HANGMAN'S FRACTURE

The combination of distraction and capital hyperextension results from judicial hanging with the noose placed in the submental position (injury mechanism A, Fig. 5-5*A*). Falls with a rostrally oriented force vector applied to the submental position can uncommonly cause the same injury.[12,13]

POSTERIOR DISLOCATION OF C1 ON C2

Posterior C1-C2 dislocations (Fig. 5-6) are rare.[14] They are purported to be caused by injury mechanism A (Fig. 5-5*A*). This results in the anterior arch of C1 riding over the dens, with the result that it becomes "locked" behind the dens.

TRAUMATIC SPONDYLOLISTHESIS OF THE AXIS (HANGMAN'S FRACTURE)

The sudden capital hyperextension of the head, without an associated distraction component, causes the commonly observed hangman's fracture (traumatic spondylolisthesis of the axis) (injury mechanism B, Fig. 5-5*A*).[5]

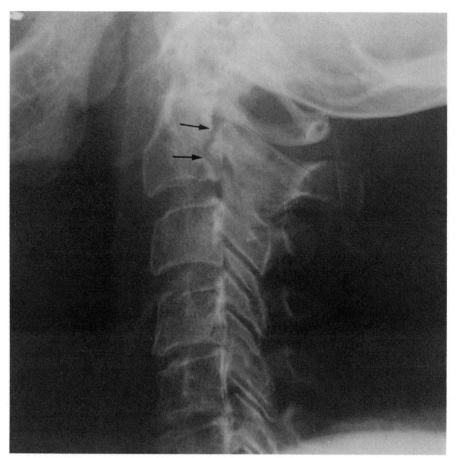

A

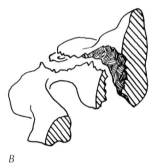

B

FIGURE 5-4 When a failure-producing load is applied, the location of the fault line depends largely on the orientation of the injury force vector. The length of the moment arm also depends on this orientation. In C2 body injuries, a common fault line occurs in the posterior coronal plane in the posterior C2 vertebral body. *A.* X-ray. *B.* Illustration. This type of fracture is called a *vertical coronally oriented C2 body fracture* (type 1 C2 body fracture).

VERTICAL CORONALLY ORIENTED POSTERIOR C2 BODY FRACTURE WITH C2-C3 EXTENSION-SUBLUXATION (TYPE 1 C2 BODY FRACTURE WITH C2-C3 EXTENSION-SUBLUXATION)[10]

Slightly less capital extension, combined with a small axial load component (injury mechanism C, Fig. 5-5*A*), may result in an injury slightly different from the traumatic spondylolisthesis of the axis. In this case the bony fault travels through the posterior C2 vertebral body instead of the pars interarticularis of C2, which is typical for traumatic spondylolisthesis of the axis. This fracture is a posterior C2 body fracture with C2-C3 extension-subluxation (type 1 C2 body fracture). It has been called an atypical traumatic spondylolisthesis of the axis by Burke and Harris,[4] and by Effendi and coworkers.[5] However, it is *not* atypical and is not a spondylolisthesis of the axis (hangman's fracture). It has an appearance similar to that of the type 1 C2 body fracture (Fig. 5-4).

VERTICAL CORONALLY ORIENTED POSTERIOR C2 BODY FRACTURE WITH C2-C3 EXTENSION-SUBLUXATION AND ANTERIOR TEARDROP (TYPE 1 C2 BODY FRACTURE WITH C2-C3 EXTENSION-SUBLUXATION AND ANTERIOR TEARDROP)[10]

A force vector applied to the high forehead region may result in the application of an axial load and capital hyperextension forces to the upper cervical spine (injury mechanism D, Fig. 5-5*A*). In this case the C2 body fails in a location similar to the location of the posterior C2 body fracture with C2-C3 subluxation. The direction and magnitude of the force applied, however, result in disruption of the disk interspace and hyperextension of the spine at the C2-C3 level. This causes an opening of the anterior disk interspace and a teardrop avulsion fracture of the anterior caudal aspect of the C2 vertebral body. The vertically oriented axial load causes significant compression of the C2-C3 disk interspace with a shearing mechanism applied to the ventral and dorsal

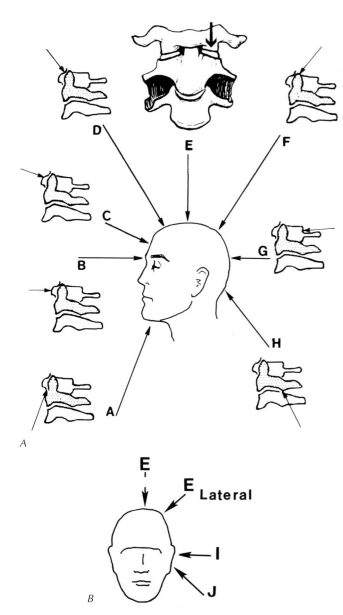

FIGURE 5-5 The mechanism of injury (orientation of injury force vector) partly dictates the type of injury incurred. *A.* Sagittal plane injury. *B.* Coronal plane injury.

aspects of the vertebral body because of the variable resistance encountered (the perimeter of the disk interspace is more rigid). This is called a posterior C2 body fracture and subluxation with an anterior teardrop (type 1 C2 body fracture). It resembles other type 1 C2 body fractures, except for the addition of the anterior teardrop component (Fig. 5-4).

TYPE 1 C2 BODY FRACTURE VARIANTS: HORIZONTAL CAUDAL C2 BODY FRACTURES

Type 1 C2 body fracture variants include the isolated extension teardrop and hyperextension dislocation injuries

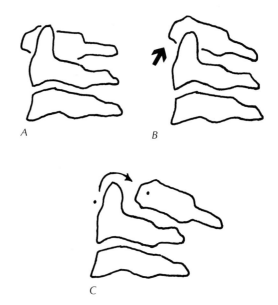

FIGURE 5-6 The mechanism of injury of a posterior C1-C2 dislocation. Note the requirement for at least some distraction *(heavy straight arrow)* to cause the anterior arch of C1 to slide over the dens *(curved arrow).*

described by Burke and Harris (injury mechanisms C and D, Fig. 5-5*A*).[4] With these fracture variants, the vertical coronal posterior C2 body component is not observed. Therefore, the whole C2 body extends—instead of the aspect of the vertebral body located ventral to the fault, as in the formal type 2 C2 body fracture. This extension results in C2-C3 disk interspace disruption (with the hyperextension dislocation injury) and a teardrop or avulsion injury to the ventral caudal aspect of the C2 vertebral body (Fig. 5-7).

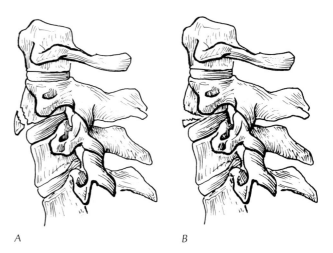

FIGURE 5-7 The mechanism of injury of type 1 C2 body fracture variants. *A.* Isolated extension teardrop fracture. *B.* Hyperextension dislocation. *(From J. T. Burke and J. H. Harris.[4])*

These variants are more common than other C2 body fractures.[4] They are called *horizontal caudal C2 body fractures.*

C1 BURST FRACTURE (JEFFERSON FRACTURE)

Axial loads applied to the vertex of the calvarium (injury mechanism E, Fig. 5-5A) can cause several types of injury. The most common of these is the C1 burst fracture (Jefferson fracture) (Fig. 5-1). The bursting of the C1 ring occurs because of the radially oriented resultant forces applied by the condyles of the occiput and the facet joints of C2. Their oblique orientation causes the laterally directed resultant force. This causes a fracture about the ring of C1 in four locations. If the total lateral displacement of the C1 facet joints on C2 exceeds 7 mm (adding together the lateral displacements of the right and left sides), the fracture may be unstable. This is due to the rupture of the transverse ligament of the atlas (Fig. 5-8).

OCCIPITAL CONDYLE FRACTURE (TYPES 1 AND 2)

There are several types of occipital condyle fracture[15,16]; types 1 and 2 usually are incurred via an axially applied load (injury mechanism E, Fig. 5-5A; see also Fig. 5-9). A type 1 fracture is a medial disruption of the condyle (impacted occipital condyle) caused by a resultant force that is applied medially on account of the oblique orientation of the occipital condyle–C1 facet (Fig. 5-13A). This is relatively uncommon, most likely because the C1 arch usually is a weaker link and so tends to fail first (Jefferson fracture). The type 2 occipital condyle fracture (an extension of a basilar skull fracture) most likely also results from an axially applied load (Fig. 5-9B).[15,16]

VERTICAL SAGITTALLY ORIENTED C2 BURST-PEDICLE FRACTURE (TYPE 2 C2 BODY FRACTURE)

Axial loads applied to the skull's vertex (injury mechanism E, Fig. 5-5A and B) may uncommonly cause a C2 body

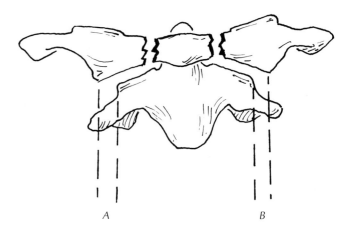

FIGURE 5-8 A greater-than-7-mm lateral displacement of the C1 facet on the C2 facet [adding the right (A) and left (B) displacements] implies disruption of the transverse ligament of the atlas and significant instability.

fracture. If other spinal elements do not fail first (resulting in an occipital condyle fracture, a Jefferson fracture, or a subaxial cervical spine burst fracture), the load applied to the articular pillars of C2 may result in a comminuted sagittal fracture of the C2 body. This injury is best visualized via an anteroposterior "view" (Fig. 5-10). With this fracture the C2 body fails along the lateral aspect of the vertebral body, in the region of the pedicle's junction with the vertebral body. Because part of the posterior wall of the C2 vertebral body is thrust into the spinal canal by virtue of the predominant axial load applied, the fracture is, by the definition of Denis,[17] a burst fracture.

The C1 burst fracture (Jefferson fracture) and the type 1 and type 2 occipital condyle fractures are caused by the same mechanism of injury. If the C1 ring and the occipital condyle are strong, the better part of an applied axial load is accepted by C2. If not, the mechanism of injury may result in a Jefferson fracture, or, less commonly, an occipital condyle fracture. With pure axial loads the majority of the load is borne by the facet joints; with the addition of hyperexten-

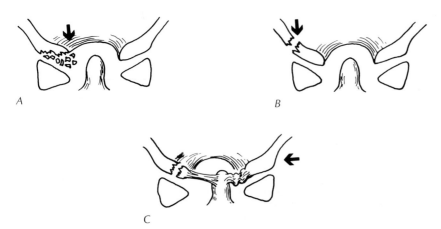

FIGURE 5-9 Occipital condyle fractures. A. Type 1. B. Type 2. C. Type 3. Types 1 and 2 are caused by axial loading. Type 3 is caused by a lateral blow. *(From P. A. Anderson and P. X. Montesano.*[15]

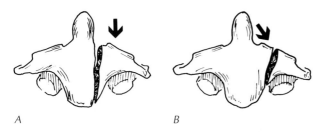

FIGURE 5-10 *A.* The mechanism of injury of a vertical sagittally oriented C2 burst-pedicle fracture (type 2 C2 body fracture). Note the absence of bony support immediately below the lateral mass of C2 (shaded area). *B.* A more lateral orientation of the axial load (see Fig. 5-5*A* and *B*) may result in a more laterally situated fracture.

sion or flexion components, a large portion of the load is borne by the odontoid process. In the case of non-axially applied loads, the odontoid process functions as a lever or moment arm by accepting the load and applying a bending moment. Only when isolated axial loads are applied to the C2 vertebra does the odontoid process not function as a lever arm. The addition of a flexion or extension component results in the stressing of a substantially weaker link (Fig. 5-3).

The addition of a lateral component to the axial load may shift the location of the fracture laterally (Fig. 5-5*A* and *B*), causing a more laterally situated sagittal C2 fracture.[10] This fracture may pass through the foramina transversaria and along the pars interarticularis of C2.

C1 ARCH FRACTURE

Axial loads, with or without a hyperextension component (injury mechanisms C, D, and E, Fig. 5-5*A*), may result in a fracture through the weakest point of the ring of C1. This weak point is near the course of the vertebral artery; its fracture is commonly associated with other upper cervical spine injuries (e.g., hangman's fracture). Hyperflexion may result in the same injury, via the ligamentous attachments to C1 (Fig. 5-1).

VERTICAL CORONALLY ORIENTED POSTERIOR C2 BODY TEARDROP FRACTURE WITH C2-C3 FLEXION-SUBLUXATION (TYPE 1 C2 BODY FRACTURE WITH FLEXION-SUBLUXATION)

A dorsally applied force vector with an axial load component (injury mechanism F, Fig. 5-5*A*) may result in the opening of the dorsal aspect of the C2-C3 disk interspace (capital neck flexion), thus causing an accompanying avulsion teardrop fracture of the dorsal aspect of the caudal C2 vertebral body. Since the C2-C3 disk interspace is slanted in a downward direction, its orientation is nearly in line with the applied-force vector. This, then, results in a subluxation between C2 and C3. This fracture resembles other type 1 C2 body fractures (Fig. 5-4).

HORIZONTAL ROSTRAL C2 BODY FRACTURE (TYPE 3 C2 BODY FRACTURE)

A dorsal blow to the head (injury mechanism G, Fig. 5-5*A*) may result in true neck flexion. Previously reported data[8] show that if the C2 region fails there occurs a horizontal fracture through the rostral portion of the body of C2. This has been called a "type 3 odontoid process fracture."[18] This fracture, however, is—by the definition of Anderson and D'Alonzo[18]—through the region of the C2 body, not the odontoid process.[10,16] Therefore it should be considered not an odontoid process fracture, but rather a C2 body fracture (horizontal rostral C2 body fracture; type 3 C2 body fracture).

RUPTURE OF THE TRANSVERSE LIGAMENT OF THE ATLAS

If the odontoid process does not yield to a failure-producing force applied by injury mechanism G (Fig. 5-5*A*), the transverse ligament of the atlas may rupture (Fig. 5-11).[8,19] The

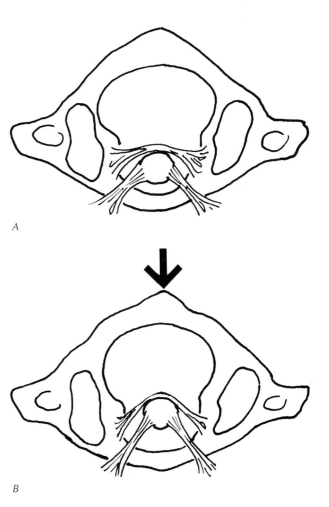

FIGURE 5-11 The mechanism of injury of a rupture of the transverse ligament of the atlas. The transverse ligament of the atlas (*A*) stretches if a dorsal force vector (*arrow*) is applied to the ring of C1, usually via the calvarium (*B*).

ligament usually is a stronger link than the rostral portion of the C2 vertebral body; hence the lesser incidence of this injury. MRI may be used to demonstrate disruption of the transverse ligament of the atlas.[20]

VERTICAL CORONALLY ORIENTED POSTERIOR C2 BODY FRACTURE WITH FLEXION-DISTRACTION (TYPE 1 C2 BODY FRACTURE WITH FLEXION-DISTRACTION)

If a capital flexion injury is combined with a distraction component, usually caused by a deceleration over a fulcrum (e.g., an automobile's shoulder harness), a flexion-distraction force complex is applied (injury mechanism H, Fig. 5-5A). This results in a bending moment about the ventral caudal aspect of C2, an opening of the disk interspace dorsally, maintenance or exaggeration of disk height, and preservation of anterior soft tissue integrity (as evidenced by the lack of demonstration of anterior soft tissue injuries on MRI). This is called a *vertical coronally oriented C2 body fracture with flexion-distraction* (type 1 C2 body fracture with flexion-distraction). Its radiographic appearance is similar to those of other type 1 C2 body fractures (Fig. 5-4).

Comment Vertical coronally oriented C2 body fractures have multiple mechanistic etiologies. These include hyperextension with an axial load, hyperflexion with an axial load, and flexion-distraction (Fig. 5-12). The complex etiology of C2 body fractures is the source of the confusion surrounding this aspect of spinal trauma.

DENS FRACTURE

The type 2 odontoid process fracture of Anderson and D'Alonzo[18] may be more appropriately called a *dens fracture*.[16] It most probably results from a lateral blow to the head (injury mechanism I, Fig. 5-5B),[8] perhaps combined with vertical compression.[21]

OCCIPITAL CONDYLE FRACTURE (TYPE 3)

A lateral blow to the head (injury mechanism I, Fig. 5-5B) uncommonly results in a medial avulsion of the occipital condyle. This is called a *type 3 occipital condyle fracture*.[15] It is an avulsion injury caused by shearing forces that put tension on the occipital condyle via the alar and capsular ligaments (Fig. 5-9).[15,16]

ATLANTOOCCIPITAL DISLOCATION

A lateral deceleration injury (with or without a hyperextension component) involves an applied lateral bending-rotation-distraction force complex (injury mechanism J, Fig. 5-5B). This may result in atlantooccipital dislocation, although some authors have postulated hyperextension-distraction mechanisms (Fig. 5-13).[3,22]

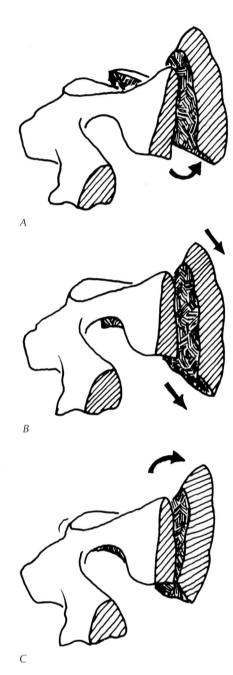

A

B

C

FIGURE 5-12 Various mechanisms of injury of vertical coronally oriented C2 body fractures (type 1 C2 body fractures). A. Hyperextension with varying degrees of axial loading (injury mechanisms C and D, Fig. 5-5A), resulting in a bending moment (*arrow*). B. Axial loading with some flexion (injury mechanism F, Fig. 5-5A), resulting in a translational deformation (*arrows*). C. Flexion-distraction (injury mechanism H, Fig. 5-5A), resulting in a bending moment (*arrow*).

AVULSION FRACTURES OF THE DENS

A distraction of the spine, not unlike the one that might be incurred with a judicial hanging (injury mechanism A, Fig. 5-5A) or with a force vector having a lateral component

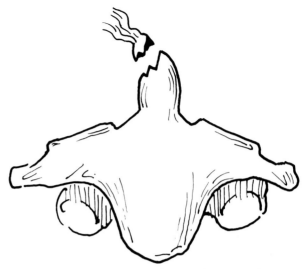

FIGURE 5-14 The mechanism of injury of a dens avulsion fracture.

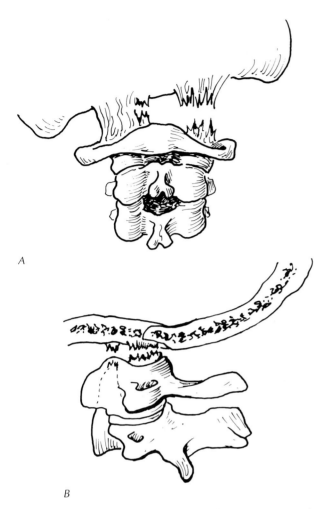

A

B

FIGURE 5-13 The mechanism of injury of an atlantooccipital dislocation: lateral (*A*) and extension-distraction (*B*).

(injury mechanism J, Fig. 5-5*B*), may result in an avulsion of the tip of the dens (Fig. 5-14).

ROTATORY SUBLUXATION INJURIES

If a torque (bending moment) is created about the long axis of the spine (about the dens), a rotational injury may occur.[23] This may result in rotatory subluxation of C1 on C2. This is

clearly the weakest link in the occiput-C1-C2 ligamentous complex. This is confirmed by the substantial rotory movement allowed about the dens (see Chap. 1).

LOSS OF STRUCTURAL INTEGRITY OF THE SUBAXIAL CERVICAL, THORACIC, AND LUMBAR SPINE

Relevant Anatomy

The anatomy of the entire subaxial spine is relatively monotonous compared to the significant level-to-level anatomic variations seen in the upper cervical spine. Subaxial injuries are less various, in number of definable injury patterns and types, than upper cervical injuries. For this reason they are grouped together here.

Factors Determining Type of Injury

Denis described several fracture types, and accompanying modes of failure, for the subaxial spine (Table 5-1).[24] This

TABLE 5-1 Basic modes of failure of the three columns in the four types of spinal injury

Type of fracture	Column		
	Anterior	Middle	Posterior
Compression	Compression	None	None or severe distraction
Burst	Compression	Compression	None
"Seatbelt"	None or compression	Distraction	Distraction
Fracture-dislocation	Compression rotation shear	Distraction rotation shear	Distraction rotation shear

SOURCE: From F. Denis.[24]

scheme of definitions of fracture types is the most widely used today. In contrast to the Denis scheme, however, injury types will be described here on the basis of *mechanism of injury*.[2] The difference between the two schemes is subtle; it may be most clearly discerned in the differentiation of ventral wedge compression and burst fractures. The presence or absence of retropulsed bone and/or disk fragments in the spinal canal is not used herein as a criterion for fracture type definition, as in Denis's scheme. [Denis's concepts are not to be disregarded, however. His three-column concepts are used in this text (see Chap. 3) for determination of spinal stability and instability.]

The way in which a load is applied partly determines the bending moment applied (see Chap. 2). This, in turn, determines the stresses placed on a given spinal segment. These are discussed below, with regard to each fracture type.

The fracture pattern is influenced by the position of the point of force application in relation to the instantaneous axis of rotation (IAR). The point of force application directly affects the type and extent of injury by virtue of its role in determining the bending moment. Likewise, an alteration of the IAR can affect the bending moment significantly. The type and extent of force application, the mode of failure, and the fracture incurred are altered by these factors. A mechanism of injury that not only applies a load to the spine but also alters the bending moment can significantly affect the stresses applied to the spinal elements (see below).

Applied-Force Vectors

The magnitude and characteristics of the failure-producing force and the resultant configuration of the injured spinal level (as well as the need for spinal decompression) dictate the management scheme and, thus, are used as criteria for injury type definition. As a result, the scheme used here limits the definition of the burst fracture; when one uses this scheme, the incidence of burst fracture is less and the incidence of wedge compression fracture greater than when one uses the scheme of Denis.[24]

Types and Mechanisms of Injury

VENTRAL WEDGE COMPRESSION FRACTURES

Ventral wedge compression fractures are the product of an axial load and a ventrally oriented bending moment (to failure); that is, the axial load is eccentrically placed (anterior to the IAR) (Fig. 5-15). This results in a flexion deformity of the fractured bone (an asymmetry of vertebral body height in which the ventral height is less than the dorsal height).[25-30] The cervical spine, thoracic spine, and thoracolumbar junction are prone to such injuries, because of the flexibility of the cervical spine and the often-assumed relatively flexed posture of the cervical and thoracic spine and thoracolumbar junction at the moment of impact. The sig-

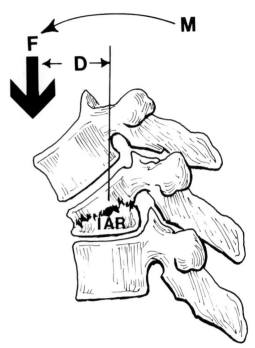

FIGURE 5-15 A depiction of the injury force vector causing a ventral wedge compression fracture. F = applied force vector; D = length of moment arm (from IAR to plane of F); M = bending moment.

nificant flexibility often counterbalances the influence of the natural lordotic posture of the cervical spine. However, if the person has not assumed a posture of flexion, the biomechanics of the natural lordotic posture prevail, and a burst fracture may occur (see below). The thoracic and thoracolumbar regions of the spine have a natural kyphotic curvature that, by its nature, exposes the spine to an increased chance of a flexion component in the injury. An eccentric load application is often encouraged by a flexed posture, whether it be secondary to a "natural" kyphosis or to a superimposed flexion (Fig. 5-16).

The mid- to low cervical and lumbar regions of the spine have intrinsic lordotic curvatures. In addition, the lumbar spine, because of the massive size of the vertebral bodies, is relatively unyielding. These factors minimize the likelihood of a significant flexion component in a spinal fracture in these regions. That is, the bending moment is nil, or nearly nil. Therefore, an isolated axial load is often applied to the mid- to low cervical and lumbar regions. As mentioned, in the cervical region, however, the frequent assumption of a kyphotic posture at the moment of impact (e.g., during "spear" tackling in football) results in a higher incidence of wedge compression fractures in the cervical region than in the lumbar region.

Nevertheless, ventral wedge compression fractures do occur in the mid- to low lumbar region. Because of the reasons outlined above, they more frequently occur near the upper limits of the lumbar spine, because of the lessening of

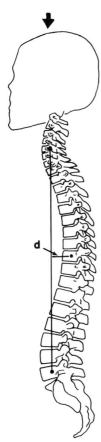

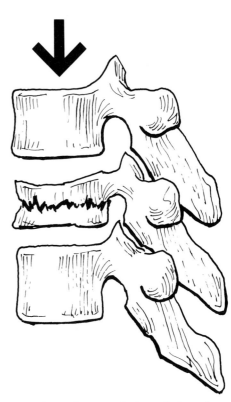

FIGURE 5-17 The mechanism of injury of a burst fracture: true axial loading without a bending moment (*d* = 0).

FIGURE 5-16 A kyphotic posture (as is present in the thoracic spine) increases the length of the natural moment arm (*d*) and, thus, the magnitude of the bending moment resulting from an eccentrically placed (with respect to the IAR) axial load (*arrows*).

the natural lordotic curvature observed as one ascends the lumbar spine. Retropulsion of bony and/or disk fragments into the spinal canal may occur.

BURST FRACTURES

If a true axial load (to failure) is applied to the subaxial spine, wedging of the resultant vertebral body fracture (i.e., asymmetry of vertebral body height loss) is unlikely. Typically, a symmetric compression of the vertebral body results—a burst fracture.[1,25–29,31–33] This ''pancaking'' of the vertebral body often causes retropulsion of bony fragments into the spinal canal and dural sac compression.[24,34] This retropulsion is a requirement in Denis's definition of burst fracture. It is a manifestation of an axial load that is not eccentrically placed with regard to the IAR (Fig. 5-17).

The latter point is crucial. If a force is transmitted in a rostral-to-caudal direction along the axis of the spine—delivering an axial load—the vector of the force passes through, or close to, the IARs of all vertebral bodies. Since a vertebral body rotates about the IAR, the location of the IAR dictates the vertebral body's response to the applied force.

If a force vector passes precisely through the IAR of a vertebral body that is stressed to failure by the force, a burst fracture will result. This is so because no eccentric component to the force vector is present; the moment arm length of this force vector (perpendicular distance from the force vector to the IAR; see Chap. 2) is zero (Fig. 5-17).

If a force vector passes in a plane that is adjacent to the IAR, bending of the spine will occur if the force is less than that required to produce failure. The concave side of the curvature induced is directed toward the orientation of the force vector (Fig. 5-18A). If the force applied is sufficient to cause failure, a fracture may result. This fracture will be eccentrically located with respect to the IAR and will result in an eccentric collapse of the vertebral body (wedge compression fracture), the direction of which is dictated by the location of the force vector (Fig. 5-18B). From these biomechanical facts one can easily categorize vertebral body fractures by mechanism of injury; or, more appropriately, by the configuration of the vertebral body after fracture.

Burst fractures, because they are caused only by relatively isolated axial loads, occur most frequently in the upper and midcervical and lumbar regions. In the lumbar region the relatively high incidence of burst fractures is due to the relatively limited flexibility of the lumbar spine, compared with the cervical spine, and to the substantial lordotic posture present in the lower lumbar spine. In the lower lum-

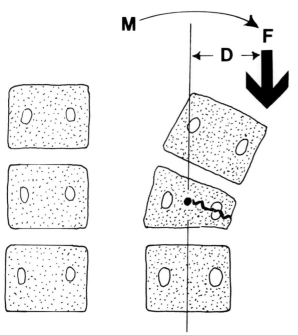

FIGURE 5-18 Eccentrically applied loads cause bending of the spine. The bending occurs in the direction of the eccentrically applied load (*F, large arrow*) with respect to the IAR (*dot*). If failure of the vertebral body occurs, it will be oriented in the same direction. *D* = length of moment arm (from IAR to plane of *F*); *M* = bending moment.

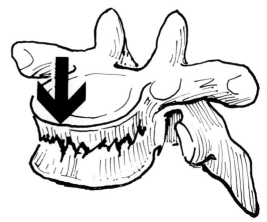

FIGURE 5-19 The mechanism of injury of a combination ventral and lateral wedge compression fracture. The arrow depicts an eccentrically applied load.

bar spine, however, these fractures are less common, because of the spinal column's increased intrinsic compression-resisting ability (secondary to increased bony and muscle mass in this region) (see Chap. 1).[32,35] In the cervical region the flexibility of the spine contributes to an increased incidence of flexion components in injuries; wedge compression fractures account for a greater percentage of the overall fracture rate in this region.

LATERAL WEDGE COMPRESSION FRACTURES

Few vertebral body fractures are pure. That is, most fractures are combinations of fracture types resulting from multiple injury mechanisms. Thus far, the discussion of the two fracture types—wedge compression and burst fractures—has centered on sagittal plane deformations. Coronal plane deformations, however, often occur simultaneously. Anteroposterior x-rays often demonstrate asymmetric loss of height of the vertebral body between the right and left sides. In such cases a lateral wedge compression fracture component coexists with the sagittal plane fracture component (Fig. 5-19). But lateral wedge compression fractures also occur as isolated injuries. These injuries are caused by axial loads placed eccentrically with respect to the IAR (similar to, but different in location from, the axial loads associated with ventral wedge compression fractures) (Fig. 5-18).

The mechanism of injury in lateral wedge compression fractures may be secondary to the "buckling" of the spine that follows the application of an axial load. This buckling results in an "effective" lateral bending moment (Fig. 5-20). An axial load combined with a lateral bending moment may result in the same vertebral body deformity seen in the axial buckling injury. This buckling may also occur in the sagittal plane, with a resultant compression fracture.

FLEXION-DISTRACTION (CHANCE) FRACTURES

Axial loading is the most common primary mechanism of spinal column injury. Rarely a distraction component plays a role, particularly in the subaxial spine. This is because few traumatic injuries involve distraction of the spine. One type of trauma that does involve distraction occurs when a lap belt is worn without a shoulder harness by a motorist involved in a deceleration accident. Distraction and flexion of the lumbar spine result.[25,36–39] These effects are secondary to the restriction of pelvic and lumbosacral movement with accompanying unrestricted distraction and forward flexion of the remainder of the spine (flexion bending moment). This injury was first described by Chance and, thus, commonly bears his name.[36] It may be broken down into two basic types: (1) A diastasis (fracture cleavage) through the pedicles and (2) a fracture through the vertebral endplate (Fig. 5-21). Variations may occur. Regardless of the type of Chance fracture, the mechanism of injury is the same.

POSTERIOR ELEMENT FRACTURES

So far, this chapter has focused on the effects of pure axial loads (force vector passing through the IAR) and loads that are predominantly axial but have slight eccentric components (force vector passing close to, but not through, the IAR). The majority of the failure-producing axial load force

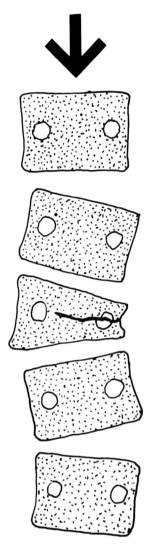

FIGURE 5-20 A depiction of spine "buckling" secondary to axial load application as an etiology of a wedge compression fracture.

vectors are oriented in a plane anterior or anterolateral to the IAR. If, indeed, they are located posterior to the IAR (i.e., if there is an extension component), an excessive compressive force is applied to the posterior elements at the affected spinal level; this increases the chance of posterior element failure (Fig. 5-22).

Posterior element fractures are fairly common, especially in the cervical spine, where the spine naturally assumes a lordotic posture and the vertebral segments are relatively small. The lumbar spine, which also assumes a lordotic posture, has a lower incidence of posterior element fractures because of the more massive nature of the vertebrae and the somewhat sagittal orientation of the facet joints. In the cervical region, spinal extension thrusts the opposing facet surfaces together, thus subjecting the facets and pars interarticularis to significant stress (Fig. 5-22*A*); rotation causes them to slide past each other (Fig. 5-22*B*).

Because of the relative lack of flexibility and the vertical orientation of the lumbar facets, their fracture, particularly as an isolated entity, is relatively uncommon. A hyperextension injury results in the facet joints' sliding past each other, because of their vertical orientation (Fig. 5-22*C*). Fractures of the lamina and pars interarticularis may result.[25] At the same time, the relative restriction of rotation of the lumbar spine minimizes the chance that rotation would cause injury to the facet joint(s).

Rotatory components may also induce posterior element injuries by forcing opposing inferior and superior articulating facet joints against each other with such force that failure occurs (Fig. 5-22*C*). Often, the forces applied are of such magnitude that vertebral body fracture or disk interspace disruption occurs also. Posterior element lumbar spine fractures are most commonly associated with other injuries to the spinal column complex—for example, compression fractures, rotational injuries, and translational injuries. A violent rotational component in the injury may result in disruption of posterior elements, as well as disruption of the integrity of the ventral axial-load-resisting substructure.[30]

Fractures of the spinous process and lamina fractures may occasionally result from extreme flexion or extension. Similarly, extreme lateral bending may cause transverse process fracture(s) on the convex side of the bend (Fig. 5-23).

LIGAMENTOUS INJURIES

In the lumbar spine, ligamentous injuries are common but are usually associated with other bony injuries. In the cervical spine, isolated ligamentous injuries are common. This is manifested by the high incidence of positive MRI scans in the face of negative x-ray or CT after cervical spine injury.[40,41] T2-weighted MRI images are the most useful in this regard.

The cervical spine's higher incidence of isolated ligamentous injuries is due, in part, to its substantial flexibility (Fig. 5-23). This flexibility allows greater strain to be placed on the ligaments. The more massive and less flexible lumbar spine does not rely so heavily on ligamentous support; in fact, the posterior ligaments, particularly the interspinous and supraspinous ligaments (especially in the low lumbar region), are weak or essentially nonexistent. Therefore, isolated ligamentous injuries are less frequent in this region.

FACET DISLOCATION

Facet dislocations occur frequently in the cervical region and less frequently in the upper thoracic region. They are rare in the lumbar region. Their more common occurrence in the cervical and thoracic spine is due to the relatively coronal orientation of the facet joints in these regions. An exaggerated flexion can exceed the normal limits of mobil-

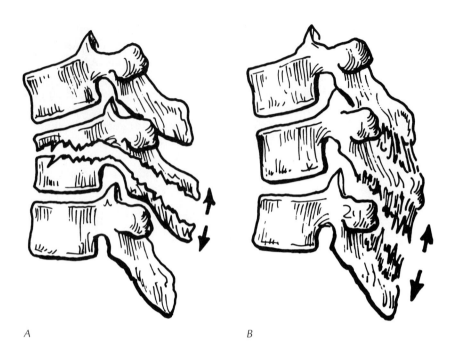

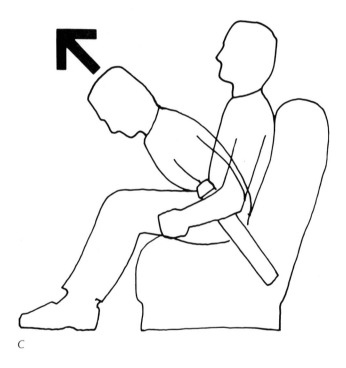

FIGURE 5-21 There are two fundamental types of Chance (flexion-distraction) fracture. *A*. Diastasis fracture through the pedicles and vertebral body. *B*. Fracture through the vertebral endplate or disk. *C*. The mechanism of injury is depicted.

ity of the facet joints. This causes the joints themselves to become dysfunctional by fracture, perching, or locking (Fig. 5-24). Obviously, these deformations affect stability.

The associated force vectors contribute to the complexity of the resultant injury pattern. A true flexion moment most commonly results in bilateral facet dislocation. A flexion moment combined with a rotational component most commonly results in unilateral facet dislocation. Either of the mechanisms or hyperextension, if combined with an axial load, may result in facet fracture (Fig. 5-25).

LOSS OF STRUCTURAL INTEGRITY OF THE SACRUM AND SURROUNDING BONY ELEMENTS

Sacral fractures are uncommon as isolated entities. They are usually associated with disruption of the pelvic ring in at least one other location. Two basic types of sacral fracture occur: vertical and horizontal. They involve three zones of the sacrum, and so have been classified accordingly (Fig. 5-26).[17] Zone 1 injuries involve fractures (usually vertical) through the ala and do not involve the neuroforamina. They

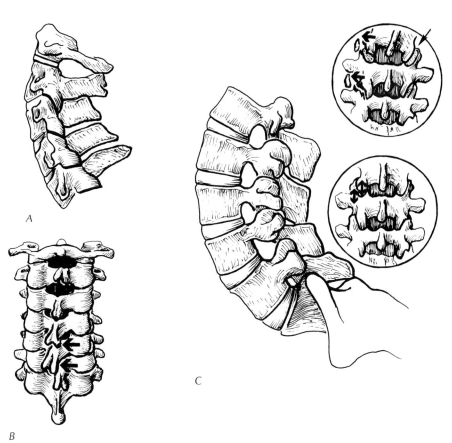

FIGURE 5-22 The mechanism of injury of posterior element fractures. Cervical spine extension forcibly approximates the facet joints and/or the laminae (A); cervical rotation causes the coronally oriented facet joints to slide past each other (B). The former may produce fracture; the latter may produce isolated ligamentous disruption or dislocation. In the lumbar region, the facet joints are able to slide past each other during extension, thus minimizing the chance for facet fracture by this mechamism (B). Lumbar rotation, however, results in one facet's abutting against another. This results in facet fracture if the force is substantial (C, upper inset). Conversely, extension or flexion causes the sagittally oriented facet joints to slide past each other (C, lower inset).

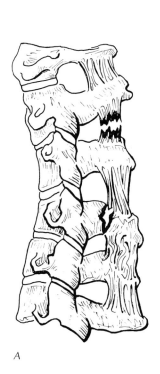

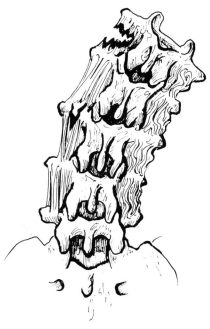

FIGURE 5-23 Extreme flexion may cause spinous process fractures or ligamentous disruption (A). Extreme lateral bending may cause a transverse process fracture or ligamentous disruption (B).

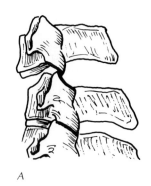
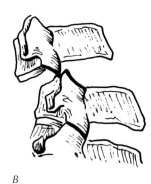

A

B

FIGURE 5-24 Cervical spine facet injuries: perched (*A*) and locked (*B*).

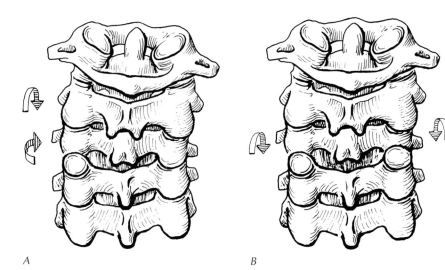

A

B

FIGURE 5-25 Flexion plus rotation (*curved arrows*) causes unilateral cervical facet joint dislocation (*A*). Pure flexion (*curved arrows*) causes bilateral cervical facet joint dislocation (*B*).

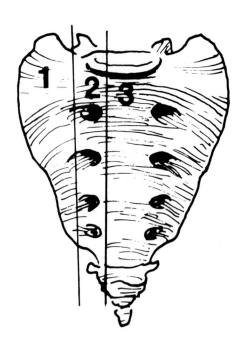

FIGURE 5-26 Sacral fractures and the three zones, or injury patterns.

usually result from lateral compression forces and are relatively stable if there is no significant translational component. Zone 2 injuries too are generally vertical and involve the ventral neuroforamina. Zone 3 injuries are vertical and/or horizontal and involve the sacral spinal canal; thus, neurological injury (particularly bladder dysfunction) often accompanies these fractures. Sacral anatomy has been nicely reviewed by Esses and coworkers.[42]

REFERENCES

1. McAfee PC, Yuan HA, Frederickson BE, et al: The value of computed tomography in thoracolumbar fractures. *J Bone Joint Surg* 1983; 65A:461–473.
2. Benzel EC: Biomechanics of lumbar and lumbosacral spine fracture, in Rea GL, Miller CA (eds): *Spinal Trauma: Current Evaluation and Management.* AANS Publications 1993:165–195..
3. Bucholz RW, Burkhead WZ: The pathological anatomy of fatal atlanto-occipital dislocations. *J Bone Joint Surg* 1979; 61A:248–250.
4. Burke JT, Harris JH: Acute injuries of the axis vertebra. *Skeletal Radiol* 1989; 18:335–346.
5. Effendi B, Roy D, Cornish B, et al: Fractures of the ring of the axis: A classification based on the analysis of 131 cases. *J Bone Joint Surg* 1981; 63B:319–327.
6. Francis WR, Fielding JW: Traumatic spondylolisthesis of the axis. *Orthop Clin North Am* 1978; 9:1011–1027.
7. Francis WR, Fielding JW, Hawkins RJ, et al: Traumatic spondylolisthesis of the axis. *J Bone Joint Surg* 1981; 63B:313–318.
8. Mouradian WH, Fietti VG, Cochran GVB: Fractures of the odontoid: A laboratory and clinical study of mechanisms. *Orthop Clin North Am* 1978; 9:985–1001.
9. Williams TG: Hangman's fracture. *J Bone Joint Surg* 1975; 57B:82–88.
10. Benzel EC, Hart BL, Ball PA, et al: Vertical C2 body fractures. (Submitted)
11. Kesterson L, Benzel EC, Orrison W, et al: Evaluation and treatment of atlas burst fractures (Jefferson fractures). *J Neurosurg* 1991; 75:213–220.
12. Levine AM, Edwards CC: Treatment of injuries in the C1-C2 complex. *Orthop Clin North Am* 1986; 17:31–44.
13. Wood-Jones F: The ideal lesion produced by judicial hanging. *Lancet* 1913; 1:53.
14. Patzakis MJ, Knopf A, Elfering M, et al: Posterior dislocation of the atlas on the axis: A case report. *J Bone Joint Surg* 1974; 56A:1260–1262.
15. Anderson PA, Montesano PX: Morphology and treatment of occipital condyle fractures. *Spine* 1988; 13:731–736.
16. White AA, Panjabi MM: *Clinical Biomechanics of the Spine* (2d ed). Philadelphia: Lippincott, 1990:130–342.
17. Denis F, Davis S, Comfort T: Sacral fractures; an important problem. Retrospective analysis of 236 cases. *Clin Orthop* 1988; 227:67–81.
18. Anderson LD, D'Alonzo RT: Fractures of the odontoid process of the axis. *J Bone Joint Surg* 1974; 56A:1663–1674.
19. Fielding JW, Cochran GVB, Lawsing JF, et al: Tears of the transverse ligament of the atlas. A clinical and biomechanical study. *J Bone Joint Surg* 1974; 56A:1683–1691.
20. Dickman CA, Mamourian A, Sonntag VKH, et al: Magnetic resonance imaging of the transverse atlantal ligament for the evaluation of atlantoaxial instability. *J Neurosurg* 1991; 75:221–227.
21. Altoff B: Fracture of the odontoid process. An experimental study. *Acta Orthop Scand* 1979; 177(suppl):61–95.
22. Montane I, Eismont FJ, Green GA: Traumatic occipitoatlantal dislocation. *Spine* 1991; 16:112–116.
23. Garber JN: Abnormalities of the atlas and the axis: Vertebral, congenital and traumatic. *J Bone Joint Surg* 1964; 46A:1782–1791.
24. Denis F: The three-column spine and its significance in the classification of acute thoracolumbar spine injuries. *Spine* 1983; 8:817–831.
25. Bucholz RW, Gill K: Classification of injuries to the thoracolumbar spine. *Orthop Clin North Am* 1986; 17:67–83.
26. Holdsworth FW: Fractures, dislocations and fracture dislocations of the spine. *J Bone Joint Surg* 1970; 52A:1534–1551.
27. Jelsma RK, Kirsch PT, Rice JF, et al: The radiographic description of thoracolumbar fractures. *Surg Neurol* 1982; 18:230–236.
28. Keene JS: Radiographic evaluation of thoracolumbar fractures. *Clin Orthop* 1984; 189:58–64.
29. Kelly RP, Whitesides TE Jr: Treatment of lumbodorsal fracture-dislocations. *Ann Surg* 1968; 167:705–717.
30. Whitesides TE Jr: Traumatic kyphosis of the thoracolumbar spine. *Clin Orthop* 1977; 128:78–92.
31. Cope R, Kilcoyne RF, Gaines RW: The thoracolumbar burst fracture with intact posterior elements. Implications for neurologic deficit and stability. *Neuro-Orthopedics* 1989; 7:83–87.
32. Court-Brown CM, Gertzbein SD: The management of burst fractures of the fifth lumbar vertebra. *Spine* 1987; 12:308–312.
33. McEnvoy RD, Bradford, DS: The management of burst fractures of the thoracic and lumbar spine. Experience in 53 patients. *Spine* 1985; 10:631–637.
34. Hashimoto T, Kaneda K, Abumi K: Relationship between traumatic spinal canal and neurologic deficits in thoracolumbar burst fractures. *Spine* 1988; 13:1268–1272.
35. De SD, McCreath SW: Lumbosacral fracture-dislocations. A report of four cases. *J Bone Joint Surg* 1981; 63B:58–60.
36. Chance GQ: Note on a type of flexion fracture of the spine. *Br J Radiol* 1948; 21:452–453.
37. Gertzbein SD, Court-Brown CM: Flexion-distraction injuries of the lumbar spine. *Clin Orthop* 1988; 227:52–60.
38. Rennie W, Mitchell N: Flexion distraction fractures of the thoracolumbar spine. *J Bone Joint Surg* 1973; 55A:386–390.
39. Smith WS, Kaufer H: Patterns and mechanisms of lumbar injuries associated with lap seat belts. *J Bone Joint Surg* 1969; 51A:239–254.
40. Benzel EC, Hart BL, Ball PA, et al: MRI for the evaluation of patients with non-obvious cervical spine injury. (Submitted)
41. Orrison WW, Hart BL, Benzel EC, et al: MRI, CT and plain film comparison in acute cervical spine trauma. (Submitted.)
42. Esses SI, Botsford DJ, Huler RF, et al: Surgical anatomy of the sacrum. *Spine* 1991; 16:283–288.

Chapter 6

Spinal Deformities

INTRODUCTION

Spinal deformities can result from unstable motion segments, or, conversely, can cause them. The classification of spinal deformities can be complex. For example, the use of the long axis of the spine as a reference has traditionally caused the term *rotation* to be used only for rotation about this axis; that is, rotatory deformations of the spine are traditionally thought of as those deformations that involve rotation, or twisting, of one or more of the vertebrae about the long axis of the spine. Although this usage of the term *rotation* is, for the most part, maintained in this chapter, the more all-encompassing usage of the term is also used (i.e., meaning rotation about *any* axis). The latter usage comprehends flexion, extension, and lateral bending.

Translation and rotation can occur, respectively, along and about each of the three axes of the Cartesian coordinate system. Therefore, six fundamental movements can occur; hence the six fundamental types of spinal deformation: (1) rotation about the long axis of the spine, (2) rotation about the coronal axis of the spine, (3) rotation about the sagittal axis of the spine, (4) translation along the long axis of the spine, (5) translation along the coronal axis of the spine, and (6) translation along the sagittal axis of the spine. Each of these movements or deformations can occur in either of two directions (Fig. 6-1). Each deformity type may involve only one spinal segment or multiple segments. Spinal deformities are most often combinations of two or more of the types. They may result from either acutely or chronically applied loads.

ROTATION DEFORMATION

Rotation deformations are manifestations of an asymmetric load or a rotatory load (torque) applied to a spinal segment (Fig. 6-2). Rotation deformations about an axially oriented axis (coronal or sagittal) can occur at the level of the verte-bral body (via asymmetric loss of vertebral height, as in posttraumatic kyphosis) (Fig. 6-2*B*) or at the level of the disk interspace (via asymmetric disk interspace height loss, as in degenerative scoliosis) (Fig. 6-2*C*).[1–4] Segmental spinal rotatory deformation can also occur about the long axis of the spine (Fig. 6-3).

The often-unrecognized coupling phenomenon, whereby one spinal movement or deformation (e.g., lateral bending) obligates another (e.g., rotatory deformation about the long axis of the spine), commonly results in subtle or not-so-subtle rotatory deformities about the long axis of the spine. The concept of spinal coupling is reemphasized here in order to underscore its importance in complex spinal surgery. As discussed in Chap. 2, the phenomenon of coupling is significant clinically. It plays roles both in the prevention of spinal deformation (by contributing to movement restriction) and in the exaggeration of the complexity of the deformation itself (when a deformity indeed occurs).

Rotation Deformation about the Long Axis of the Spine

The application of a rotatory or torsional load to the spine [either acutely, via trauma, or chronically, via gradual deformity progression (commonly complicated by the coupling phenomenon)] can cause the spinal segments above the unstable segment to rotate in a direction *opposite* to the direction of rotation of the segments below the unstable segment. This usually occurs about the long axis of the spine (Fig. 6-3). In traumatic permanent deformation, ligamentous and bony elements (e.g., facet joints) are often disrupted. Classic examples of such acute injuries are the unilateral cervical locked facet (rotation combined with flexion) and posttraumatic fracture-dislocation with an accompanying rotatory component (see Chap. 5). These two injuries exemplify the fact that rotatory deformation about the long axis is seldom an isolated entity.

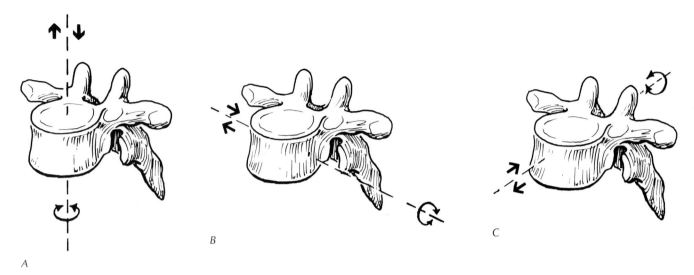

FIGURE 6-1 The six fundamental segmental movements, or types of deformation, of the spine along or about the IAR are (1) rotation about the long axis of the spine (*A*), (2) rotation about the coronal axis of the spine (*B*), (3) rotation about the sagittal axis of the spine (*C*), (4) translation along the long axis of the spine (*A*), (5) translation along the coronal axis of the spine (*B*), and (6) translation along the sagittal axis of the spine (*C*).

Rotatory Deformation about the Coronal and Sagittal Axes of the Spine

The application of eccentrically placed loads in a spinal segment creates a bending moment upon that segment. The applied bending moment may result in failure of the spinal segment with accompanying deformation along one or both of the axially oriented axes (Fig. 6-2). This deformation results in rotation of the segments above and below the involved segment(s); relatively speaking, the segments above and below rotate toward each other. This rotation can take the form of kyphosis (flexion rotation deformation), lordosis (extension rotation deformation), scoliosis (lateral bending rotation deformation), or some combination of these. A classic rotation deformation about an axially oriented axis, resulting from asymmetric load application, is that caused by a wedge compression fracture (Figs. 6-2 and 6-4). An anterior wedge compression fracture results in a flexion rotation deformation about an axially oriented axis.

It is mainly this type of deformation that leads to aberrant force application to the spine, by creating a moment arm through which externally applied forces can have pathological effects. In this way a deformation can cause or create an unstable motion segment (deformation progression) by

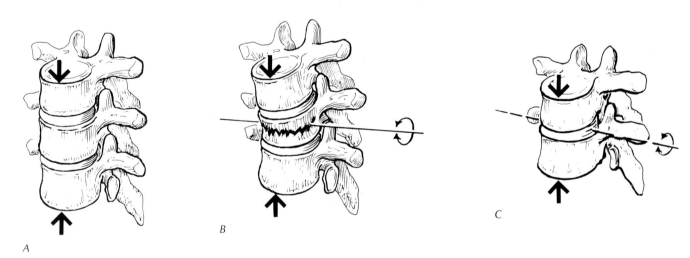

FIGURE 6-2 A depiction of the forces (*A*) and the resultant rotation deformation (*B*) about a coronally oriented axis of the spine, resulting in a wedgelike deformation. Rotation deformations about an axially (coronally or sagittally) oriented axis can occur at the level of the disk interspace as well (*C*). Curved arrows depict bending moments. Straight arrows depict applied forces.

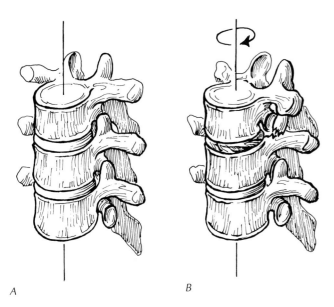

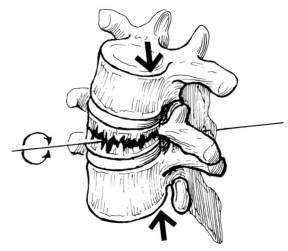

FIGURE 6-4 Rotation deformation can occur about the coronal axis of the spine (anterior wedge compression fracture, as in Fig. 6-2) and about the sagittal axis (lateral wedge compression fracture, as here). Curved arrow depicts bending moment. Straight arrows depict applied forces.

FIGURE 6-3 A twisting of the spine about its long axis (*A*) can result in a rotatory deformation about this axis (*B*). Curved arrow depicts applied bending moment.

leading to the application of excessive stresses to the affected segment(s) via the concocted moment arm (see Chaps. 4 and 5).

TRANSLATIONAL DEFORMATION

Translational deformation of the spine occurs along an axis defined by the direction of the deformation-inducing force vector.[1,3,4] This may result in shearing, compression, or distraction of spinal elements. Translational deformation differs from rotational deformation, which is created by an applied bending moment due to a force vector applied at some distance from the axis of deformation.

Translational deformation can occur in any plane. It can be acute or chronic. Classic examples of this type of deformation are burst fractures (deforming force vector applied along the longitudinal axis of the spine) and fracture-dislocations and the various spondylolistheses (deforming force vector applied along one of the axially oriented axes of the spine) (Fig. 6-5). Note that the vertical orientation of the lumbosacral intervertebral joint in most persons converts axially applied loads to translation-deformity-enhancing

FIGURE 6-5 A burst fracture results from translation of the upper and lower endplates of a vertebral body toward each other along the long axis of the spine. This results from two parallel and coincident opposed force vectors (*arrows*) (*A*). Axially oriented translational deformation, resulting in a fracture-dislocation, occurs via two parallel, but noncoincident opposed force vectors (*arrows*) (*B*).

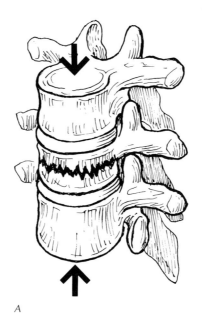
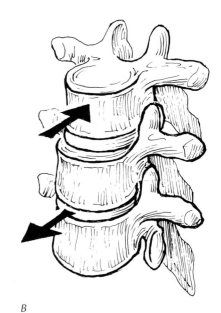

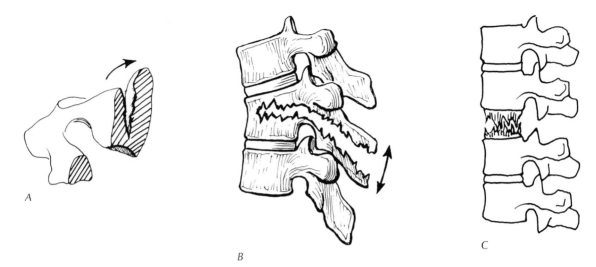

FIGURE 6-6 Flexion-distraction of the spine can result in a type 1 C2 body fracture in the cervical region (*A*) or a Chance fracture in the thoracic or lumbar region (*B*). Excessive spinal traction can also result in distraction of spinal elements (*C*).

force vectors (see Chaps. 1 and 5). This translational stress is encouraged by the upright posture.[5]

Translational Deformation along the Long Axis of the Spine

Distraction deformation of the spine is uncommon, particularly in a chronic form. Flexion-distraction injuries (see Chap. 5) result in distraction of the spine, usually with an accompanying flexion component (Fig. 6-6).[1–4] Extension or lateral bending mechanisms may become clinically manifest as well. Since axial loads are borne by the spine during the activities of daily living, compression of the spine is common. Distraction of the spine during the activities of daily living, particularly on a chronic or ongoing basis, is uncommon. The exposure of the spine to distraction forces can occur iatrogenically—for example, via the application of spinal traction, the use of inversion boots (hanging by one's feet), or the application of excessive distraction forces via spinal implants. The amount of distraction necessary to achieve a clinical effect can be calculated on a theoretical basis.[6]

The application of a true axial load to the spine along an axially oriented axis can result in failure of a component of a spinal segment (bone or soft tissue), with a resultant loss of height of that component.[1,3,4] In order for this to occur the force vector of the applied load must be in line with the IAR (along the neutral axis of the spine), thus applying an isolated axial load with no applied bending moment. The opposed forces are *coincident*. Translational deformation along the long axis of the spine occurs via two parallel coincident forces applied along the neutral axis of the spine (Fig. 6-5).

Translational Deformation along the Coronal and Sagittal Axes of the Spine

Translation and shearing of the spinal elements along the coronal or sagittal axis of the spine result in what have been called *spinal dislocations* or *listheses* (Fig. 6-5*B*). They result from the application of parallel, but not aligned, force vectors applied in opposite directions. The opposed forces are *noncoincident*.

COMBINATION DEFORMATIONS

Most spinal deformations are manifestations of more than one type of deformation. For example, a compression deformation (translational deformation along the long axis of the spine) is often accompanied by a rotational deformation (rotational deformation about the coronal axis of the spine). This results in a wedge compression fracture (Fig. 6-4; see also Chap. 5). Type 1 C2 body fractures (flexion-distraction) and Chance fractures (flexion-distraction) are other examples of combination deformations (Fig. 6-6).

DEFORMATION PROGRESSION

In order for deformation progression to occur, at least one unstable spinal segment must be present. This instability may be either acute or chronic (see Chap. 3). Instability as an isolated entity, however, is not sufficient to create a deformation or to cause it to progress. Deformation creation or progression requires the application of pathological (excessive) stresses to the spine, and/or the application of nonpathological stresses to an already deformed spine. The

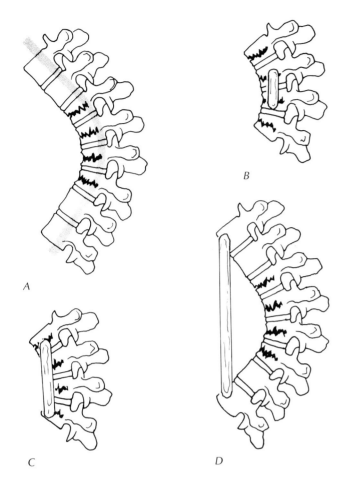

A

B

C

D

FIGURE 6-7 A spinal deformity (A) may be inappropriately managed by placement of a ventral spinal weight-bearing strut near the neutral axis *(shaded area, B),* rather than ventral to the neutral axis. This is problematic because the strut does not span the entire length of the injured and deformed portion of the spine. A longer strut may be required (C). The Cobb's angle may be misleading in this regard (see Chap. 3). The location of the neutral axis obviously influences this process. The ventral weight-bearing strut should not be placed behind or too close to the neutral axis, as is the case in B; rather, it should be placed well ventral to the neutral axis throughout its extent. This may require an even longer construct that extends well beyond the length depicted in C; this is depicted in D.

former can create a deformity by bending, twisting, etcetera. The latter can exaggerate an already existing spinal deformation via the action of what would normally be *non-pathological* stresses upon the *pathological* moment arm of the already-present deformation.

Awareness of the complexities of deformation formation and progression is critical to the design of an appropriate management scheme. Knowledge of the approximate loca-

tions of the IAR and the neutral axis is very useful in the consideration of operative indications and construct design.[7]

Deformation and deformation progression can present problems to the spine surgeon. The presence of spinal deformation can lead to further progression despite spinal fusion. Knowledge of the location of the neutral axis, Cobb's angle, and the radius of curvature plays a vital role in the decision-making process (Fig. 6-7).

Ventral fusions placed to prevent kyphotic deformation progression are best placed well ventral to the neutral axis. This mandates the use of a longer strut (Fig. 6-7). Similarly, dorsal fusions are best placed well dorsal to the neutral axis to prevent kyphotic deformation progression.[5] *The farther from the neutral axis a graft is placed, the more effective it becomes in preventing kyphotic deformation progression. On the other hand, in a spine with minimal deformation, axial loads are best borne by a graft placed close to the neutral axis and in line with the IARs at each segmental level. This is addressed in greater detail in Chap. 10.*

STABLE DEFORMATIONS

The definition of a stable deformation can be made, in the strictest sense, only by serial observation of the patient, clinically and radiographically, over an extended period. The essential findings are the absence of radiographic evidence of deformation progression and the accompanying absence of progressive neurological deficit or pain related to instability. Bone scanning or MRI may be helpful in difficult cases where long-term follow-up is not available or is not a reasonable clinical alternative.

REFERENCES

1. Benzel EC: Biomechanics of lumbar and lumbosacral spine fracture, in Rea GL, Miller CA (eds): *Spinal Trauma. Current Evaluation and Management.* AANS Publications, 1993:165–195.
2. Chance GQ: Note on a type of flexion fracture of the spine. *Br J Radiol* 1948; 21:452–453.
3. Holdsworth FW: Fractures, dislocations and fracture dislocations of the spine. *J Bone Joint Surg* 1970; 52A:1534–1551.
4. White AA, Panjabi MM: *Clinical Biomechanics of the Spine* (2d ed): Philadelphia: Lippincott, 1990:30–342.
5. Farfan HF: The biomechanical advantage of lordosis and hip extension for upright activity: Man as compared with other anthropoids. *Spine* 1978; 3:336–342.
6. Miller LS, Cotler HB, De Lucia FA, et al: Biomechanical analysis of cervical distraction. *Spine* 1987; 12:831–837.
7. White AA, Panjabi MM, Thomas CL: The clinical biomechanics of kyphotic deformities. *Clin Orthop Rel Res* 1977; 128:8–17.

Chapter 7

Neural Element Injury

MECHANISMS OF NEURAL ELEMENT INJURY

External influences can cause a cell to become dysfunctional, or to die, by one or a combination of three mechanisms: (1) cell disruption, (2) cell distortion, and (3) metabolic derangements. Disruption of the cell usually results in its death. Cell distortion and metabolic derangements can cause temporary dysfunction or death of the cell. Cell disruption can result from the initial injury (primary injury), or secondarily, from the exaggeration of cell distortion that can result from delayed CNS tissue shifts—such as those related to edema or hematoma formation (ongoing primary injury). Cell disruption (death) can also be caused by metabolic derangements, such as extracellular osmotic shifts and autodestructive processes that can follow the primary injury (secondary injuries). Thus, cell distortion and metabolic derangements can lead to cell disruption.[1,2]

The surgical decompression of a mass lesion (bone, disk, hematoma, etc.) can relieve distortion of the cell and can also relieve metabolic derangements. Augmentation of tissue perfusion pressure, alone, can result in an improved metabolic milieu.

The spine surgeon can do nothing to affect the primary insult (injury), other than to participate in consumer safety and injury prevention programs. Conversely, the secondary injury response to neural injury can be interrupted, at least in part, by pharmacologic interventions.[3] It is not the purpose of this chapter to delve into the neurochemistry and neuropharmacology of neural injury; suffice it to say that the possibility of minimizing neural injury by pharmacologic means should not be underestimated.

As mentioned above, an ongoing primary injury with an obligatory ongoing secondary injury response may frequently follow a neural insult. This ongoing primary injury may be the result of such factors as persistent extrinsic neural element impingement and ischemia. Complex biocellular and biomechanical events may contribute to neurological impairment.[1,2,4–8] These may be closely interrelated. Therefore, the biomechanics of the spine and spine pathol-

ogy, as well as the biomechanics of neural decompression, fusion, and instrumentation, play a role in the prevention of an ongoing primary injury. The timing of surgery may or may not play a role in the propagation of the ongoing primary injury process.

There are four fundamental mechanisms of injury related to persistent neural element distortion: (1) extrinsic neural element compression, (2) simple distraction, (3) tethering of the neural elements over extrinsic masses in the sagittal plane ("sagittal bowstring" effect), and (4) tethering of the neural elements over extrinsic masses in the coronal plane ("coronal bowstring" effect) (Fig. 7-1). Each must be considered and accounted for before surgical intervention, both so that the neural elements are adequately decompressed by the operative intervention and so that operative intervention itself does not cause neural element distortion.

Extrinsic Neural Element Compression

Spinal cord compression is often considered the most important cause of neurological dysfunction associated with degenerative disease and trauma. In the case of degenerative spine diseases, compression often results from an annular constriction of the neural elements. This constriction is a result of a combination of factors, such as ventral osteophyte, dorsolateral facet, and dorsal hypertrophied ligamentum flavum compression. In the case of trauma, compression is often related to impingement onto the neural elements by an extrinsic mass located only on one side—usually ventral—of the neural elements.

The spinal cord consists predominantly of long tracts with relatively little gray matter. In this respect it differs substantially from brain CNS tissue. Differences in blood supply, sensitivity to injury, myelination, and the surrounding bony and soft tissue elements make brain injuries and spinal cord injuries very different with regard both to theory and to management. Nevertheless, neurons in general can withstand significant external pressure and remain func-

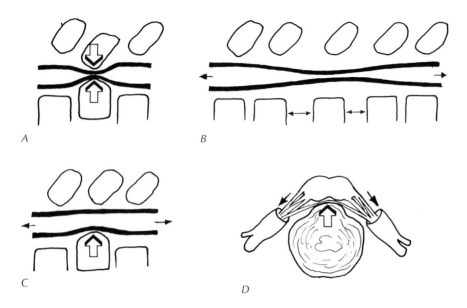

FIGURE 7-1 The four mechanisms of neural element distortion–related injury: neural element compression (*A*), simple distraction resulting in spinal cord stretching and narrowing (*B*), tethering over an extrinsic mass in the sagittal plane ("sagittal bowstring" effect) (*C*), and tethering of neural elements over an extrinsic mass in the coronal plane ("coronal bowstring" effect); and an axial depiction (*D*). Solid arrows depict "distractive" forces; hollow arrows depict forces applied directly to the dural sac.

tional. With compressive lesions, therefore, the cause of neurological dysfunction is often not clear.

As mentioned above, distortion and metabolic derangements are not well tolerated by the cell. Although the mechanism of injury of a compressive lesion may appear to be pure compression, distortion and ischemia may play significant roles. Degenerative spine diseases, such as cervical spondylosis, may appear to be causing only compression of the spinal cord via annular constriction.[9] In reality, however, the distortion of neural elements, combined with their exposure to repetitive movement (trauma), can result in persistence of distortion and in repeated insults.[10–16]

A compressive lesion can cause asymmetric deformation of the spinal cord (Fig. 7-2), thus causing not only increased tissue pressure but also distortion (and focal distortion) of the neurons. This causes neuronal dysfunction over and above that caused by compression alone.

Finally, ischemia related to decreases in tissue perfusion pressure can also cause neuronal impairment. The importance of this, however, is not clear. Also important is the fact that the spinal cord responds differently to ischemia than does the brain.

Simple Distraction

Simply distracting a neural element may result in electrophysiological and metabolic dysfunction or cell death. Distraction has two fundamental potentially harmful effects: (1) neuronal distortion and (2) impediment of the blood supply (Fig. 7-3).

Cusick and coworkers and Brieg have studied spinal cord distraction in detail.[17–20] Distraction alone may require the application of a considerable force to cause neural dysfunction. However, a combination of injury mechanisms—such as is often seen in cases of trauma—may exaggerate the

neural injury. For example, in distraction of the spinal cord over an impinging mass (tethering), much less force is required to cause a given neuronal impairment than in simple distraction (Fig. 7-1*C*).

"Sagittal Bowstring" Effect

An underestimated cause of neurological dysfunction is the tethering of the spinal cord over extrinsic structures. In the sagittal plane this usually involves either anterior or posterior structures; most often, extrinsic masses located anterior to the spinal cord are implicated. The neurological deficit in a patient with a focal kyphosis is related, in part, to spinal cord tethering in the sagittal plane (*"sagittal bowstring" effect*—Fig. 7-4*A*).[21] This explains why some patients may

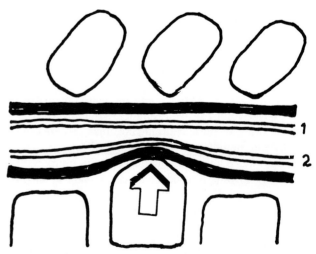

FIGURE 7-2 Spinal cord compression. Some neural elements are compressed (1); others are compressed and distorted (2).

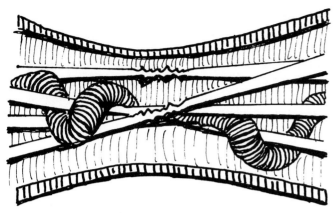

FIGURE 7-3 Spinal cord distraction can distort and disrupt both neurons and the blood supply to the spinal cord.

be neurologically worsened after posterior decompression procedures (Fig. 7-4B). Morgan and coworkers documented this clinically in patients with posttraumatic ventral mass lesions.[22] The neurological dysfunction in these cases may be related to vascular compromise in the spinal cord, as is probably the case with simple distraction.

The neurological ineffectiveness of operative procedures using posterior distraction for thoracic and lumbar spine trauma has been clearly documented by Dickson and coworkers.[23] They demonstrated, in patients who underwent posterior distraction fixation (Harrington distraction rods) combined with a posterior fusion without decompression, that the patients so treated enjoyed no greater neurological recovery than those treated without surgery. How-

ever, several reports have documented the "anatomical efficacy" of posterior distraction procedures[24-29] and nonoperative management.[30]

Retropulsed bone and disk fragments can be reduced if the posterior longitudinal ligament is intact (Fig. 7-5A). The attempted reduction of ventral spinal masses by this posterior distraction technique is called *ligamentotaxis.* The rationale for this treatment option assumes that, in addition to the presence of an intact posterior longitudinal ligament, the bone and disk fragments are mobile in an anteroposterior orientation (i.e., that they can be relocated) and that the anterior longitudinal ligament does not impede spinal distraction (Fig. 7-5B). One must keep in mind that (1) this is unlikely, since most injuries are compression injuries, with relative preservation of the anterior longitudinal ligament; and (2) the anterior longitudinal ligament is much stronger than the posterior longitudinal ligament (see Chap. 1).

Other authors have shown that ventral decompression operations are effective in improving neurological function.[31-33] Both ventral decompression and posterior distraction operations, when combined with instrumentation and fusion, effectively restore spinal stability and, in many cases, relatively normal spinal canal dimensions. What, then, is the cause of the discrepancy in neurological outcome between the two types of procedure? First, and most obvious, the normal spinal canal dimensions may not have been completely restored. Even small ventral masses may have great significance in the face of spinal cord distraction. Second, the act of reducing retropulsed bone and disk frag-

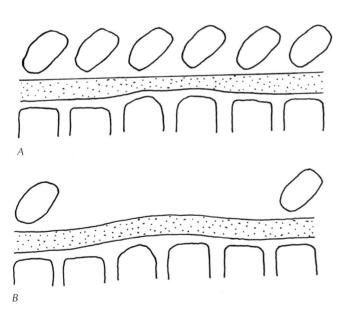

FIGURE 7-4 *A.* A kyphosis associated with cervical spondylosis causes neural injury, in part, by tethering the spinal cord over a ventral mass via the "sagittal bowstring" effect. *B.* Posterior decompression (e.g., via laminectomy) may worsen deformation.

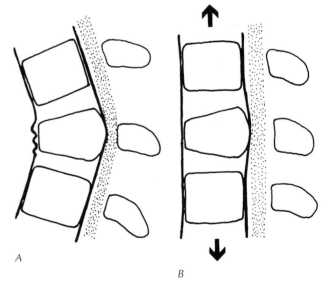

FIGURE 7-5 *A.* Spinal distraction can be used as a mechanism of reducing (relocating) ventral retropulsed bone and/or disk fragments (ligamentotaxis). *B.* Both an intact posterior longitudinal ligament and an anterior longitudinal ligament that does not effectively impede distraction are required for this technique to be anatomically effective.

ments may, by its nature, cause significant tethering during the act of reduction. It seems likely, therefore, that the reason why Dickson and coworkers saw no neurological "advantage" in their posterior distraction procedures was the collective effect of a number of potential sequelae of the biomechanics of the distraction process.

Of course, some patients may have been improved neurologically by effective decompression of the spinal cord with minimal distraction-related distortion or tethering. In others, neurological improvement may be impeded by the tethering of the spinal cord over an incompletely reduced mass (Fig. 7-5). The adverse nature of this type of outcome may not be immediately obvious on neurological examination. It may manifest itself, however, in any early plateauing of neurological recovery—that is, an incomplete recovery. Finally, the patient may be worsened by this treatment regimen. The cumulative import of these various neurological outcomes may indeed be as Dickson and coworkers observed: that there is no neurological advantage over nonoperative management.[23]

During the operative decision-making process one must take care not to misinterpret axially oriented imaging studies, such as CT. Axial images alone can be very misleading with regard to sagittal neural element and extrinsic mass relationships. This is particularly so if sagittal-plane spinal deformation is present and if thick axial CT cuts are used (Fig. 7-6).

It is obvious from the foregoing that the anatomic restoration of spinal canal dimensions is not the only important consideration in a spinal decompression and stabilization operation. One must also consider the mechanism by which the restoration of spinal canal dimensions and the relationship of neural elements to spinal elements is to be achieved, so that the neurological outcome can be optimized. *In general, the ultimate goal in surgery for spinal decompression and stabilization is to obtain, and maintain, a nonpathological relationship between the bone and soft tissues of the spine and the neural elements. The restoration of normal spinal alignment is not absolutely necessary in all cases.*

"Coronal Bowstring" Effect

The spinal cord can be tethered in the coronal plane as well as in the sagittal plane.[21] Coronal plane tethering ("coronal bowstring" effect) is caused by the tethering of the spinal cord ventrally by the lateral extensions of the spinal cord proper—that is, by nerve roots or the dentate ligaments (Fig. 7-7A). If "coronal bowstringing" is present, a laminectomy may be ineffective in relieving spinal cord distortion (Fig. 7-7B).[34] Thus an anterior decompressive procedure or a laminectomy, combined with an untethering procedure, is required to adequately relieve the spinal cord distortion. This might be achieved by anterior decompression of the spinal cord or by sectioning of the dentate ligament (Fig. 7-7C).[34] Kahn detailed the anatomic and biomechanical factors involved.[10] In theory, at least, these factors may have clinical roles. This is corroborated by the often-observed cervical spondylosis–related flattening of the spinal cord that may persist following laminectomy.

TWO MECHANISMS OF IATROGENIC NEURAL ELEMENT INJURY

Inappropriate Width of Decompression

The width of decompression is critically important. For example, a laminectomy that is not wide enough to adequately decompress the spinal canal may result in persistent neurological dysfunction. Conversely, a laminectomy that is too wide or that is performed in conjunction with a wide foraminotomy may result in spinal instability. A laminectomy, therefore, should be extended laterally to the lateral-most aspect of the dural sac. This almost always results in adequate preservation of the stability contributions of the facet joint.[35]

Inappropriate Length of Decompression

Similarly, a laminectomy can be too long or too short. If it is too long, development of spinal instability or deformation is encouraged. This phenomenon may be observed in situations where thoracic laminae are removed during a cervical laminectomy. The incidence of postoperative kyphotic deformities may be unacceptable in this patient population. Therefore, unless absolutely necessary, a laminectomy should not be extended inferiorly to include the removal of T1 without some compensatory maneuver, such as fusion.[21]

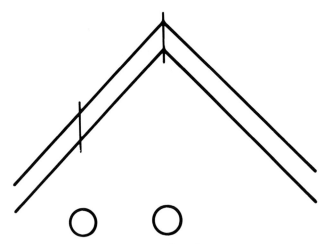

FIGURE 7-6 Misinterpretation of axially oriented images can lead the surgeon to believe that no significant neural impairment exists. Without a sagittal "view" of the spine, spinal canal dimension assessment may be inaccurate. In this exaggerated example, axial-plane spinal canal dimensions (*circles*) are not altered from location to location, while sagittal-plane spinal canal deformation by the kyphosis is significant.

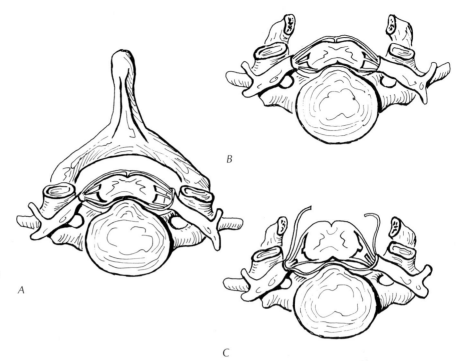

FIGURE 7-7 Coronal plane tethering ("coronal bowstring" effect). *A.* The nerve roots or, more commonly, the dentate ligaments may tether the spinal cord in the coronal plane. *B.* Laminectomy may not relieve the distortion. *C.* Sectioning of the offending cause of the tethering (dentate ligaments) may relieve this type of distortion. Anterior decompression is a more commonly considered approach.

On the other hand, a laminectomy that is not extended far enough rostral and caudal to an extrinsic mass located ventral to the spinal cord may result in worsening of the pre-operative neurological deficit. Dorsal kinking (distortion) of the spinal cord may ensue. This kinking may result from unopposed dorsally directed forces (ventral mass), combined with acute-angle deformation of the spinal cord at the margins of the short laminectomy (Fig. 7-8).[21]

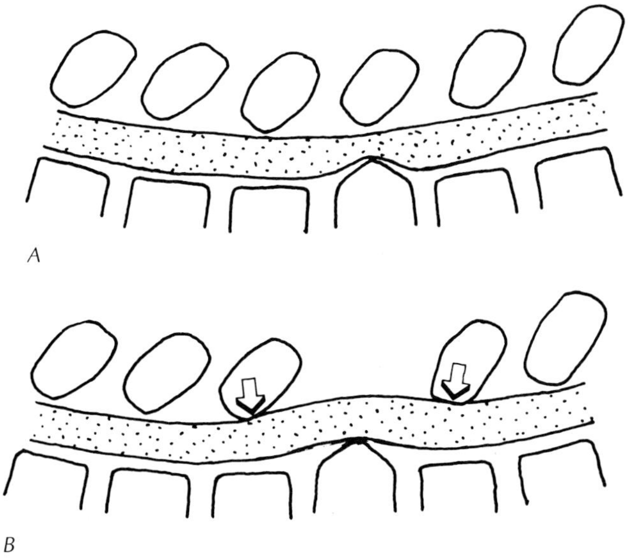

FIGURE 7-8 Kinking of the spinal cord may occur after laminectomy if an inadequate length of the spinal canal is decompressed.

Extensive laminectomies can be used if accompanied by fusion. This is especially important in the presence of a kyphotic posture of the spine (as in the cervicothoracic region). A laminectomy may be safely extended into this region if a fusion (usually with accompanying instrumentation) is also performed.

SPINAL CORD INJURY SYNDROMES

The aforementioned spinal cord distortions may result in a variety of spinal cord injury syndromes. Their anatomic and biomechanical bases are predictable; the consideration of these may aid the spine surgeon clinically.

Complete Myelopathy

The mere definition of *complete myelopathy* is often controversial. Although this definition appears simple on the surface, several factors have confused the issue. The definition of a complete myelopathy, in the purest sense, dictates that no evidence of long-tract neural transmission occurs across the injury site. Although this is a simple concept, its substance may be difficult to document clinically. Some authors have observed a high incidence of significant neurological recovery following the incurrence of a complete myelopathy; others have observed none at all. Those who have observed such recovery have often attributed it to a variety of interventions.[2,35] On the other hand, the recovery may have been simply a manifestation of the natural history of the injury-recovery process.

Theoretically, at least, the anatomic correlate of a complete myelopathy is spinal cord transection. Most authors concede that spinal cord transection is, at this time, a neurologically irreversible process. Therefore, in the case of complete myelopathy, the only factor that eliminates the neurological examination as the ultimate prognosticator is the adequacy of the examination itself.

Careful, often serial, examinations of the patient are mandatory. Each should include a meticulous sensory examination, with particular attention to saddle sensation (lower sacral sensation). The examination must also take into account the patient's ability to cooperate with the examination process. Inebriation, intoxication, shock, stress, and head injury—to name a few examples—all may impair the patient's ability to cooperate. Since sensory function is assessed subjectively, the importance of meticulous serial examinations cannot be overstated.

The issue of the definition of complete myelopathy is further confused by some authors' inclusion of patients with some sensory preservation. These patients have some sensory sparing (motor-complete myelopathy). They have no preserved motor function, but sensory fibers are obviously intact. The preservation of any function below the level of injury has been shown to confer a chance for neurological recovery not observed in patients without this function.[31,33] For this reason alone, the grouping together of patients with complete and motor-complete myelopathies is inappropriate. Careful serial examinations may be necessary to categorize these patients appropriately.

Anterior Spinal Cord Injury Syndrome

A ventral injury to the spinal cord can result in dysfunction of the ventral spinal cord tracts. This involves mainly the dysfunction of the spinothalamic (pain and temperature) and corticospinal (motor) tracts, with preservation of the

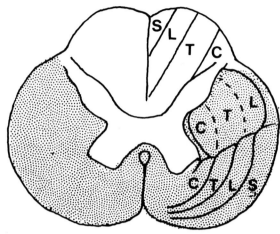

FIGURE 7-9 Anterior spinal cord injury syndrome (*shaded area*). The shaded areas depict the injured portion of the spinal cord.

posterior columns (joint position sense and gross touch) (Fig. 7-9). The preservation of at least some sensation changes the overall prognosis significantly.[31,33] The extent of posterior column function may be impressive in the face of complete or near-complete loss of motor function and pain and temperature sensation.

Brown-Séquard Syndrome

Hemisection of the spinal cord can result in the loss of ipsilateral motor function and contralateral pain and temperature function—the Brown-Séquard syndrome (Fig. 7-10A). Blunt injuries can cause this syndrome, most often in a modified form; penetrating impalement injuries are most often implicated.[36]

In the face of this clinical syndrome, the clinician must carefully assess the imaging studies for evidence of a later-

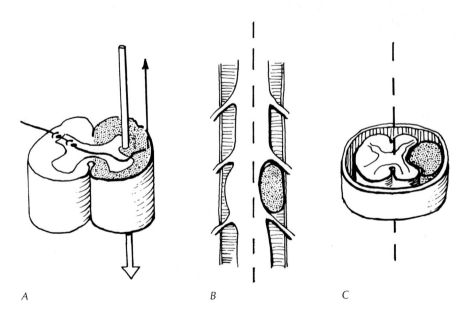

A   *B*   *C*

FIGURE 7-10 Brown-Séquard syndrome. *A.* The shaded areas depict the injured portion of the spinal cord. The crossed ascending pain and temperature fibers (spinothalamic tract, *solid arrow*) and the uncrossed descending motor fibers (corticospinal tract, *hollow arrow*) are disrupted. *B* and *C.* A laterally impinging mass may be missed by sagittal imaging through the dotted line. Therefore, coronal (myelogram or MRI, *B*) or axial (CT or MRI, *C*) images may be critically important.

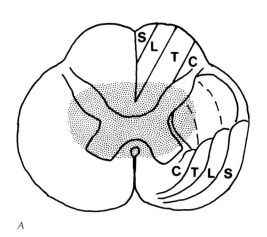
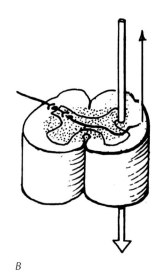

FIGURE 7-11 Central spinal cord injury syndrome. *A.* The shaded areas depict the injured portion of the spinal cord. *B.* The somatotopic distribution of the spinal cord's long tracts predisposes the patient subjected to such an injury to a unique clinical syndrome. This is manifested by the loss of crossing pain and temperature fibers (spinothalamic fibers, *solid arrow*), resulting in "shawl distribution" sensory loss; and a loss of medial descending motor fibers (corticospinal tract, *hollow arrow*), resulting in loss of motor function to the hands and arms (served by the most medially located fibers in the corticospinal tract).

A

B

ally impinging mass. In this case, anteroposterior (e.g., AP myelogram) and axial imaging techniques (CT) may provide vital information that sagittal images might miss (Fig. 7-10*B* and *C*).

Central Spinal Cord Injury Syndrome

Annular constriction of the spinal cord can lead, in certain situations, to an injury to the central portion of the spinal cord. The mechanism of this injury is not entirely clear; but a stenotic spinal canal, combined with a superimposed deforming insult, appears to be a common recurring element in this clinical syndrome. The superimposed deforming insult may be the result of excessive flexion, extension, or translation, or of ventral impingement. Whatever the nature of the deforming insult, the central portion of the spinal cord is injured, most likely by ischemia, contusion, or hematoma formation.[10,12–16]

Because of the somatotopic distribution of the spinal cord's long tracts (Fig. 7-11*A*), a central injury to the cervical spinal cord results in a characteristic clinical picture: a loss of motor and sensory function in the upper extremities that is out of proportion to the loss in the lower extremities (Fig. 7-11*B*).

REFERENCES

1. Benzel EC, Rodriguez DJ, Wild G, et al: The focal and systemic metabolic response to spinal cord injury. *Neurosurgery* (in press).
2. Benzel EC, Wild GC: Biochemical mechanisms of neural injury, in Barrow D (ed): *Perspectives in Neurological Surgery*. St. Louis: Quality Medical Publishing, 1991:95–126.
3. National Acute Spinal Cord Injury Study Group: A randomized controlled trial of methylprednisolone or naloxone in the treatment of acute spinal cord injury. *N Engl J Med* 1990; 332:1405–1411.
4. Benoist G, Kausz M, Rethelyi M, et al: Sensitivity of the short-range spinal interneurons of the cat to experimental spinal cord trauma. *J Neurosurg* 1979; 51:834–840.
5. Dohrmann GJ, Panjabi MM, Banks D: Biomechanics of experimental spinal cord trauma. *J Neurosurg* 1978; 48:993–1001.
6. Hung T-k, Lin H, Bunegin L, et al: Mechanical and neurological response of cat spinal cord under static loading. *Surg Neurol* 1982; 17:213–217.
7. Tunturi AR: Elasticity of the spinal cord dura in the dog. *J Neurosurg* 1977; 47:391–396.
8. Tunturi AR: Elasticity of the spinal cord, pia, and denticulate ligament in the dog. *J Neurosurg* 1978; 48:975–979.
9. Shapiro K, Shulman K, Marmarou A, et al: Tissue pressure gradients in spinal cord injury. *Surg Neurol* 1977; 7:275–279.
10. Kahn EA: The role of the dentate ligaments in spinal cord compression and the syndrome of lateral sclerosis. *J Neurosurg* 1947; 4:191–199.
11. Nurick S: The pathogenesis of the spinal cord disorder associated with cervical spondylosis. *Brain* 1972; 95:87–100.
12. Payne EE, Spillane JD: The cervical spine. An anatomico-pathological study of 70 specimens (using a special technique) with particular reference to the problem of cervical spondylosis. *Brain* 1957; 80:571–596.
13. Reid JD: Effects of flexion-extension movements of the head and spine upon the spinal cord and nerve roots. *J Neurol Neurosurg Psychiatry* 1960; 23:214–221.
14. Stoops WL, King RB: Neural complications of cervical spondylosis: Their response to laminectomy and foraminotomy. *J Neurosurg* 1962; 19:986–989.
15. Taylor AR: The mechanism of injury to the spinal cord in the neck without damage to the vertebral column. *J Bone Joint Surg* 1951; 33B:543–547.
16. Wilkinson HA, LeMay ML, Ferris EJ: Clinical-radiographic correlations in cervical spondylosis. *J Neurosurg* 1969; 30:213–218.
17. Breig A: *Adverse Mechanical Tension in the Central Nervous System. An Analysis of Cause and Effect: Relief by Functional Neurosurgery*. Stockholm: Almqvist and Wiksell, 1978: 1–264.
18. Breig A: *Biomechanics of the Central Nervous System*. Chicago: Year Book Medical, 1960: 1–183.
19. Cusick JF, Ackmann JJ, Larson SJ: Mechanical and physiological effects of dentatotomy. *J Neurosurg* 1977; 46:767–775.
20. Cusick JF, Myklebust J, Zyvoloski M, et al: Effects of vertebral column distraction in the monkey. *J Neurosurg* 1982; 57:651–659.
21. Benzel EC: Cervical spondylotic myelopathy: Posterior surgical approaches, in Cooper PR (ed): *Degenerative Disease of the Cervical Spine*. AANS Publications, 1992: 91–104.
22. Morgan TH, Wharton GW, Austin GN: The results of laminectomy in patients with incomplete spinal cord injuries. *Paraplegia* 1971; 9:14–23.

23. Dickson JH, Harrington PR, Erwin WD: Results of reduction and stabilization of the severely fractured thoracic and lumbar spine. *J Bone Joint Surg* 1978; 60A:799–805.

24. Bradford DS, Akbarnia BA, Winter RB, et al: Surgical stabilization of fracture and fracture dislocations of the thoracic spine. *Spine* 1977; 2:185–196.

25. Convery FR, Minteer MA, Smith RW, et al: Fracture-dislocation of the dorsal-lumbar spine. Acute operative stabilization by Harrington instrumentation. *Spine* 1978; 3:160–166.

26. Jacobs RR, Asher MA, Snider RK: Dorso-lumbar spine fractures: Recumbent versus operative treatment. *Paraplegia* 1980; 18:358–376.

27. Kelly RP, Whitesides TE: Treatment of lumbo-dorsal fracture-dislocation. *Ann Surg* 1968; 167(5):705–717.

28. Rosenthal RE, Lowery ER: Unstable fracture-dislocations of the thoracolumbar spine: Results of surgical treatment. *J Trauma* 1980; 20:485–490.

29. Yosipovitch Z, Robin GC, Makin M: Open reduction of unstable thoraco-lumbar spinal injuries and fixation with Harrington rods. *J Bone Joint Surg* 1977; 59A:1003–1014.

30. Chakera TMH, Bedbrook G, Bradley CM: Spontaneous resolution of spinal canal deformity after burst-dispersion fracture. *AJNR* 1988; 9:779–785.

31. Benzel EC, Larson SJ: Functional recovery after decompressive operation for thoracic and lumbar spine fractures. *Neurosurgery* 1986; 19:772–778.

32. Benzel EC, Larson SJ: Recovery of nerve root function after complete quadriplegia from cervical spine fractures. *Neurosurgery* 1986; 19:809–812.

33. Benzel EC, Larson SJ: Functional recovery after decompressive spine operation for cervical spine fractures. *Neurosurgery* 1987; 20:742–746.

34. Benzel EC, Lancon J, Kesterson L, et al: Cervical laminectomy and dentate ligament section for cervical spondylotic myelopathy. *J Spinal Disord* 1991; 4:286–295.

35. Raynor RB, Pugh J, Shapiro I: Cervical facetectomy and its effect on spine strength. *J Neurosurg* 1985; 63:278–282.

36. Benzel EC, Ball PA: Controversies: Penetrating injuries, in Garfin SR, Northrup B (eds): *Principles and Techniques in Spine Surgery.* New York: Raven Press, 1993: 269–278.

Part III

Spine Surgery

Chapter 8

Surgical Approaches to the Subaxial Spine

The surgical approaches to spinal decompression, fusion, and instrumentation vary widely. This chapter focuses on surgical approaches to the subaxial spine for the explicit purpose of the placement of instrumentation. The "angle of view" is emphasized and illustrated. In nearly all cases the surgical approaches traditionally used for decompression and for fusion are used for instrumentation. Differences and additional concerns do exist, however. It is these differences and concerns that will be addressed here.

THE ANTERIOR AND LATERAL APPROACHES TO THE CERVICAL SPINE

The traditional anterior approach to the cervical spine allows a wide exposure of the ventral cervical vertebral bodies. For the purpose of instrumentation placement, this approach provides an appropriate exposure of the spine.

Usually, a nearly horizontal incision placed along a skin crease is used. If a lengthy exposure of the ventral cervical spine is desired, a diagonal incision along the anterior border of the sternocleidomastoid muscle is used. Blunt and careful sharp dissection is accomplished along the medial border of the sternocleidomastoid muscle; between the trachea and esophagus medially; and the carotid artery, jugular vein, and vagus nerve laterally.

Subperiosteal dissection, starting at the midline and extending laterally to the lateral-most extent of the vertebral body, is performed bilaterally and past the rostral and caudal extents of the planned vertebral exposure as defined by x-ray localization (Fig. 8-1A).[1-3] Two points are crucial: (1) the attainment of more than adequate exposure, both laterally and rostrally-caudally; and (2) the maintenance of this exposure with appropriate self-retaining retraction. The former is achieved via meticulous sharp and blunt dissection with minimal soft-tissue stretching. The latter can be

achieved via either of two types of retractor systems:(1) patient-mounted systems, and (2) table-mounted systems. The former causes an asymmetric, and often excessive, application of pressure to the soft tissues. The latter may eliminate this complication while providing greater exposure. As with all instrumentation techniques, a thorough knowledge of the anatomic and biomechanical nuances of implant-bone interface sites is imperative.

Ventral cervical spine exposure via the anterior approach does not result in de-innervation of muscles. Although the longus colli muscles are injured, they are injured symmetrically along the midline raphe. Furthermore, their importance to the prevention of spinal deformity is not known, but most likely is minimal.

Lateral exposure of the cervical spine can be gained via an approach described by Verbiest.[4] Usually going through the same tissue planes as depicted in Fig. 8-1A, this approach is used to gain access to the lateral-most aspect of the spine, overlying the vertebral arteries. Retraction of the sympathetic chain medially with the longus colli muscle often preserves the function of this structure (Fig. 8-1B).

THE ANTEROLATERAL TRANSTHORACIC APPROACH

The anterolateral approach to the thoracic spine can be used for anterolateral exposure from about T5 to T10. Intercostal muscle incision, with or without rib resection, gives access to the thoracic cavity. Careful lung retraction provides a wide view of a lengthy portion of the spine. Postoperatively, the remaining ribs may be bound together by strong circumferential sutures to augment chest wall stability (perhaps at the cost of an exaggerated tendency toward spinal deformation).

Exposure from the left is impeded by the aorta, and expo-

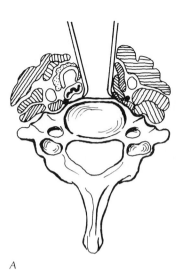
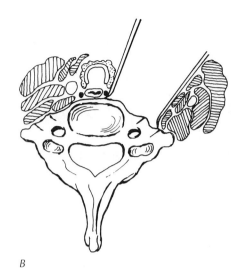

A   *B*

FIGURE 8-1 The anterior and anterolateral (*A*) and lateral (*B*) approaches to the subaxial cervical spine, seen in axial views. Note the subperiosteal dissection, the placement of retractors, and the exposures thus gained. Dots depict sympathetic chain and ganglia.

sure from the right by the vena cava. These structures pose a risk related to vascular injury and from an intraoperative exposure point of view (Fig. 8-2). The anterolateral approach, in addition, poses problems with visualization of the entirety of ventrally placed construct components and with adequacy of purchase site integrity and number of purchase site options. Furthermore, the dural sac is not decompressed until all ventral structures have been removed. This may pose a slight hazard in dural sac–decompression operations.[1]

The transthoracic exposure, by definition, is asymmetric. The intercostal muscle incision minimally disrupts stability.

Rib resection, with postoperative binding-together of the remaining ribs, predisposes to a spinal deformation about the coronal plane (scoliosis). In some cases it may be appropriate to consider the use of intraoperative stabilization techniques to augment stability.

THE TRANSDIAPHRAGMATIC APPROACH TO THE THORACOLUMBAR SPINE

The transdiaphragmatic approach to the spine allows for an anterolateral exposure of the thoracolumbar junction. Other than the lateral extracavitary approach, the transdiaphragmatic is the only approach that provides a ventral exposure of this region of the spine (Fig. 8-3).[1]

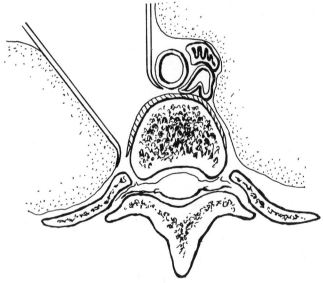

FIGURE 8-2 The anterolateral transthoracic approach to the spine, seen in an axial view. The exposure gained is slightly lateral to that gained in the cervical region with the anterior approach.

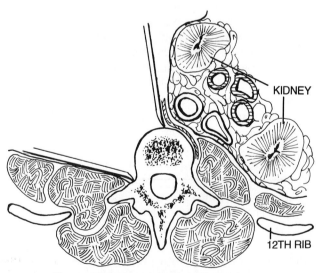

KIDNEY

12TH RIB

FIGURE 8-3 The transdiaphragmatic approach to the thoracolumbar spine, seen in an axial view. Note the significant soft tissue violation required for this approach.

Rib resection may be required for this approach. The lower ribs, however, have a minimal impact on stability. Asymmetric loss of muscle integrity in the anterolateral upper abdominal wall, too, has a minimal impact.

THE ANTEROLATERAL EXTRAPERITONEAL APPROACH TO THE UPPER AND MIDLUMBAR SPINE

The anterolateral extraperitoneal approach to the upper lumbar spine is essentially the same approach used by surgeons to gain access to the sympathetic chain in the lumbar paravertebral region.[1,3] This exposure allows access to the anterolateral spinal canal from L2 to below the pelvic brim (although, with greater difficulty, the upper vertebrae lumbar may be exposed). The dissection proceeds in an anatomic manner by muscle-splitting incisions through the external oblique, internal oblique, and transversalis muscles, along the muscle fibers of each muscle layer, into the retroperitoneal space and then to the spine. If high lumbar exposure is necessary, the diaphragmatic crus may be separated from the anterior longitudinal ligament of the vertebral column. The sympathetic chain can be visualized in the groove between the psoas muscle and the vertebral body.

A major advantage of this approach is the straightforward nature of the exposure, which is familiar to most spine and vascular surgeons. However, it offers a disappointingly narrow longitudinal exposure. This exposure is limited superiorly by the crus of the diaphragm and inferiorly by the pelvic brim. This approach also makes it difficult to expose the neuroforamina without psoas muscle retraction (which is difficult) or resection. The advantages and disadvantages of this approach are similar to those of the anterior transthoracic approach (Fig. 8-4).

This exposure asymmetrically de-innervates and injures muscle, albeit minimally. A unilateral injury to the psoas muscle from lateral subperiosteal exposure along the vertebral body can cause hip flexor weakness; also, it may affect spinal stability directly, through disruption of muscular spinal support (asymmetrically), and indirectly, through induced hip flexor weakness.

PELVIC BRIM EXTRAPERITONEAL APPROACH

The approach to the intrapelvic portion of the lumbosacral spine is challenging. An incision beginning lateral to, and slightly above, the anterior superior iliac spine can be carried medially and inferiorly, parallel and cephalad to the iliac crest and inguinal ligament. This gives access to the muscular plane below this level. An incision along the external oblique muscle fibers and across the internal oblique and transversus abdominis muscle fibers, in turn, gives access to the extraperitoneal pelvic structures. Extraperitoneal structures are swept from the pelvic floor posterior to the peritoneum and renal fascia.

The advantages of this approach include relatively good exposure of the intrapelvic lumbar plexus from an anterior and lateral orientation. On the other hand, it offers a limited overall exposure; and the intrapelvic sciatic nerve and lower sacral plexus are difficult, if not impossible, to visualize adequately through this approach. Although spinal instrumentation can be applied throughout this exposure, the depth of the exposure, combined with equivocal instrumentation purchase sites, essentially dictates that other approaches be used for spinal instrumentation (Fig. 8-5).[5]

The effects of this approach on stability are similar to those of the anterolateral extraperitoneal approach (see above).

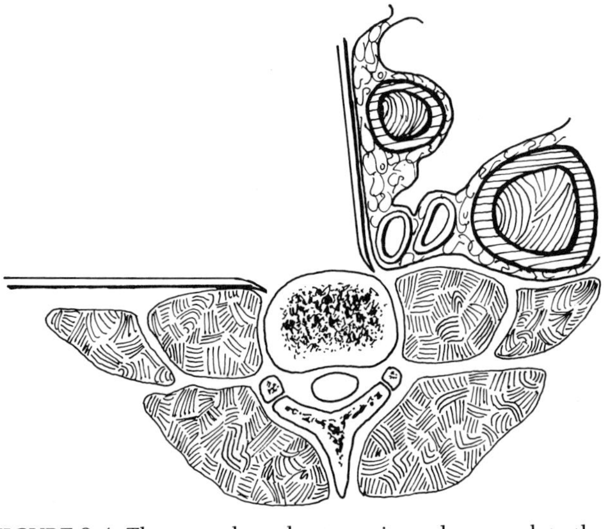

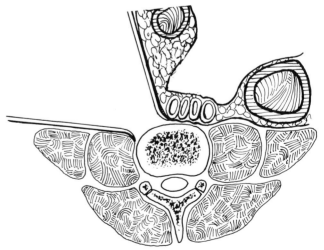

FIGURE 8-4 The anterolateral extraperitoneal approach to the lumbar spine, seen in an axial view.

FIGURE 8-5 The pelvic brim extraperitoneal approach to the low lumbar spine, seen in an axial view. Note that the vertebral body exposure is less than that achieved with more rostal approaches; this is due to the confining iliac vessels.

THE TRANSPERITONEAL APPROACH

Much of the exposure achieved by the preceding two techniques may be realized via the transperitoneal approach (Fig. 8-6).[1] After performance of a standard midline laparotomy incision and entry into the peritoneal cavity, the small intestine is packed into the upper abdomen and retracted to the right. The sigmoid colon is retracted laterally, and a longitudinal incision is made in the posterior peritoneum, in the midline, so as to expose the desired aspect of the retroperitoneal space. Occasionally the left nerve roots cannot be easily visualized in this manner; if need be, the colon may be retracted medially and mobilized from left to right after incision along the line of Toldt. Care should be taken to avoid injury to the ureters. The sacral promontory is a consistent, easily identifiable landmark that should be used to identify the L5-S1 interspace.

An excellent exposure of the retroperitoneal space is achieved through the transperitoneal approach. Lower retroperitoneal structures are more easily visualized than the more proximal structures (more easily, especially, on the right, because of the presence of the sigmoid colon on the left). The disadvantages are the requirement of a laparotomy and the potential for neural and vascular injury. The approach is very useful, however, when a wide exposure is needed, as for tumors of neural origin or for "re-do" surgical procedures.

Vertical midline or horizontal abdominal incisions minimally affect stability. In the immediate postoperative period the loss of abdominal strength can adversely affect spinal flexion; this phenomenon, however, is short-lived.

THE LATERAL EXTRACAVITARY APPROACH TO THE THORACIC AND LUMBAR SPINE

The lateral extracavitary approach to the spine, as originally described by Capener and popularized by Larson and coworkers, is now commonly used for surgical decompression of the thoracic and lumbar spine.[6,7] All regions of the thoracic and lumbar spine can be approached with this operation, although surgical exposure of the low lumbar region via the lateral extracavitary approach requires significant dorsal ilium resection.

The advantages of this approach include the lack of any need for intrathoracic or intrapelvic dissection and the ability to extend the dissection farther laterally than would be possible with a wide foraminotomy approach. Furthermore, the lateral extracavitary approach allows the performance of a ventral dural sac decompression, the placement of posterior spinal instrumentation, and subsequent fusion—in that order—through the same incision (Fig. 8-7). The disadvantages include the difficulties of dissecting across tissue planes and the resultant soft tissue trauma incurred.

The lateral extracavitary approach to the spine involves significant asymmetric muscle dissection, de-innervation, and potential injury. This can affect stability adversely. The postoperative unilateral loss of paraspinous, quadratus lumborum, psoas, latissimus dorsi, trapezius, or intercostal muscle function may place untoward asymmetric stresses on the spine. This should be taken into account during the operative decision-making process.

THE LATERAL TRANSCAVITARY APPROACH TO THE THORACIC SPINE

The lateral transcavitary approach allows true lateral exposure of the spine without the problems of anatomic visualization associated with the lateral extracavitary approach. Its angle of visualization is somewhat between that of the exposures given by the transthoracic and lateral extracavitary approaches. The advantage of being able to observe the pathological anatomy through the undisturbed parietal pleura of the lung, and the slightly more ventral exposure than that provided by the lateral extracavitary approach, may often outweigh the disadvantage of pleural invasion (Fig. 8-8).

The effects of the lateral transcavitary approach on stability are the same as those of the lateral extracavitary approach to the thoracic and lumbar spine (see above).

THE POSTERIOR APPROACHES TO THE SPINE

Posterior approaches to the spine generally are direct; thus, midline incisions are usually used. In the thoracic and lumbar regions (particularly the low thoracic region), alternative incisions may be used. In the thin, poorly nourished, and/or insensate patient, a paramedian incision may help avoid wound healing problems by minimizing externally applied incisional pressure. Subperiosteal dissection is then performed in the traditional manner after one has gained access to the midline along a subcutaneous plane. A variety of techniques of site preparation for instrumentation insertion are then employed, depending on the implant selected (Fig. 8-9). An extreme lateral exposure may also be gained.[8,9]

Posterior spinal exposure is usually, but not always, symmetric. The farther the dissection proceeds laterally, the greater the chance of paraspinous muscle de-innervation. In addition, the subperiosteal dissection causes muscle injury and dysfunction. In the lumbar region this is of relatively little significance, most likely because of the persisting lordosis. In the cervical and upper thoracic spine, however, this muscle dysfunction can contribute to flexion deformation—especially in the cervical region in patients with an "effective"kyphosis (see Chap. 6). Paraspinous muscle deinnervation and injury may play a significant contributing role in this process.

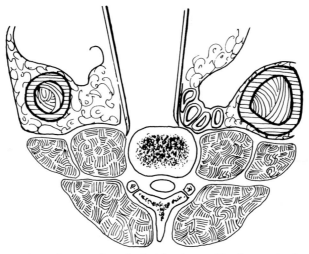

FIGURE 8-6 The transperitoneal approach to the low lumbar and lumbosacral spine, seen in an axial view.

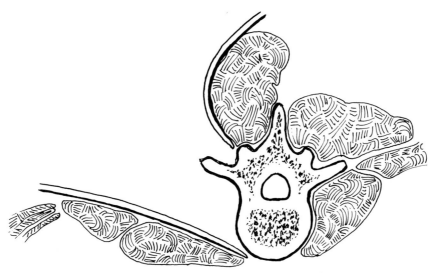

FIGURE 8-7 The lateral extracavitary approach to the thoracic and lumbar spine, seen in an axial view.

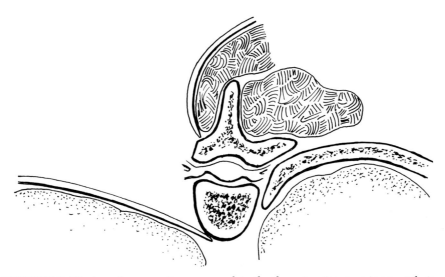

FIGURE 8-8 The lateral transcavitary approach to the thoracic spine, seen in an axial view.

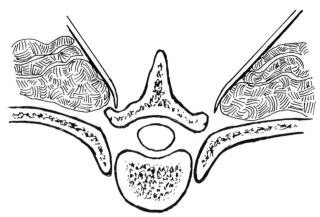

FIGURE 8-9 The posterior approach to the subaxial spine, seen in an axial view.

SELECTING THE MOST APPROPRIATE SURGICAL APPROACH

The choice of the most appropriate surgical approach for any given surgical endeavor depends largely on the "view" that is needed of the spine. This also dictates the degree of exposure, as well as the adequacy of dural sac decompression (Figs. 8-10 and 8-11).

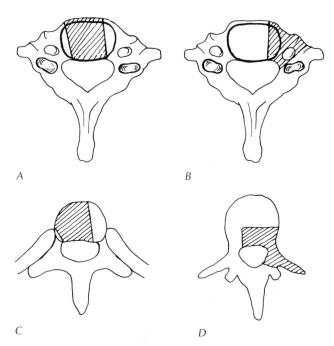

FIGURE 8-10 The anterior and lateral operative exposures of the dural sac, seen in axial views. *A.* Anterior cervical. *B.* Lateral cervical. *C.* Anterolateral transthoracic, transdiaphragmatic thoracolumbar, anterolateral extraperitoneal lumbar spine, extraperitoneal low lumbar spine, pelvic brim extraperitoneal low lumbar spine, and transperitoneal low lumbar spine. *D.* Lateral extracavitary and lateral transcavitary thoracic and lumbar spine. Hatched area indicates areas of bone removal to gain access to dural sac or vertebral artery.

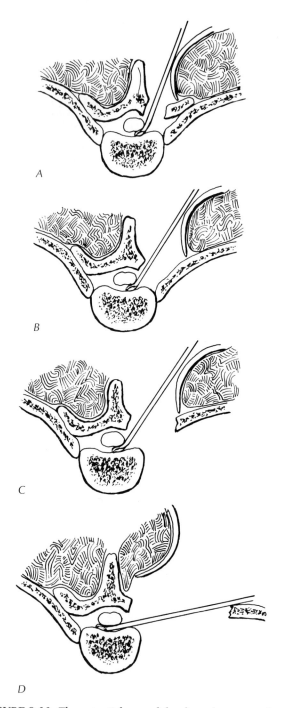

FIGURE 8-11 The potential ventral dural sac decompression achieved via a reversed-angle curette through the posterior surgical exposures, seen in axial views. *A.* Laminectomy. *B.* Transpedicle approach. *C.* Costotransversectomy approach. *D.* Lateral extracavitary approach (for comparison). Note that the main difference between the costotransversectomy approach and the lateral extracavitary approach is in the direction of the retraction of the erector spinae muscle (medial for the lateral extracavitary, lateral for the costotransversectomy). Also note that an approximately 20- to 40-degree "angle of view" advantage for ventral dural sac decompression is realized with the lateral extracavitary approach, versus the costotransversectomy approach. Resection of the erector spinae muscle eliminates much of this difference.

REFERENCES

1. Johnson RM, Southwick WO: Surgical approaches to the spine, in Rothman RH, Simeone FA (eds): *The Spine*, vol 1 (2d ed). Philadelphia: Saunders, 1982; 171–187.
2. Smith GW, Robinson RA: The treatment of certain cervical spine disorders by anterior removal of the intervertebral disc and interbody fusion. *J Bone Joint Surg* 1958; 40A:607–624.
3. Southwick WO, Robinson RA: Surgical approaches to the vertebral bodies in the cervical and lumber regions. *J Bone Joint Surg* 1957; 39A:631–643.
4. Verbiest H: A lateral approach to the cervical spine: Technique and indications. *J Neurosurg* 1968; 28:191–203.
5. Benzel EC: Surgical exposure of the lumbosacral plexus and proximal sciatic nerve, in Benzel EC (ed): *Practical Approaches to Peripheral Nerve Surgery*. Park Ridge, IL: American Association of Neurological Surgeons, 1992: 153–170.
6. Capener N: The evolution of lateral rhachotomy. *J Bone Joint Surg (BR)* 1954; 36:173–179.
7. Larson SJ, Holst RA, Hemmy DC, et al: Lateral extracavitary approach to traumatic lesions of the thoracic and lumbar spine. *J Neurosurg* 1976; 45:628–637.
8. Jane JA, Haworth CS, Broaddus WC, et al: A neurosurgical approach to far-lateral disc herniation. *J Neurosurg* 1990; 72:143–144.
9. Maroon JC, Kopitnik TA, Schulhof LA, et al: Diagnosis and microsurgical approach to far-lateral disc herniation in the lumbar spine. *J Neurosurg* 1990; 72:378–382.

Chapter 9

Destabilizing Effects of Spinal Surgery

Spinal surgery *by its nature* destabilizes the spine, whether by iatrogenic destruction of spinal ligaments, muscle injury, muscle de-innervation, or reduction of intrinsic bony integrity. The destabilizing effects of spinal surgery must always be taken into account.

Anterior and posterior spinal surgical procedures affect spinal stability in different ways. This is dictated mainly by the nature of the spinal structures violated by the surgical exposure in each type of procedure. Pathological (intrinsic) or iatrogenic (surgical) reduction of spinal stability, if biomechanically significant, must be compensated for by one or a combination of three therapeutic maneuvers: (1) postural, nonoperative management (including external spinal splinting) that provides time for bony and ligamentous healing to offset acute disruption of spinal integrity; (2) ventral spinal bony strut or instrumentation placement; and (3) posterior instrumentation placement. The role that any of these therapeutic maneuvers plays in any clinical situation depends on the bias of the surgeon and on the nuances of the clinical situation at hand. The effect of iatrogenic spinal destabilization is specifically addressed in this chapter.

ANTERIOR SPINAL DECOMPRESSION

Ligamentous Disruption

A significant portion of the contribution to ligamentous stability by ventral ligamentous structures is via the anterior and posterior longitudinal ligaments and the anulus fibrosus. The disruption of the anterior or posterior longitudinal ligament or the anulus fibrosus, either by the offending pathological process or by the surgical approach, can substantially reduce the intrinsic stability of the spine.

MRI techniques have provided a diagnostic tool for the assessment of the integrity of ligamentous structures (see Chap. 3).[1] This assessment, however, is static; it informs the clinician only of the extent of anatomic *continuity* of the ligament, revealing nothing about the ligament's strength. Dynamic x-ray (flexion and extension views of the spine)

can demonstrate the lack of integrity if excessive movement occurs. However, if subluxation or excessive movement does not occur during dynamic x-ray studies, the presence of spinal *stability* is not established. Spinal guarding and splinting, or inadequate imaging techniques, can lead to erroneous interpretations in this regard (see Chap. 3). These factors notwithstanding, the ligamentous contribution to stability can usually be reasonably assessed preoperatively.

The extent of the disruption of ventral ligamentous structures by an operative exposure is difficult to assess. Biomechanical laboratory information in this regard is lacking. However, several facts about the anatomy and strength characteristics of the anterior and posterior longitudinal ligaments should suffice for most clinical decision-making processes, particularly when combined with information gained from intraoperative observations.

The anterior longitudinal ligament is a strong ligament. It is also relatively wide (see Chap. 1). If it is not disrupted prior to surgery the surgical exposure (even a wide anterior exposure) does not usually disrupt the entire ligament. Therefore, in most cases, the contribution of the anterior longitudinal ligament to postoperative spinal stability is significant. Thus the tension-band nature of the anterior longitudinal ligament is partly preserved, as is its contribution to the limitation of extension. Therefore, it is a limiting factor in ligamentotaxis (see Chap. 7).

The posterior longitudinal ligament, on the other hand, is weaker than the anterior longitudinal ligament in all regions of the spine. Furthermore, it is waisted (narrower) in the mid-vertebral-body region at each segmental level. The posterior longitudinal ligament in the mid-vertebral-body region is narrower, at each spinal level, than the dural sac. Therefore, at any level of the spine, a vertebrectomy that adequately decompresses the dural sac is almost certain to totally disrupt the posterior longitudinal ligament, at any level of the spine. Thus the tension-band nature of the posterior longitudinal ligament is disrupted. Therefore, its contribution to the limitation of flexion (and distraction) is impaired.

One may have a "feeling" for the extent of ligamentous stability at the time of surgery, following dural sac decompression (vertebrectomy). The application of traction, spinal distraction by instruments such as vertebral body spreaders, or other intraoperative spinal manipulation can provide the surgeon with vital information regarding spinal laxity. This may help to determine whether a spinal implant is necessary as an adjuct to interbody fusion. For example, excessive laxity, as determined by intraoperative distraction maneuvers, may indicate that an interbody bone graft alone will not suffice.

In order for an interbody strut graft to be immediately effective as a stabilization aid, it must be securely positioned in the mortises of the vertebral bodies (i.e., the vertebral bodies above and below the strut). This allows a semi-rigid fixation of the vertebral bodies abutting the strut (Fig. 9-1A).

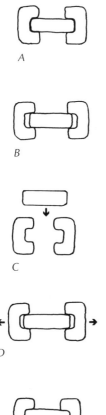

A

B

C

D

E

FIGURE 9-1 *A.* An anterior vertebral body strut graft firmly positioned in relatively deep mortises. *B.* Ligamentous laxity results in an inability of the abutting vertebral bodies to apply enough force to the strut graft to secure its position. Distraction followed by bone graft placement into well-formed mortises (*C*) and (*D*), followed by the relaxation of distraction (*E*), provides the foundation for a well-conceived interbody fusion, if adequate ligamentous resistance to distraction is present.

If ligamentous integrity is not adequate, as demonstrated by excessive laxity during intraoperative stress maneuvers, the strut graft is not securely affixed in the mortises of the vertebral bodies above and below the strut (Fig. 9-1B). The resistance to distraction provided by intact ligaments allows the vertebral bodies to "clamp down" on the strut graft. This "clamping-down" effect is an integral part of most interbody fusion techniques. Spinal distraction, followed by the placement of a well-fashioned strut graft into well-fashioned mortises and then by the relaxation of the distraction, allows the "clamping-down" properties of the ligaments to become manifest and leads to a strong construct (Fig. 9-1C, D, and E). Thus a spinal implant, prolonged bed rest, or a bracing adjunct to the decompression-fusion procedure is usually necessary when this ligamentous resistance to distraction is lost. Many spinal implants placed in a distraction mode, including Harrington distraction rods and interbody strut grafts, rely on intrinsic spinal resistance to distraction in order to obtain optimal security of fixation.

Disk interspace disruption is a cause of spinal instability. It can be easily assessed by MRI (Fig. 9-2). However, as an isolated entity, it does not substantially affect the decision-making process, except by necessitating a period of external spinal bracing.[1] The contribution of the anulus fibrosus to spinal stability, although significant, parallels that of the immediately adjacent anterior and posterior longitudinal ligaments. Its contribution cannot be separated from that of these ligaments. Therefore, no separate biomechanical consideration is warranted. It is worthy of emphasis, however,

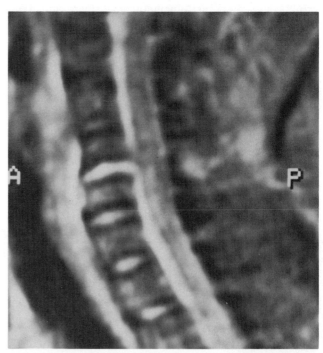

FIGURE 9-2 An MRI scan of a patient with a posttraumatic disk interspace disruption.

that the anulus fibrosus–anterior longitudinal ligament–posterior longitudinal ligament complex provides substantial stability to the spine.

Bony Disruption

Like instability from the loss of ligamentous integrity, diminished integrity of the vertebral body—whether due to the spinal pathological process or to surgical bone removal—reduces spinal stability. MRI, useful in the determination of ligamentous integrity, is less so in the determination of the bony contribution to stability; plain x-ray and CT are better in this regard.[2] However, the use of sagittal CT reconstructions or sagittal MRI scans to depict the sagittal plane anatomy cannot be overvalued.

The extent of anterior spinal decompression obviously affects spinal stability. A spine that has undergone a complete vertebrectomy obviously is less intrinsically stable than one that has undergone an incomplete vertebral body resection. This is true of both anterior and lateral approaches to the vertebrectomy. Rarely, however, is the entire vertebral body resected. The fraction of the vertebral body, as well as the anatomic position (in the anteroposterior plane) of the portion of the vertebral body resected, significantly affects spinal stability. For example, a standard anterior cervical corpectomy resects the vertebral body incompletely over the entire rostral-caudal dimension of the vertebral body (Fig. 9-3*A*). Similarly, anterolateral (Fig. 9-3*B*) and lateral extracavitary (Fig. 9-3*C*) decompressions incompletely resect the vertebral body over the entire rostral-caudal dimension of the vertebral body (see Chap. 8). The fraction of the bone remaining in the anterior portion (versus the posterior portion) of the vertebral body partly determines the extent of ventral spinal stability.

The location of the segment resected also affects the extent of iatrogenic spinal destabilization. To illustrate this point, consider the vertebral body to be a cube composed of 27 equal-sized cubical segments. Also assume that posterior column stability is present (Fig. 9-4). The surgical removal of the middle third (i.e., the middle layer of nine cubes) of the vertebral body as viewed in the sagittal plane grossly

destabilizes the spine (Fig. 9-5*A*); whereas the surgical removal of the middle third as viewed in the coronal plane does not (Fig. 9-5*B* and *C*). In the former case, the anterior and middle columns of Denis[3] are disrupted in the entire cross section of the vertebral body, resulting in loss of stability. In the latter case, only one-third of the integrity of the anterior and middle columns of Denis has been disrupted.

Partial vertebrectomies, as viewed in the sagittal plane, also vary in their destabilizing effects by virtue of the portion of the vertebral body removed. For example, the removal of the ventral section (the ventral nine cubes) will most likely have a significant effect on stability; whereas the removal of both the middle and posterior sections may not result in a significantly unstable situation if the following things remain intact: (1) the anterior section, (2) the anterior longitudinal ligament, (3) posterior column ligamentous integrity, and (4) posterior column bony integrity (Fig. 9-6). Minimizing the extent of vertebral body resection minimizes iatrogenic destabilization by the surgical procedure. In the case of true anterior surgical approaches, a narrow trough of vertebral body resection results in less vertebral body resection and a lesser width of anterior longitudinal ligament disruption. On the other hand, a narrow vertebral body resection may often result in inadequate spinal canal exposure and dural sac decompression (Fig. 9-7). In a similar vein, a natural tendency is for the surgeon to more-than-adequately decompress the spinal canal opposite the side of the patient on which he or she is standing, and to inadequately decompress the dural sac on the ipsilateral side (Fig. 9-8). An "Erlenmeyer flask decompression," therefore, warrants consideration. This type of decompression compensates for several of the problems outlined here. It involves a narrow decompression ventrally and a wider decompression dorsally (Fig. 9-9*A*); hence it allows a wide decompression of the dural sac and neuroforamina. This is accomplished by the surgeon's compensating for the known natural tendency to inadequately decompress the dural sac on the near side of the patient, by decompressing the dural sac from both sides of the table. This provides a good view of each side of the exposed spinal canal (wide decompression) while allowing minimal ventral vertebral body resec-

FIGURE 9-3 Axial views of the extents of bone removal in (*A*) an anterior cervical decompression, (*B*) an anterolateral thoracic or lumbar decompression, and (*C*) a lateral extracavitary thoracic or lumbar decompression.

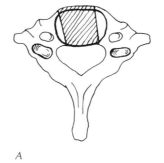

A

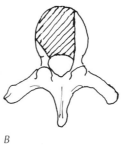

B

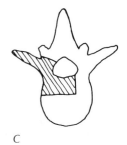

C

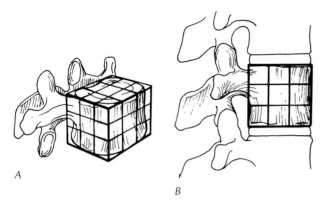

FIGURE 9-4 A vertebral body seen, for theoretical purposes, as a cube composed of 27 equal smaller cubes (3 × 3 × 3). A. Oblique view. B. Lateral view.

tion to suffice (minimizing iatrogenic destabilization of the spine) (Fig. 9-9B). The minimization of ventral vertebral body resection also provides greater lateral support for the strut graft (see Chap. 10 and Fig. 9-9B).

Lateral approaches to ventral dural sac decompression (e.g., via lateral extracavitary decompression of the spine) may also unnecessarily destabilize the spine if excessive vertebral body resection is accomplished. As mentioned above, if the ventral aspect of the vertebral body is surgically undisturbed and the posterior elements have not been violated, substantial stability may be present. Therefore, the minimization of bone removal should aid in the acquisition of postoperative stability. The preservation of the integrity

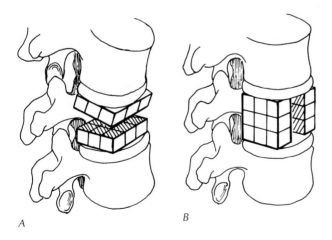

FIGURE 9-5 Resections of portions of the "cubic" vertebral body depicted in Fig. 9-4. A. Resection (or disruption) of the middle axial (horizontal) third of the vertebral body in its sagittal dimension, as might occur following trauma. B. Resection of the middle sagittal (vertical) third of the vertebral body. Note that the resection depicted in A destabilizes the spine, whereas that depicted in B does not. This is in spite of the fact that the bony resections are of similar magnitudes (i.e., similar volumes of bone are resected).

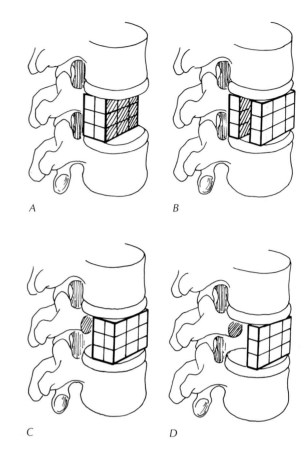

FIGURE 9-6 Resections of portions of the "cubic" vertebral body depicted in Fig. 9-4. Partial vertebrectomy involving removal of the ventral portion in the coronal plane of the vertebral body (A) affects stability more than resection of the middle (B) or posterior portion (C) of the vertebral body in the coronal plane. This assumes that an intact posterior column is present. In fact, resection of *both* the middle and posterior thirds of the vertebral body (in the presence of an intact posterior column and an intact anterior third of the vertebral body) may not significantly disrupt spinal integrity (D).

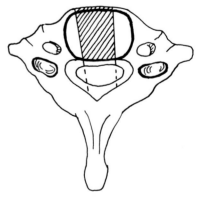

FIGURE 9-7 A narrow cervical vertebrectomy. Note that the width of the dural sac is greater than the width of the trough.

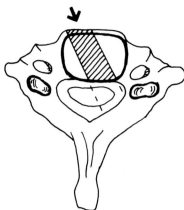

FIGURE 9-8 The end result of the natural tendency of the surgeon to waiver from midline, most commonly erring toward the side opposite the side of the patient that the surgeon is standing on.

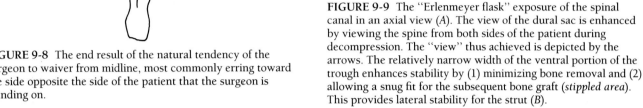

A   *B*

FIGURE 9-9 The "Erlenmeyer flask" exposure of the spinal canal in an axial view (*A*). The view of the dural sac is enhanced by viewing the spine from both sides of the patient during decompression. The "view" thus achieved is depicted by the arrows. The relatively narrow width of the ventral portion of the trough enhances stability by (1) minimizing bone removal and (2) allowing a snug fit for the subsequent bone graft (*stippled area*). This provides lateral stability for the strut (*B*).

of the ventral and lateral lateral parts of the vertebral body is particularly important.

The depiction of the vertebral body by its division into thirds in each plane (for a total of 27 cubic segments), used earlier in this chapter, is also useful in conceptualizing the destabilizing nature of a surgical procedure via the lateral extracavitary approach (Fig. 9-10). Dural sac decompression should involve the most dorsal plane, only on the side of the exposure (Fig. 9-10*B*). The middle and ventral planes may be considered for the bone graft. If ventral iatrogenic destabilization is to be minimized, the ventral plane (the ventral nine cubes) should not be surgically disrupted. Therefore, in this hypothetical case, the ventral plane should be left intact and the middle plane used as a site for interbody fusion placement (Fig. 9-10*C*). This makes further sense if one considers also that the middle plane is most likely in line with the IAR and therefore is in an optimal

position for axial load-bearing by the surgically placed strut graft (see Chap. 2).

POSTERIOR SPINAL DECOMPRESSION

Laminectomy, too, reduces the intrinsic stability of the spine. Morgan and coworkers documented a high incidence of postlaminectomy neurological worsening following spine trauma.[4] This is related to one or a combination of three factors: (1) intraoperative neurotrauma, (2) the creation of a sharp angulation of the dural sac at the limits of a decompression [which may result in neural distortion (see Chap. 7)], and (3) the destabilization of the spine (exaggerating a preexisting spinal deformity). The latter entity occurs with greater frequency as the width of the laminectomy is increased.[5] A slight increase in a flexion deformity created

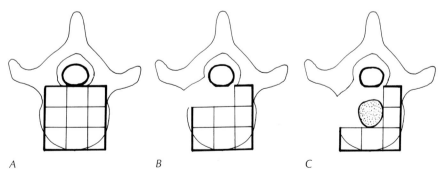

A   *B*   *C*

FIGURE 9-10 The 27-cube hypothetical cubic vertebral body can be used to depict the bony resection accomplished via a lateral extracavitary decompression of the thoracic or lumbar dural sac. *A*. A preoperative view of the spine. *B*. The restriction of bony resection to the most dorsal aspect of the vertebral body

allows substantial preservation of bony integrity. Further bony resection is then required for strut graft placement. *C*. The final extent of bone removal, with the bone graft (*stippled area*) in place.

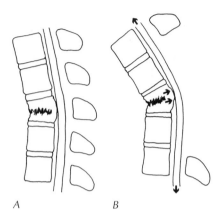

A   *B*

FIGURE 9-11 A flexion-deformity exaggeration following a laminectomy, *A*. Preoperative sagittal view. *B*. Postoperative sagittal view. Note the neural distortion by distraction (*vertical arrows*) and tethering over the ventral compression (*horizontal arrows*).

by the destabilizing effects of a laminectomy, in the presence of a ventral mass lesion, results in neural distortion both via flexion and via distraction over the ventral fulcrum (Fig. 9-11). The creation of a sharp angulation of the dural sac at the limits of a laminectomy is also a manifestation of a poorly conceived operation (see Chap. 7). Both of the latter two factors, therefore, are preventable.

Iatrogenic spinal destabilization is often predictable. However, since the extent of the instability created is not *always* obvious—especially during or shortly after surgery—it is difficult to be sure that no iatrogenic spinal destabilization has occurred. Unacceptable iatrogenic destabilization can be prevented by either or both of two techniques: (1) limited spinal integrity disruption, and (2) the addition of a stability augmentation procedure (e.g., the placement of a spinal implant). Recognition of any need for the latter is imperative—but the need is not always obvious.

Three etiologies are involved in iatrogenic destabilization via the posterior approach. The first involves lack of recognition of the presence of ventral spinal instability. The configuration of the spine may play a role in the contribution of ventral instability to the extent of iatrogenic destabilization by the posterior approach. Almost regardless of the minimal extent of iatrogenic dorsal destabilization, the presence of ventral spinal instability predicts a poor outcome from a structural point of view.

The second etiology involves the resection of the interspinous ligaments. Although the interspinous ligaments are relatively weak, they have a biomechanical advantage by virtue of the long moment arm (reaching from the spinous

process to the IAR) (see Chap. 3). One must keep in mind that the interspinous ligament is usually absent at the L5-S1 level and deficient at the L4-L5 level.

The third etiology is surgical facet joint disruption. Regardless of the region of the spine involved, excessive facet joint resection can result in instability. In the cervical spine the extent of tolerable resection has been documented to be about one-third to one-half of the facet joint (see Chap. 3).[5] In the lumbar region, facet disruption is associated with a greater incidence of glacial instability. There is controversy about the desirability of intraoperative management with fusion, with or without instrumentation when there is a preexisting translational deformity.[6,7] It should be kept in mind, however, that degenerative lumbar spondylolisthesis rarely progresses past a 30-percent translational deformation of the vertebral body.[8] Therefore, the virtue of *routine* fusion and instrumentation following spinal canal decompression must be questioned.

The combination of a vertically oriented facet joint and an exaggerated lordotic posture predisposes the spine to translational deformation. The relatively vertical orientation of the disk interspace causes an applied axial load to result in the application of a shearing force to the spine. Vertically oriented facet joints are poorly postioned to inhibit this translational deformation. Patients injured by such applied forces may benefit from fusion and instrumentation if laminectomy is performed, particularly if further facet joint disruption is surgically created.

REFERENCES

1. Benzel EC, Hart BL, Ball PA, et al: MRI for the evaluation of patients with non-obvious cervical spine injury. (Submitted)
2. Orrison WW, Hart BL, Benzel EC, et al: MRI, CT and plain film comparison in acute cervical spine trauma. *Neurosurgery* (in press).
3. Denis F: The three column spine and its significance in the classification of acute thoracolumbar spine injuries. *Spine* 1983; 8:817–831.
4. Morgan TH, Wharton GW, Austin GN: The results of laminectomy in patients with incomplete spinal cord injury. *Paraplegia* 1971; 9:14–23.
5. Raynor RB, Pugh J, Shapiro I: Cervical facetectomy and its effect on spine strength. *J Neurosurg* 1985; 63:278–282.
6. Herkowitz HN, Kurz LT: Degenerative lumbar spondylolisthesis with spinal stenosis: A prospective study comparing decompression with decompression and intertransverse process arthrodesis. *J Bone Joint Surg* 1991; 73A:802–808.
7. Shenkin HA, Hash CJ: Spondylolistheis after multiple bilateral laminectomies and facetectomies for lumbar spondylosis: Follow-up review. *J Neurosurg* 1979; 50:45–47.
8. Rosenberg NJ: Degenerative spondylolisthesis: Surgical treatment. *Clin Orthop Rel Res* 1976; 117:112–120.

Chapter 10

Spinal Fusion

THE BONE GRAFT

Ultimately, the bone graft and the resulting bony fusion are the constructs that lend stability to the spine. No matter how secure an internal fixation device may appear to be, it will eventually fail unless bony fusion and stability are achieved. There is a proverbial "race" between the failure of the instrumentation construct and the acquisition of bony union. After fusion the instrumentation construct and its interface with bone become progressively weaker, and the bony union becomes stronger (Fig. 10-1). Therefore, *most* posterior and anterior internal fixation techniques should be applied in conjunction with a bone graft.

Anterior interbody bone grafts offer superior ultimate strength characteristics.[1-3] They are placed in the weight-bearing region of the spine along the axis of the instantaneous axis of rotation (IAR). Weight-bearing itself promotes healing and bony fusion.[4] Care must be taken, however, to prevent progressive deformation following the placement of an anterior interbody fusion. Stauffer and Kelly have reported a high incidence of angular deformities following the placement of anterior fusions for cervical spine trauma.[5] Posterior stabilization procedures may be necessary (either alone or in combination with an anterior decompression and fusion) in order to achieve acceptable stability and neural element decompression. Anterior plating techniques, likewise, may be used for this purpose. Their use for this purpose, without posterior stability augmentation, must be considered carefully, since their ability to resist flexion is much less than their ability to resist extension.

Posterior bone grafts generally are not, by themselves, weight-bearing. Spine flexion (which causes flexion ventral to the IAR) causes distraction of the segments to be fused (dorsal to the IAR) (see Chap. 1). Unless anterior axial-load-resisting support is provided (i.e., via an anterior intervertebral bone strut graft), or already exists (e.g., in patients with cervical locked facets without vertebral body fracture), posterior bone grafts should be avoided unless an accompanying instrumentation construct provides the needed support. If the bone graft is applied in association with a tension-band fixation-in-flexion construct (such as with interspinous wiring), anterior support must be provided if ventral weight-bearing ability is suspect.

Frequently, stabilization procedures are performed after decompressive operations. The reduction of a ventral mass impinging on the spinal cord, therefore, frequently requires an operative approach in addition to a posteriorly placed instrumentation device. Furthermore, so that the dural sac is decompressed prior to spinal manipulation, the ventral (decompression) aspect of the operation should be performed first (before placement of the posterior instrumentation device).[6] In situations where spinal distraction is the desired mode of application, the interbody bone graft should not be placed until posterior instrumentation devices have been applied (for fear of adversely altering spinal biomechanics by loosening the already placed bone graft).[6] Theoretically, in this case, the most appropriate order of procedures should be: first, decompression of neural elements and "loosening" of the spine (by diskectomy and corpectomy); second, placement of the posterior internal fixation devices; and third, placement of the anterior bone graft (Fig. 10-2A–D).[6] If spinal compression is the desired mode of application, it may be desirable to place the interbody bone graft strut first (Fig. 10-2E–H).

ANTERIOR SPINAL FUSION

Much thought should be given to the selection of the specific location of bone graft placement, particularly in the sagittal plane. The location of the anterior interbody bone graft significantly affects the biomechanical efficacy of the construct. In general, for the optimization of axial-load-resisting ability and torso support, the optimal location for interbody bone graft placement is in the vicinity of the IAR in the sagittal plane. This, generally, is also the location of the *neutral axis* (particularly if posterior spinal element stability is deficient). The neutral axis is that region of the spine

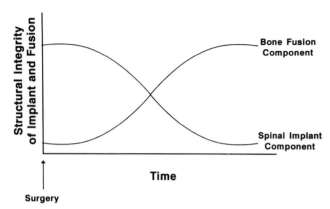

Surgery

FIGURE 10-1 The relationship between bone fusion acquisition and spinal implant integrity changes with time following surgery.

where flexion and extension do not significantly displace points located within the limits of the axis (see Chap. 6). Usually it is located at the junction of the anterior and middle columns of Denis.[7] If posterior spinal element stability is adequate, a slightly more ventral location for interbody bone graft placement may be optimal (see Chap. 6 and Fig. 10-3). In this situation, axial loads can be more effectively distributed between the strut graft and the existing posterior element structures.[8,9]

The placement of a ventral interbody fusion can offer a

substantial increase in axial-load-resisting ability.[2] The bony strut itself and the sites of attachment to the vertebral bodies (purchase sites) must be strong enough to offer such support. The needed strength may be lacking, for example, when thin iliac crest, rib, or morselized bone is used as the graft material. Yet stronger fusion masses, such as fibula, may penetrate (farther than is desired) through the accepting purchase sites in the rostral and caudal vertebral bodies—much as a toothpick might penetrate a piece of expanded polystyrene foam. On the other hand, a bone graft that is of lesser integrity than the vertebral body may itself fail. Therefore—provided that there are not other extenuating circumstances—the bone graft should be of similar consistency and integrity to the bone of the vertebral bodies that accept it (Fig. 10-4). An exception to this may be the case where the endplates of the vertebral body themselves may be used for axial-load-resisting support (Fig. 10-5).

The acute stabilizing effect of an interbody bone graft depends partly—among many other factors—on the angle that the disk interspace makes with the horizontal plane when the patient is in the upright position. If the angle is zero (i.e., if the interspace is parallel with the horizontal plane), axial loads will not produce any shear forces at the level of the fusion. If, on the other hand, the disk interspace and fusion site is more vertical (as in the lumbar spine, and particularly at the lumbosacral junction), a shear force is added to the axial load (Fig. 10-6). The axial load promotes

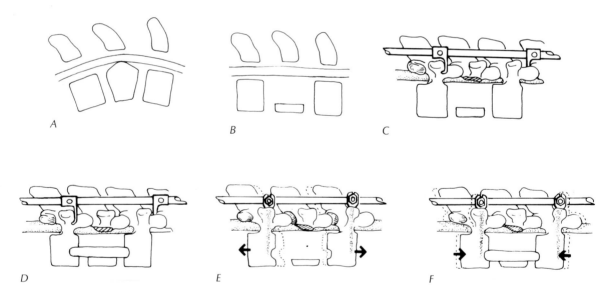

FIGURE 10-2 In most anterior interbody bone grafting situations, the appropriate order of procedural components is as follows: first, neural element decompression and spinal alignment (*A* and *B*); second, spinal stabilization (*C*); and third, placement of the bone graft (*D*). An obvious exception is the situation where it is mandatory to place the bone graft prior to the securing of the instrumentation construct. This technique, in fact, may be used to advantage in situations where the dynamics of spinal reconstruction may be enhanced by the application of bone-

healing-enhancing forces intraoperatively. In this situation the decompression may be accomplished first (*B*). Then the pathological segments may be distracted by the implant (*arrows*, panel *E*—in this case, a pedicle fixator), and the bone graft inserted. Finally, the construct may then be compressed onto the bone graft (*arrows*, panel *F*). This allows load-sharing between the ventral interbody bony structures and the posterior instrumentation construct.

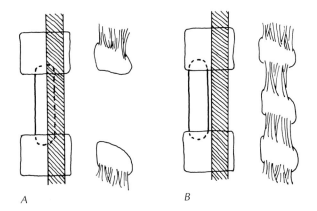

A　　　　　　*B*

FIGURE 10-3 The neutral axis of the spine is the region where normal weight-bearing may be expected to cause minimal distraction or compression of points within the region defined by the neutral axis. Therefore, interbody bone grafts should optimally be placed within, or slightly anterior to, this region— particularly if posterior stability is not adequate (*A*). If posterior stability is adequate, a more ventral location may be optimal; this allows sharing of the axial load between the anterior strut and the intact posterior spinal elements (*B*). The neutral axis is depicted by the shaded area.

bone healing; the shear forces disrupt it. This may explain, in part, the not-uncommon fusion failures observed with the posterior lumbar interbody fusion (PLIF) technique, particularly in the low lumbar region.

Anterior interbody fusion operations, including the PLIF operation, can use the phenomenon of *parallelogram distraction* to their advantage. This phenomenon takes advantage of the inherent strength of the fibro-ligamentous complex surrounding the vertebral body and connecting one vertebra to its neighbor—that is, the anulus fibrosus and the anterior and posterior longitudinal ligaments. Spondylolisthesis, by its nature, results in a parallelogram-like distortion of these structures and the adjacent vertebral bodies

(Fig. 10-7*A*). This is accompanied by a stretching of the fibro-ligamentous complex surrounding the vertebral body or, more likely, by an associated compensatory loss of disk interspace height. By taking advantage of the integrity of the fibro-ligamentous complex, the surgeon can distract the spine, thereby reducing the translational deformation in the sagittal plane. A bone graft can then be used to "hold" this alignment of the vertebral bodies, by acting as a spacer, until bony union takes place (Fig. 10-7*B*).

Inadequate mortise construction and bone graft fitting are perhaps the most common preventable errors leading to anterior interbody bone graft failure. *The mortise must be cut relatively deeply, and the bone graft must fit snugly into the mortise in such a manner that dislodgement is very unlikely* (Fig. 10-5).

The use of a fibular strut graft for interbody bone grafting may have the advantage of providing sufficient length for long fusions in selected cases. One must recognize, however, that the fibula has a much greater cortical-to-medullary bone ratio than does the vertebral body; thus the aforementioned telescoping complication can occur. This, in turn, can result in graft collapse or cut-out (Fig. 10-4). Placement of the graft near the endplate, for additional axial-load-bearing support, may help prevent such complications (Fig. 10-5). Note that fusion healing in this circumstance may be less vigorous, because of the smaller area of contact between the graft and the vertebral body. The meticulous removal of all soft tissue from the terminal 1 to 2 cm of the bone graft will minimize this problem.

POSTERIOR SPINAL FUSION

Posterior spinal fusions are not well situated mechanically to resist axial loads. That is, they do not offer substantial acute axial support of the spine. Posterior spinal fusions can provide this acute support of the spine only if secured in

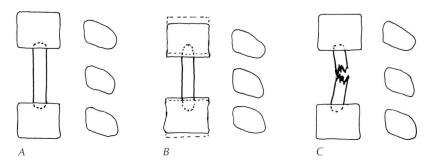

A　　　　　　　　*B*　　　　　　　　*C*

FIGURE 10-4 The importance of matching the integrity of the bone graft bed (the vertebral body) and that of the bone graft in anterior interbody fusions cannot be overemphasized. If a bone graft that is denser than the vertebral body is used, the tendency of the graft to "knife" its way through the vertebral body is significant (*A* and *B*). Conversely, if the bone graft is less dense

and weaker than the vertebral body, the bone graft may fail under the forces exerted on it (*C*). Therefore, a bone graft that is of similar density to the vertebral body is optimal. It is neither the weakest nor the strongest link in the "stability linkage system."

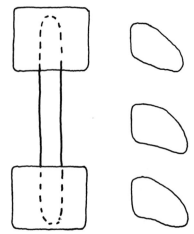

FIGURE 10-5 The vertebral body itself may be used for support of applied axial loads when anterior interbody bone grafts are used. If the medullary bone of the bone graft is too weak to resist the applied axial loads, the graft itself may be placed on or near the endplates of the vertebral body, as depicted. The endplate provides a resistance to spinal column collapse that the soft medullary bone of the vertebral body cannot. A drawback of this approach is the theoretical possibility of a decreased fusion rate due to the lack of bone graft–vertebral body contact at the terminus of the fusion construct. This is enhanced by meticulous circumferential removal of surface soft tissue from the distal 1 to 2 cm of the graft.

some way to the spine, as in posterior wiring and fusion procedures. These are most often used in the cervical region.[10] These fusion operations, however, are not practical in the lumbar region, because of the size of the spinal segments and the obligatory stresses placed on the spine in that region.

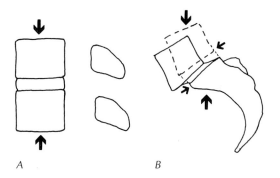

FIGURE 10-6 The vertebral body and the disk interspace most commonly accept axial loads when the torso assumes the upright position (A). The low lumbar spine, particularly at the lumbosacral junction, is prone to translational deformation with the bearing of axial loads. This is because of the orientation of the disk interspaces in this region, as depicted in this exaggerated example. This places a shear stress at the level of the disk interspace (B). Vertical arrows represent applied axial loads; oblique arrows represent resultant shear forces.

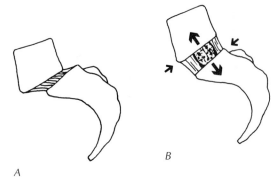

FIGURE 10-7 If the anulus fibrosus and the anterior and posterior longitudinal ligaments collectively provide sufficient integrity to the spine, the parallelogram distraction phenomenon can be used to advantage. A translational deformity of the spine (A), without loss of bony integrity and in the presence of intact ligamentous integrity, can be corrected by simple distraction of the spine. Note that laxity of the ligaments allows the translational deformity to occur. This laxity results partly from a loss of disk interspace height. Simply distracting the disk interspace and maintaining the distraction with a bone graft spacer allows the ligaments to tether the spine so that the translational deformity is reduced (B). Arrows depict distraction and the resultant shear forces. These forces are directed opposite those that caused the deformation (see Fig. 10-6).

Forces that enhance bone healing participate significantly in the fusion process. They explain the difference between the fusion rates of anterior interbody and posterior non-weight-bearing fusions (fusion being significantly more rapid in the former than in the latter). This is so because of the bone-healing-enhancing forces' ability to encourage fusion.[4]

If an axial load is borne by a spine with an accompanying posterior fusion, the bone fusion mass itself does not bear a load. In fact, the fusion mass is usually placed under some tension (distraction) during axial load-bearing.

BONE AS A SPINAL INSTRUMENT

Can bone alone function as a spinal instrument? When can the bony fusion do it all, and when is supplementation of the bony fusion with a spinal implant necessary? These questions are particularly worthy of consideration in this era of concern about the financial costs of treatment.

Bone can, indeed, function as a spinal instrument. Cloward has clearly documented this throughout his career.[11] Bone fusions can support the spine and simultaneously resist deformation (Fig. 10-7). Their ability to do so in the immediate postoperative period is usually unidirectional; that is, bone grafts by themselves apply predominantly unidirectional forces to the spine. These forces are almost always distractive (or, more appropriately, axial-load-

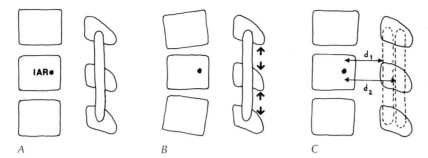

FIGURE 10-8 *A.* Acutely, a posterior bone graft (*shaded area*) does not resist axial loads well. *B.* Flexion causes distraction of all points dorsal to the IAR. This causes a posterior bone graft to be exposed to bone-healing-inhibiting (distracting) forces (*arrows*). *C.* Upon maturation of a posterior fusion, the graft itself can resist significant flexion deformation if adequate axial-load-resisting abilities are present. This is accomplished by application of a flexion-resisting moment arm. The longer the moment arm, the greater the ability to prevent flexion deformation. Short and long moment arms are represented by d_1 and d_2, respectively.

resisting) in nature. A bone graft placed between two vertebral bodies functions as a buttress that supports the spine in axial loading (Figs. 10-3–10-5). As mentioned above, this buttressing is most effective when the bone graft is placed in the plane of the IAR.

Thus the location of the bone graft with respect to the IAR is of great importance. The closer the bone graft is to the IAR, the greater the axial-load-resisting ability. Bone grafts placed in the interbody region resist axial loads well, whereas bone grafts placed in the region of the posterior elements resist axial loads poorly. Once a posterior bone graft has solidly fused, however, it resists flexion well (Fig. 10-8). Its superiority, in this regard, over an anterior interbody graft should be considered. In fact, the further dorsal to the IAR (or neutral axis) an interbody bone graft is placed, the longer the lever arm through which it functions (see Chap. 6 and Fig. 10-8).

Unless an anterior interbody bone graft and its acceptance site are conformed with the intent of acquiring specific desired effects, the only stresses resisted by a bone graft are axial; thus the bone graft itself functions only in a distraction, or axial-load-resisting, mode (Fig. 10-9A). The creation of a deep mortise in the vertebral body can provide a translation-resisting construct if the vertebral body and the bone graft have adequate integrity, the mortise is deep, and the bone graft and the mortise are fashioned meticulously (Fig. 10-9B). This contruct, albeit relatively weak under the best of circumstances, provides a terminal three-point bending construct (see Chap. 15).

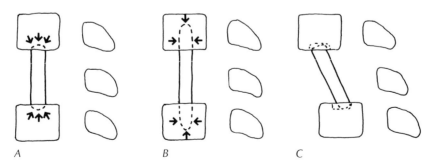

FIGURE 10-9 An interbody bone graft and its acceptance sites should be fashioned with the intent of acquiring specific desired effects. *A.* If the only stresses resisted by a bone graft are axial, the bone graft itself functions only in a distraction, or axial-load-resisting, mode. *B.* The creation of deep mortises in the vertebral bodies can provide a translation-resisting construct if the integrity of the vertebral body and the bone graft have adequate integrity, the mortises are deep, and the bone graft and the mortises are fashioned meticulously. Thus translation is inhibited by a terminal three-point bending method. *C.* If the mortise is not so constructed, a translational deformation is more likely.

REFERENCES

1. Bailey RW, Badgley CE: Stabilization of the cervical spine by anterior fusion. *J Bone Joint Surg* 1960; 42A: 565–594.
2. Benzel EC: Biomechanics of lumbar and lumbosacral spine fracture, in Rea GL, Miller CA (eds): *Spinal Trauma. Current Evaluation and Management.* Park Ridge, IL: American Association of Neurological Surgeons, 1993; 165–195.
3. Bohlman HH, Eismont FJ: Surgical techniques of anterior decompression and fusion for spinal cord injuries. *Clin Orthop Rel Res* 1981; 154:57–67.
4. Egger EL, Gottsauner-Wolf F, Palmer J, et al: Effects of axial dynamization on bone healing. *J Trauma* 1993; 34:185–192.
5. Stauffer ES, Kelly EG: Fracture-dislocation of the cervical spine. *J Bone Joint Surg* 1977; 59A:45–48.
6. Benzel EC, Larson SJ: Operative stabilization of the post-traumatic thoracic and lumbar spine: A comparative analysis for the Harrington distraction rod and the modified Weiss spring. *Neurosurgery* 1986; 19:378–385.
7. Denis F: The three column spine and its significance in the classification of acute thoracolumbar spine injuries. *Spine* 1983; 8:817–831.
8. White AA, Panjabi MM: *Clinical Biomechanics of the Spine* (2d ed). Philadelphia: Lippincott, 1990.
9. White AA, Panjabi MM, Thomas CL: The clinical biomechanics of kyphotic deformities. *Clin Orthop Rel Res* 1977; 128:8–17.
10. Benzel EC, Kesterson L: Posterior cervical interspinous compression wiring and fusion for mid to low cervical spine injuries. *J Neurosurg* 1989; 70:893–899.
11. Cloward R: Bone as a spinal instrument, in Benzel EC (ed): *Spinal Instrumentation.* Park Ridge, IL: American Association of Neurologic Surgeons, 1994:185–210.

Part IV

Spinal Instrumentation Constructs: General Principles

Chapter 11

Implant Properties

METALS

Elements and Alloys

Metallurgy is the study of metals, their material properties, and their shaping and treatment by heating and cooling. At least a rudimentary knowledge of this discipline is important for surgeons performing reconstructive spine operations; without this knowledge, inappropriate decisions may be made regarding implant or construct selection. This chapter will introduce the metallurgical principles relevant to this complex periphery of medicine.

An *element* is a simple substance that cannot be separated into simpler components by routine chemical means. An *alloy* is a metal made by the mixing and melding together of two or more metal elements, or of an element and some other substance. The mixing and melding of two or more elements of appropriate atomic numbers may yield an alloy that is useful in the manufacturer of spinal implants. These elements (with their standard abbreviations and atomic numbers, in parentheses) include aluminum (Al, 13), titanium (Ti, 22), vanadium (V, 23), chromium (Cr, 24), manganese (Mn, 25), iron (Fe, 26), cobalt (Co, 27), nickel (Ni, 28), zirconium (Zr, 40), niobium (Nb, 41), and molybdenum (Mo, 42). Titanium is the only element that is commonly used in an unalloyed ("pure") form as an implant material.

Other elements commonly found in metals are hydrogen (H, 1), carbon (C, 6), nitrogen (N, 7), and oxygen (O, 8). These latter elements are essentially contaminants. However, they may stabilize certain phases of some metals when present in small amounts. For example, small amounts of carbon and nitrogen may stabilize the alpha phase of titanium. The presence of contaminants and the unavoidable difficulty of eliminating them necessitates the grading of metals such as titanium.

"Pure" (unalloyed) titanium is available in four grades, which contain varying composition limits of multiple contaminants (including iron). Some of these contaminants are included by design; others are included because of the dif-

ficulty of removing them. Grade 1 is the most pure, and grade 4 the least pure. The strength of unalloyed titanium increases as the oxygen content increases. (The oxygen content can range from 0.18 to 0.40%.)

Although the density and modulus of elasticity of unalloyed titanium do not significantly change from grade to grade, its ultimate and 0.2 percent tensile yield strengths depend largely on its grade (Table 11-1).[1] The *modulus of elasticity* (elastic modulus) of a material describes the stress (force per unit of cross-sectional area) per unit of strain (linear deformation per unit of length) in the elastic region. A higher modulus of elasticity implies a stiffer, or more rigid, implant (see Chap. 2). The ultimate and 0.2 percent tensile *yield strengths* are the highest tolerable stress (to failure) and the stress that causes 0.2 percent deformation, respectively.

The most "pure" titanium (grade 1) is less able to tolerate "stretch" than the less pure unalloyed grades; that is, the various grades have different tensile strengths. The less-pure grades of titanium (grades 2 to 4) are similar, in this regard, to 316 stainless steel. (All have relatively high tensile strengths.) 316L stainless steel, on the other hand, is stiffer (i.e., has a higher modulus of elasticity) than all grades of unalloyed titanium. Therefore, it results in a relatively decreased transfer of stress from the implant to bone. This property augments *stress shielding* when 316L stainless steel is used with rigid systems, such as fixed-moment-arm cantilever beam constructs (see Chaps. 14 and 15).

Many alloys are used in the manufacture of spinal implants. These include 316L stainless steel (Cr 17 percent, Ni 13 percent, Mo 2.25 percent, with Fe and C), cast Co-Cr-Mo, and Ti-6A1-4V (Ti with 6 percent Al and 4 percent V). Some of their material properties are depicted in Table 11-1. Ti-6A1-4V is finding increasing use in spinal implantation.

Another alloy, vitallium, has been commonly employed. It is a trademarked alloy of Co and Cr. Finally, a new stainless steel alloy has recently been introduced. It is composed of 22 percent Cr, 13 percent Ni, and 5 percent Mn, and is

TABLE 11-1 Properties of titanium and selected alloys

Material	Density (g/cc)	Modulus of elasticity (MPa x 1000) (in tension)	Minimum ultimate tensile strength (MPa)	Minimum 0.2% yield strength (MPa)
Ti grade 1	4.51	102.7	240	170
Ti grade 2	4.51	102.7	345	275
Ti grade 3	4.51	103.4	450	380
Ti grade 4	4.51	104.1	550	483
316L stainless steel	7.95	186.4	480	170
Cast Co-Cr-Mo	8.59	248.2	655	450
Ti-6A1-4V	4.43	113.8	860	795

MPa = megapascal = 10^6 N/m^2.

called 22-13-5 stainless steel. Its modulus of elasticity in tension is similar to that of 316L stainless steel, but its ultimate tensile strength is roughly twice that of 316L stainless steel.

Surface Characteristics and Their Alteration

The surface characteristics of a spinal implant affect its performance through (1) corrosion, (2) material properties, and (3) construct-construct interface friction. Implant material selection depends, in part, on all three of these characteristics.

Corrosion, with consequent metal weakening, is a potential complication of an implant's exposure to a foreign environment—such as biological tissues. It rarely affects spinal stability, however, because bone graft incorporation usually occurs long before corrosion-related metal failure can occur. Surface corrosion resistance increases as the *anodic breakdown potential* increases (Fig. 11-1).[1] As the iron content of

an alloy is increased, the corrosion rate is increased. Corrosion resistance can be quantified by measuring the anodic polarization behavior of a specific metal against a control [e.g., a saturated calomel electrode in a physiologic (Hank's) solution]. Titanium is much more resistance to corrosion than 316L stainless steel; cast Co-Cr-Mo and Ti-6A1-4V are intermediate.

This latter quality is related to titanium's characteristic development of surface film (oxide). The surface film reforms if the metal is scratched or abraded. The surface film on titanium is both more stable and more resistant to corrosion than that associated with 316L stainless steel and other alloys. However, even a trace amount of iron decreases the stability of the protective film.

Occasionally, a limited extent of surface corrosion is desirable. As mentioned above, titanium forms a passive surface film that protects it against chemical attack. This type of protection may be enhanced, in certain circumstances, by a process called *anodizing*. Anodizing is an elec-

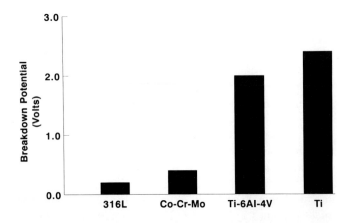

FIGURE 11-1 Breakdown potential (volts) versus metal composition for implant metals in Hanks' Solution (37°). The higher the breakdown potential, the greater the corrosion resistance. (*From J. Disegi.*[1])

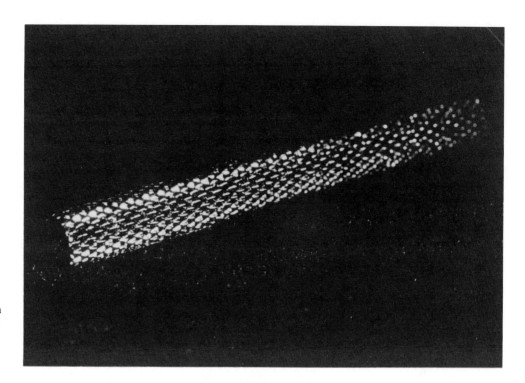

FIGURE 11-2 The knurled surface of a Cotrel-Dubousset rod gives relatively high friction between implant components if an appropriate method of attachment—such as a set screw—is used.

trolytic process that increases the thickness of a naturally occuring surface layer of oxide. This process is used to increase stability and corrosion resistance.

Corrosion occurring within crevices and small cavities on a metal's surface is called *crevice corrosion*. Titanium is much more resistant to this process than 316L stainless steel.

A form of corrosion that can occur when the protective passive film (the surface layer of oxide) is mechanically disrupted—usually via a repetetive friction mechanism—is *fretting corrosion (corrosion wear attack)*. This most commonly occurs at metal-metal interfaces. Titanium is much more resistant to fretting corrosion than 316L stainless steel. Along with metallurgical factors, the type of construct-construct interface plays a role in corrosion. The hook-rod interface of a Harrington distraction system produces much less fretting corrosion than the wire-rod interface of a Luque rod-wire system (both 316L stainless steel).[2] Ti-6A1-4V is particularly prone to fretting corrosion—a property that somewhat limits its utility. The relatively tight interfaces between components, however, considerably reduces the importance of this factor.

An accelerated form of corrosion that can occur in a mixed metal system, on account of the difference in electrochemical potential between the two metals, is *galvanic corrosion*. This phenomenon is usually clinically insignificant; for example, the use of titanium and stainless steel together causes no significant clinical sequelae. Liability considerations, however, must also be taken into account.

Osteointegration is the direct bonding of bone to an implant. The surface material properties dictate the osteointegration potential of any given material. Of all the materials commonly used for spinal implants, titanium has the greatest capacity for osteointegration. Osteointegration results in a smoother distribution of the load between the implant and bone.[3]

The surface characteristics of an implant material may affect its material properties. For example, fatigue resistance of a metal may be enhanced by the process of *shot peening*.[4] Shot peening is a surface treatment wherein small hard pellets are shot against the surface of a metal. This results in a compression deformation of the surface. This, in turn, results in an augmentation of the number of cycles required to cause failure.[5] *Fatigue* is the process of progressive permanent structural change occurring in a material subjected to repetitive alternating stresses. Fatigue resistance depends on many factors besides shot peening. In general, it increases as tensile strength increases. Annealed titanium has slightly less fatigue resistance than cold-worked 316L stainless steel (see below).

Alteration of the surface characteristics of an implant may be used to provide greater component-component friction, and thus enhanced resistance to component-component failure (see Chap. 12). An example of this is the use of a knurled surface on the Cotrel-Dubousset rod (Fig. 11-2). The combination of the set screw attachment mechanism and the coarse, rough surface of the knurled rod creates a high-friction component-component interface.

Structural Characteristics and Their Alteration

Structural characteristics of metals can be altered by a variety of processes. These include work hardening, annealing, and cold working. When a metal is permanently deformed, its yield stress (hardness) increases, while its ductility (malleability) decreases. This phenomenon is known as *work hardening.*

Annealing is a metallurgical treatment process designed to alter microstructure; in it the material is heated and cooled by a specific predetermined cycle. This creates a softer, weaker metal. *Cold working* is a metallurgical treatment process wherein the material is deformed at room temperature. This creates a harder, stronger material (i.e., tensile strength increases).

Structural Injury

Injury to implant materials can occur via several mechanisms. These include stress riser formation and notching. *Stress risers* result from the focal application of stress, usually via metal bending or contouring. This creates a focal concentration of strain that weakens the metal at a particular point—the stress riser. This weakens the construct and may result in metal fracture. A similar situation occurs via stress application in the Harrington distraction rod at the proximal ratchet. At this point the ratio of bending moment to rod diameter is at its maximum. This occasionally results in rod fracture via the focal application of forces to the rod at a specific point.

Notching is an injury to the surface of an implant that adversely affects structural integrity. This phenomenon may have significant implications for implant strength. For example, a 1 percent notch (a notch having a depth of 1 percent of the diameter of the implant) reduces fatigue resistance of 316L stainless steel wire by 63 percent, while bending, twisting, and knotting do not significantly affect fatigue resistance.[6] This has obvious implications for the handling of wire during surgery.[6-8] Twisting appears to be the optimal method of wire-to-wire approximation. The use of more than two full twists adds nothing to the security of the approximation. Commercial wire tighteners provide more consistent twists, with a concomitant decreased chance of surface injury.[8] Titanium is known to be prone to the ill effects of notching—that is, it is very notch-sensitive.[9] The braiding or weaving of small strands of wire into a cable greatly reduces the danger posed by this phenomenon.

NONMETAL MATERIALS

Many nonmetal materials have been used, or are in development for use, in the manufacture of spinal implants. These include acrylics, ceramics, polylactic acid, and hydroxyapatite. Other than acrylics, none have yet found widespread use in spine surgery. Therefore, only polymethylmethacrylate will be discussed here.

Polymethylmethacrylate

Polymethylmethacrylate (PMMA) was originally used for calvarial reconstruction and for orthopedic applications. It has also been applied in spine surgery. PMMA does not conform well to bony structures.[10] Any soft tissue surrounding the acrylic (such as fibrous tissue eschar) will loosen an initially rigid construct as it atrophies. However, PMMA has been found useful in selected clinical situations.[11]

Biomechanical testing of PMMA has been limited. Its rigid, brittle nature[12] (high modulus of elasticity) and its method of application (conformation to bony surface anatomy) are distinct characteristics not provided by most metals. It has been studied biomechanically in a clinical specimen by Panjabi and coworkers.[13] The mode of failure was wire pullout at the termini of the construct.

SUMMARY

Resistance to implant material injury or deformation depends on a multitide of factors. These factors may be broken down into 3 categories: (1) implant composition (i.e., the elements and alloys employed), (2) implant morphology (the size and shape of the implant), and (3) material treatment (work hardening, annealing, cold rolling, etc.). It behooves the surgeon to be aware of all three of these properties when considering any given type of implant.

REFERENCES

1. Disegi J: *AO/ASIF Unalloyed Titanium Implant Material* (2nd ed). 1991. AO/ASIF Materials Technical Commission: 3–25.
2. Bidez MW, Lucas LC, Lemons JE, Ward JJ, Nasca RJ: Biodegradation phenomena observed in in vivo and in vitro spinal instrumentation systems. *Spine* 1987; 12:605–608.
3. Bennett GJ: Materials and material testing, in Benzel EC (ed): *Spinal Instrumentation.* Park Ridge, IL: American Association of Neurological Surgeons 1994 (in press).
4. Collins JA: *High Cycle Fatigue in Failure of Materials in Mechanical Design: Analysis, prediction, prevention.* New York: Wiley, 1981.
5. Ashman RB: The TSRH spinal implant system, in Ashman RB, Herring JA, Johnston CE, et al (eds): *TSRH Universal Spinal Instrumentation.* Hundley and Associates, Inc., 1993:9–52.
6. Oh I, Sander TW, Treharne RW: The fatigue resistance of orthopaedic wire. *Clin Orthop Rel Res* 1985; 192:228–236.
7. Guadagni JR, Drummond DS: Strength of surgical wire fixation: A laboratory study. *Clin Orthop Rel Res* 1986; 209:176–181.
8. Schultz RS, Boger JW, Dunn HK: Strength of stainless steel surgical wire in various fixation modes. *Clin Orthop Rel Res* 1985; 198:304–307.

9. Scuderi GJ, Greenberg SS, Latta LL, et al: A biomechanical evaluation of MRI compatible wire for use in cervical spine fixation. Presented at Cervical Spine Research Society annual meeting, 1992.
10. Eismont FJ, Bohlman HH: Posterior methylmethacrylate fixation for cervical trauma. *Spine* 1981; 6:347–353.
11. Whitehill R, Cicoria AD, Hooper WE, et al: Posterior cervical reconstruction with methyl methacrylate cement and wire: A clinical review. *J Neurosurg* 1988; 68:576–584.
12. Duff TA: Surgical stabilization of traumatic cervical spine dislocation using methylmethacrylate. *J Neurosurg* 1986; 64:39–44.
13. Panjabi MM, Hopper W, White AA, et al: Posterior spine stabilization with methylmethacrylate: Biomechanical testing of a surgical specimen. *Spine* 1977; 2:241–247.

Chapter 12

Component-Component Interfaces

The locking mechanism employed between components of a spinal implant system (construct) is essential to the establishment of construct integrity. For the most part, two types of longitudinal member are clinically employed: rods and plates. The longitudinal member is connected to other implant components via one or a combination of six commonly used fundamental types of locking mechanisms: (1) three-point shear clamps, (2) lock screw connectors, (3) circumferential grip connectors, (4) constrained bolt-plate connectors, (5) semiconstrained screw-plate connectors, and (6) semiconstrained component-rod connectors (Fig. 12-1). Usually, a combination of two of these locking mechanisms, working in opposition to each other, is used at each component-component interface. This provides a pincerlike action to grip the rod or plate on opposite sides. For example, a circumferential grip connector may be used with a lock screw connector at opposing sides of a rod (Fig. 12-2). Interface friction may be enhanced by the provision of knurled surfaces, which allow seating of lock screws [e.g., Cotrel-Dubousset (CD)], or of a grid-on-grid surface (see below).

Constrained (rigid) screw-plate interfaces, such as constrained bolt-plate connectors (e.g., the Steffee plate), generally are stronger than most hook-rod or hook-screw interfaces. Other factors, however, must be considered in the implant section process.

Implant Surface Characteristics   All locking mechanism types rely on friction between the components to minimize or prevent failure at the component-component interface. Therefore, implant surface characteristics are a critical aspect of component-component interface considerations. Compatibility (or lack thereof) between the surfaces of the interfacing components is also critical. Some component-component interfaces rely mainly on torques or other forces applied; others rely more on friction between components to secure the desired interface integrity. All, however, rely on both to one degree or another.

Ways of Assessing Component-Component Interfaces   Mechanically, several laboratory techniques can be employed to assess component-component interface integrity. These include (1) axial push strength and (2) torsional strength (Fig. 12-3), which are the most widely used and the most easily reproduced.

LOCKING MECHANISMS

Three-Point Shear Clamp

The three-point shear clamp is a feature of Texas Scottish Rite Hospital (TSRH) hooks, screws, and crossmembers (*TSRH* is a registered trademark of Danek, Inc.). It provides significant resistance to axial, torsional, and bending-moment force application. It relies primarily on the force applied at the interface and secondarily on the friction between components. Security is attained via the application of a torque to a nut (bolt-plate connector) or a tangentially oriented lock screw. This tightly approximates the rod to *two* contoured surfaces (circumferential grip connectors). These combinations provide both halves of the pincer mechanism required for the attainment of security (Fig. 12-4). This is via a three-point bending–like mechanism (see Chap. 15).

Lock Screw Connectors

A lock screw connector uses a set screw mechanism to oppose the rod to the other half of the component system. Thus it provides half of the pincer mechanism required for security. The other half of the pincer mechanism is usually either a three-point shear clamp or a circumferential grip connector. The lock screw may be applied end-on or tangentially. There appears to be a mechanical advantage to tangential application (e.g., TSRH top tightening T-bolt assembly; see below). The lock screw may be seated on a knurled surface, as with the Cotrel-Dubousset (CD) system, thus relying mainly on friction between the two objects; or on a smoother surface, as with the Isola V-groove hollow ground (VHG) system, thus relying mainly on a circumfer-

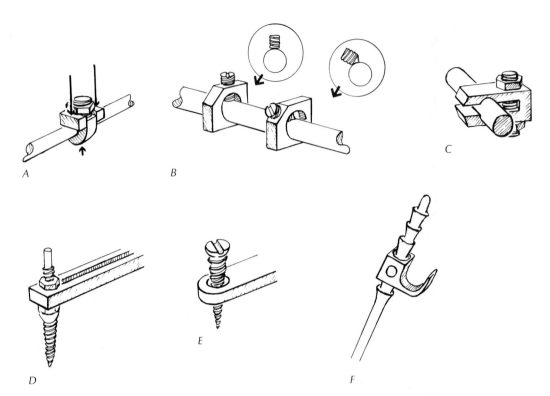

FIGURE 12-1 The six fundamental component-component locking mechanisms. *A.* Three-point shear clamp. *B.* Lock screw, seen end-on (left) and tangentially (right). *C.* Circumferential grip. *D.* Constrained bolt-plate. *E.* Semiconstrained screw-plate. *F.* Semiconstrained component-rod.

ential gripping force (Fig. 12-5). The VHG design also allows the application of a three-point bending–like complex of forces (Fig. 12-5*A*).

Circumferential Grip Connectors

Circumferential grip connectors may be used to provide both halves of the pincer [e.g., Isola crossmember, CD cross-member (device transverse traction, or DTT)], truly circumferential force application (e.g., the Synthes locking screw-plate technique) or, more commonly, only half of the pincer, as with a lock screw [e.g., Isola VHG design connector, Rogozinski connector, Puno-Winter-Byrd (PWB) connector etc.]. Representative examples are depicted in Fig. 12-6. Note that with the Isola VHG connector, a three-point shear clamp–like force application is achieved.

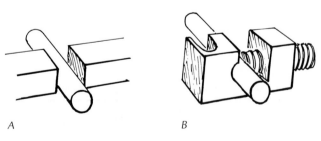

FIGURE 12-2 A rudimentary pincerlike action used to grip a rod, where the rod is simply sandwiched between two blocks (*A*). Often, each half of the pincer is of a different locking mechanism type. In this case the left portion of the pincer uses a circumferential grip, and the right an end-on lock screw mechanism (*B*).

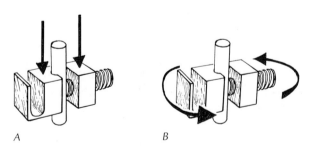

FIGURE 12-3 The axial-push-strength (*A*) and torsional-strength (*B*) methods of laboratory assessment. Arrows depict the forces applied by the testing device.

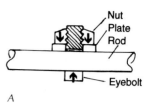

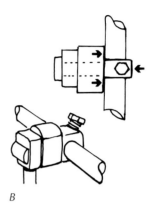

FIGURE 12-4 *A.* A three-point shear clamp with an eye-bolt connector (the combination of a three-point shear clamp and a constrained bolt-plate locking mechanism) and the forces applied when assembled. *B.* A three-point shear clamp with a tangential lock screw connector (the combination of a three-point shear clamp and a tangential lock screw connector). Arrows depict force vectors.

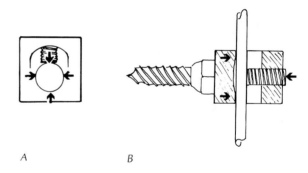

FIGURE 12-5 Lock screw connectors. *A.* An end-on lock screw (the Isola VHG lock screw design). A tangential lock screw (the TSRH top-tightening T-bolt assembly design) is depicted in Fig. 12-4*B. B.* The Isola VHG connector design applies three-point shear clamp forces. Arrows depict force vectors.

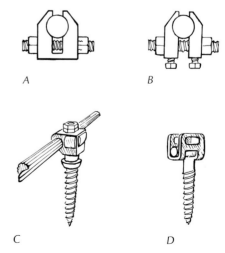

FIGURE 12-6 *A, B,* and *C.* Circumferential grip connectors in which both halves of the pincer mechanism are provided: Isola crossmember connector, CD crossmember connector, and Wiltse circumferential grip connector with linear grid-on-grid friction enhancement. *D.* The Rogozinski connector, in which only half of the pincer mechanism is provided by the circumferential grip mechanism. Another such system is the Isola VHG (see Fig. 12-5). Both of the latter systems use end-on lock screw mechanisms.

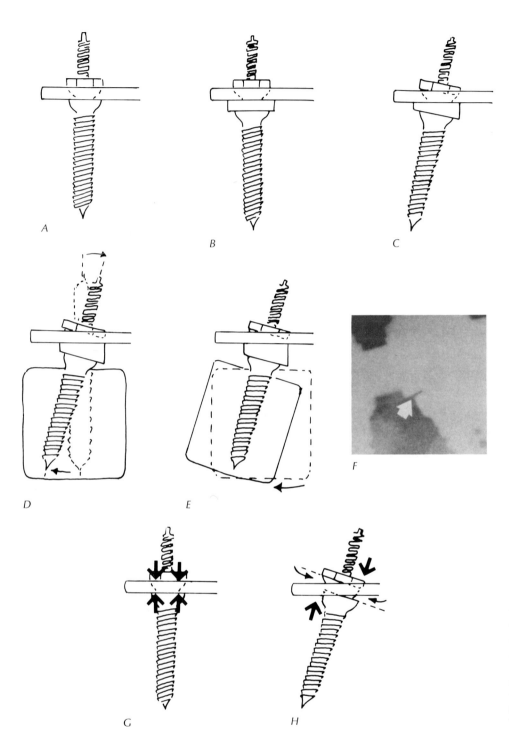

FIGURE 12-7 *A.* Constrained bolt-plate (Steffee plate) connectors. Note the rigid fixation of the screw to the plate via the bolt plate mechanism. *B* and *C.* The use of washers to compensate for screw height discrepancy and direction discrepancy, respectively. An angled washer may not accurately compensate precisely for the angle at the screw-plate junction. This may result in inadvertent application of a moment arm to the vertebral body by the screw, resulting in cutout (windshield wiper effect) (*D*) or an undesirable reorientation of the vertebral body (*E*). It may also result in inadequate tightening of the nut, which leaves a gap (*arrow*), thus fostering connector loosening (*F*). Contoured hub-plate interfaces provide some latitude in the latter regard. However, unless the screw is perpendicular to the plate (*G*), the connection has not resulted in optimal tightness and security, because of the inability to achieve an "in-line" configuration of the points of maximal contact between the plate and the hubs. Therefore, an optimally stable relationship between connector components is not achieved. Straight arrows depict points of contact of the nut and screw with the plate. Note the gaps and suboptimal contact realized when the screw is angled (*H*).

Constrained Bolt-Plate Connectors

The terms *constrained, semiconstrained, rigid, dynamic,* and *semirigid* describe different spinal implants qualitatively (see Chap. 14). They can be used to qualitatively portray and define component-component interfaces. Constrained (rigid) interfaces are stiff and do not yield, except upon failure. Semiconstrained (dynamic or semirigid) interfaces are less stiff and allow some movement at the component-component interface and between spinal segments.

Constrained (rigid) bolt-plate connectors are applicable to screw-plate systems (e.g., Steffee plate), as well as to hook-rod or screw-rod systems (Fig. 12-7A). The latter is used with the Isola (Acromed) slotted connector for attaching the screw to the rod and with the three-point shear clamp (TSRH) for attaching the eyebolt to the nut and thus achieving fixation of the hook, screw, or crossmember to the rod.

Constrained bolt-plate connectors are very rigid and are the strongest connectors available. This is particularly true at screw- or bolt-plate interfaces (e.g., Steffee plate). Component-rod interfaces are, by their nature, slightly weaker. Rod implant-implant connections that use a bolt-plate mechanism of connection (e.g., the three-point shear clamp of TSRH or the three-point shear clamp–like mechanism of the Isola VHG design) generally provide greater interface security than those that do not. The tangential lock screw mechanism of security attainment, which provides a stronger implant-implant interface than the traditional eyebolt mechanism, may provide further biomechanical advantages (see below). This implies that rod-to-implant interfaces that mimic a bolt-plate connector (three-point shear clamp) are stronger than those that do not.

Constrained screw- or bolt-plate connectors used with screw-plate systems (e.g., Steffee plate) pose problems of latitude for the surgeon. The screws must be placed in a relatively linear manner, at similar heights and in similar orientations. Furthermore, they are usually bulkier than screw-rod systems. Spacers, washers, and contoured screw hub-plate interfaces have been used to compensate for some of these problems. However, they present additional problems (Fig. 12-7*B* through *I*).

Semiconstrained Screw-Plate Connectors

Most screw-through-the-plate systems are semiconstrained. Myriad variations have been used clinically. Luque and Caspar plates, as well as a variety of other posterior cervical and anterior and pedicle fixation thoracic and lumbar plate systems, are included in this group. They have in common the allowance of toggling of the screw on the plate and, thus, the lack of a rigid binding of the screw to the plate (Fig. 12-8). Hence, truly rigid fixation is not achieved (see Chaps. 1, 14, and 15).

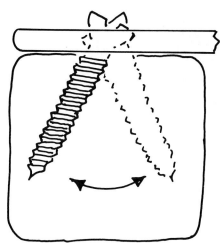

FIGURE 12-8 Semiconstrained screw-plate connectors (e.g., Luque plate). The screw is allowed to toggle in the plate, resulting in a dynamic, or nonrigid, system.

Semiconstrained Component-Rod Connectors

Semiconstrained component-rod connectors are typified by the Harrington distraction rod, the Harrington compression rod, and other relatively "loose" component-rod interfaces. The connections allow some toggling of the component on the rod (Fig. 12-9); hence, fretting and loosening at the component-rod interface are potential complications.

IMPLANT SURFACE CHARACTERISTICS

In general, friction between the components must be enhanced in order to achieve maximal torsional or axial push strength. An analogy to contact between automobile tires and terrain is appropriate here.

A mud tire has deep treads with a knobby surface. It matches well the surface of the terrain for which it is designed. A drag-racing slick is smooth and wide. It, too,

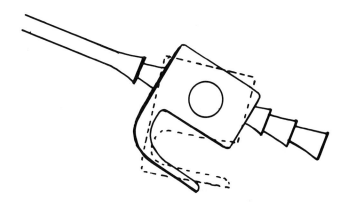

FIGURE 12-9 An exaggerated depiction of a semiconstrained component-rod connector (Harrington distraction rod and hook) in extremes of the allowed toggle.

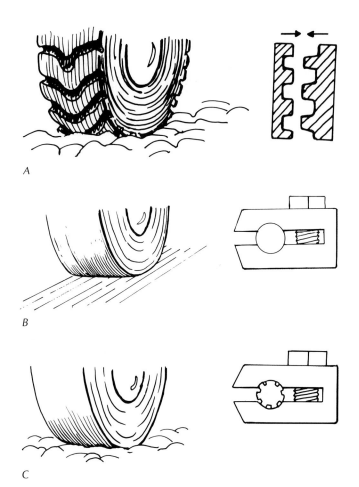

A

B

C

FIGURE 12-10 The two opposing surfaces of a component-component interface must "match" if the security of fixation is to be optimized. In each portion of this figure an analogy to tire-versus-terrain is depicted on the left, and the component-component relationship on the right (see text). *A.* A mud tire on off-road terrain, and a grid-grid interface. Note the meshing of the two surfaces. *B.* A racing slick on an asphalt road, and a circumferential grip connector on a smooth rod. In *A* and *B* the surfaces are matched, and contact between surfaces is maximized. *C.* Mixing of the two types of surface characteristics may give inadequate contact between surfaces. This is depicted with a racing slick interfacing with an off-road terrain, and a knurled rod interfacing with a smooth component.

matches well the surface of the terrain for which it is designed. In the former case, a rough surface is matched to a rough surface (as in a grid-on-grid interface—see below). In the latter case two relatively smooth surfaces are matched, with maximum surface-to-surface contact (as in a circumferential grip connection). Mixing of the two systems may result in less friction. For example, a knurled surface ("off-road terrain," or half of a grid-on-grid interface) will not allow significant friction at the interface with a smooth surface ("drag slick," or circumferential-grip half of a pin- ·

cer). The surface area of contact is diminished, and thus the desired interface friction is not achieved (Fig. 12-10).

Enhanced Friction in Grid-on-Grid Interfaces

Grid-on-grid interfaces take advantage of the friction achieved between two opposing surfaces with matching interlocking grids. These should not be considered as *connectors* in the strictest sense; rather, one might call them interface *friction enhancers*. The grids usually are either lin-

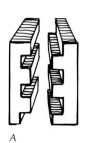

A

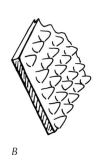

B

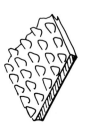

C

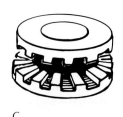

FIGURE 12-11 Different ways to enhance friction with a grid-on-grid interface: *A.* Linear type. *B.* Checkerboard type. *C.* Radial type.

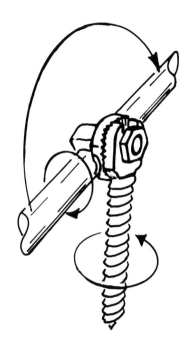

FIGURE 12-12 The TSRH variable-angle screw has the advantage of allowing multiplane 360-degree flexibility in the orientation of the screw. Three planes of movement *(curved arrows)* are depicted. This is made possible by the radial orientation of the friction enhancement grid, the rotation of the screw-rod connector, and the rotation of the screw, as depicted.

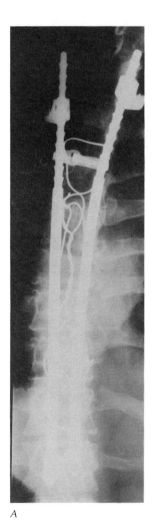

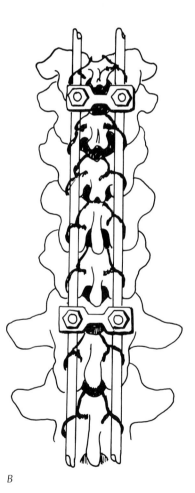

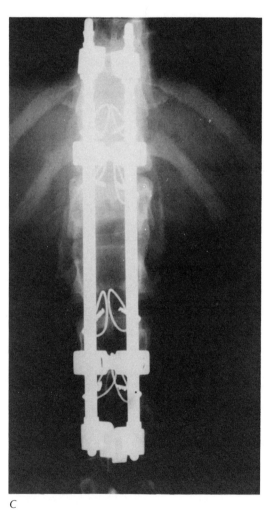

A *B* *C*

FIGURE 12-13 *A.* An x-ray of an acrylic-wire combination used as a crossmember with a Harrington distraction rod system. *B.* The use of crossmembers to increase stability and to prevent one rod's telescoping past another with the Luque sublaminar wire technique. The use of two crossmembers near the junction of thirds provides a rectangular construct that can be fabricated in situ; in this case a Harrington distraction rod system with accompanying sublaminar wires was employed with rigid crossfixation (*C*).

ear (e.g., Wiltse system), checkerboard-like (e.g., CD system), or radial (e.g., TSRH variable-angled screw) (Fig. 12-11). Besides enhancing friction, such gridded surfaces can provide other advantages (Fig. 12-12).

CROSSFIXATION

Crossfixation is defined herein as *the rigid fixation of bilaterally placed posterior fixation devices to each other in a rigid or semirigid manner so as to make the construct effectively a quadrilateral frame*. This technique has been used for some time with wire and acrylic crossfixation of Harrington distraction rods and other posterior rigid devices (Fig. 12-13A).

There are various forms of crossfixation. The CD and Isola techniques provide a less substantial crossmember than the TSRH system. The CD and Isola crossmembers, however, can be applied at any inter-rod width, whereas the TSRH crossmembers are not adjustable, but are available in multiple sizes. Others (e.g., the PWB, Rogozinski, and Wiltse devices) offer their own advantages and disadvantages.

Crossfixation gives substantially greater stiffness and stability than are achieved without crossfixation. This is especially advantageous with longer systems. The increase in stability is obvious at surgery and warrants the use of crossfixation with long instrumentation systems whenever possible.

Crossmembers may be used with Harrington distraction rods or Luque rods. This addition may enhance the stability of the construct. With the Luque rod, the often-observed telescoping of one rod on the other will be eliminated by this crossfixation technique. A rectangular construct can essentially be fabricated in situ in the operating room (Fig. 12-13B and C).

COMPARISON OF CONSTRUCT-CONSTRUCT CONNECTORS

Conversion Factors

For the uninitiated (and for those who simply have forgotten), the units or measurement of force application and load-bearing can be confusing. The pertinent terms and conversion factors are presented in Table 12-1. For the purposes of this discussion, newtons and newton-meters are used as measurements of force (weight) and of torque (bending moment), respectively.

Comparison Data

The strength of component-component locking mechanisms is difficult to assess. Comparisons between systems, therefore, are precarious. This is compounded by the fact that differences in laboratory assessment technique contam-

TABLE 12-1 Units of measure pertinent to the mechanics of spinal stabilization constructs, with conversion factors

Measure of distance

1 meter = 39.37 inches

Measures of force (weight)

1 newton = 10^5 dynes
1 pound = 16 ounces (avoirdupois)
1 pound = 4.448 newtons
1 newton = 0.225 pounds
1 kilogram = 9.8 newtons
1 kilogram = 2.2 pounds

Measures of work (energy)

1 inch-pound = quantity of energy required to raise a weight of 1 pound against gravity by a height of 1 inch
1 newton-meter = quantity of energy required to raise a weight of 1 newton against gravity by a height of 1 meter
1 erg = 1 dyne-centimeter
1 inch-pound = $\frac{1}{2}$ foot-pound
1 joule = 1 newton-meter
1 newton-meter = 0.7375 foot-pounds
1 newton-meter = 8.85 inch-pounds
1 inch-pound = 0.113 newton-meters

Measures of torque (bending moment)

Torque, like work or energy, comprehends factors of force and distance. It is essential to differentiate between these two measurements. The magnitude *and direction* of a torque depend on the axis of rotation through which the force is applied; work, or energy, is simply a quantity, with no inherent directional component.

inate the data. Nevertheless, averaged and extrapolated data from *available* manufacturer-provided information for selected component-rod systems are presented here, in order to provide at least some basis for comparison of certain component-rod locking mechanisms.

Laboratory data for many systems are unavailable or are not comparable with data for other systems. Nevertheless, the strength characteristics of several system-specific implant-rod connector systems are compared in order to illustrate *some* advantages and disadvantages of *some* connector designs. *This information was derived from multiple laboratories (often partisan), each having its own laboratory-specific characteristics. This provides, at best, a rough comparison. Where conflicting data were reported by two or more laboratories, the most favorable result is reported here (Figs. 12-14 and 12-15). Furthermore, laboratory biomechanical assessments are performed under ideal circumstances. If appropriate tightening torque (as defined by the laboratory studies) is not applied in vivo (as may often be the case), the*

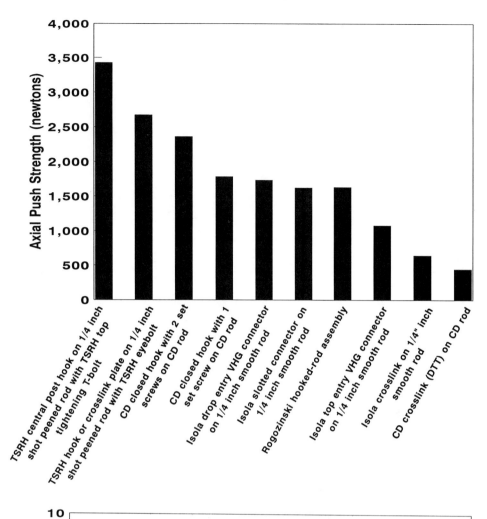

FIGURE 12-14 Selected component-rod axial push strength comparison data (see text).

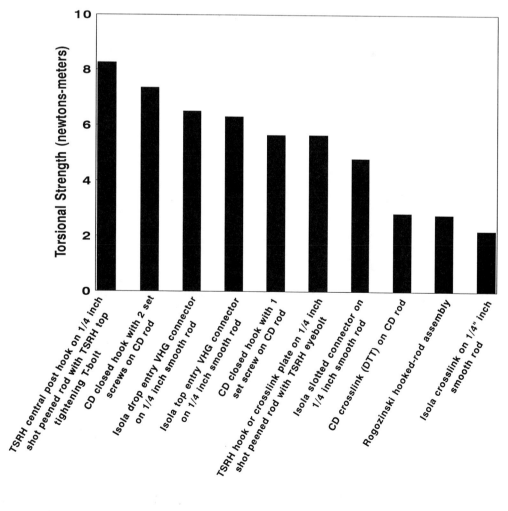

FIGURE 12-15 Selected component-rod torsional strength comparison data (see text).

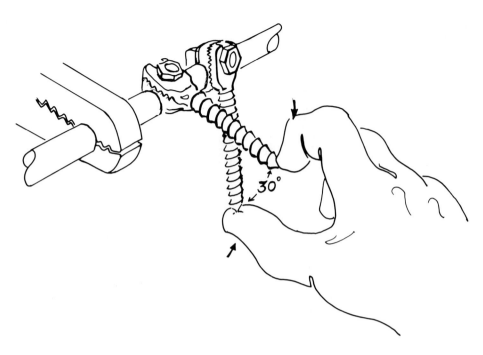

FIGURE 12-16 "Poor man's" biomechanical testing. Apply two 50-mm screws to a rod (next to each other and divergent by 30°) via the manufacturer's prescribed technique. Have an assistant hold the rod with a locking plier. Apply increasing degrees of force. This can be graded according to the force required to cause rotation of the screw on the rod. In this manner two or more systems can be compared.

application of laboratory biomechanical data to the clinical situation is meaningless. The available data are presented for axial push strength (Fig. 12-14) and torsional strength (Fig. 12-15). These methods of analysis are illustrated in Fig. 12-3.

A "best guess" as to relative torsional strength can be made manually; a "relative" grading scheme can be employed. Thus one can compare torsional strength of component-rod interfaces by using this simple "poor man's" biomechanical test (Fig. 12-16).

Chapter 13

Implant-Bone Interfaces

Various types of interface between bone and surgically applied implants are used clinically. In spinal surgery there are five fundamental types of implant-bone interface: (1) abutting (e.g., interbody bone, interbody acrylic); (2) penetrating (e.g., nail, staple, screw); (3) gripping (e.g., hook, wire; (4) conforming (e.g., posterior application of acrylic; and (5) osteointegration (e.g., titanium).

Within these categories there are subcategories and implant variations. The biomechanical principles involved range from the very simple, as with the abutting interbody implants, to the very complex nuances of screw-bone interfaces. Each category is considered separately, with accompanying theoretical and biomechanical information.

ABUTTING IMPLANT-BONE INTERFACES

The predominant location for the placement of abutting implants is the interbody region. Their application elsewhere, on or within the vertebra, makes little sense. For an abutting construct to be effective, it must "bear a load." Since the interbody region is the approximate region of the neutral axis (see Chap. 10), and since most of the axial load is borne in this region, the interbody location is the most appropriate region for placement of abutting implants.

Abutting implants, by their nature, distribute loads over a relatively large surface area. One would not usually select a slender interbody implant, for it would likely "knife" its way through the relatively soft cancellous bone of the vertebral body. The placement of the interbody implant in close approximation to the endplate (where the bone is more compact and, thus, more able to resist compression) may be desirable (see Chap. 5).

Specific information on the biomechanics of such implants is lacking. All other factors being constant, however, the larger the surface area of the contact between the implant and the bone, the more effective the implant's resistance to axial loads. The axial load–resisting capacity is, in theory, directly proportional to the surface area of con-

tact. The larger the circumference of the interbody abutting implant—be it bone, acrylic, or a metal implant (e.g., the Rezaian spinal fixator)—the more effective it is in achieving one of its most important goals: to resist applied axial loads (Fig. 13-1).

Another goal with abutting interbody implants is for the implant to remain in the desired interbody location; thus load-bearing is optimized, the chance of neural impingement is minimized, and the chance of subsequent spinal deformation is also minimized. This necessitates the use of an adjunctive implant component. For example, interbody acrylic implants may be applied with a rigid wire stabilizer that penetrates into the endplates of the adjacent and supported vertebral bodies. This minimizes the chance of implant migration. The Rezaian spinal fixator uses spikes at the terminal bone-contacting surfaces to achieve the same result. Bone graft implants are often positioned in a deep mortise or fashioned in a conical shape at the termini. These maneuvers also minimize the chance of implant (interbody bone graft) migration (Fig. 13-2).

PENETRATING IMPLANT-BONE INTERFACES

Penetrating implant-bone interfaces are of two fundamental types: (1) those without pullout-resistance attributes, and (2) those with pullout-resistance attributes. The former type includes nails, spikes, and staples. (The penetrating adjuncts of the abutting implant-bone interface implants are examples of this type.) The latter type includes screws and penetrating implants that change configuration upon placement into bone (e.g., expanding screws).

Penetrating Implant-Bone Interfaces without Pullout Resistance (Posts)

Nails, spikes, and staples are seldom used as sole methods of implant-bone interface in clinical practice. This is due partly to their relative inability to resist dislodgment; their pullout-resistance capabilities are nearly nil. They usually

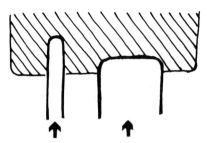

FIGURE 13-1 The surface area of the contact surface of interfaces between abutting implants and bone correlates with weight-bearing capacity. A smaller-diameter implant penetrates farther *(left)*, while a larger-diameter implant withstands axial loading more effectively *(right)*. Arrows depict load applied to bone *(hatched area)* by the implant.

function as adjuncts (stabilizers) for implants (e.g., as adjuncts for interbody axial load–bearing implants); as the cantilever components of rigid, constrained implant systems for axial load–bearing (fixed moment arm cantilever beam; see Chap. 15); or as the cantilever components of terminal three-point bending constructs (posts) (see Chap. 15) (Fig. 13-3).

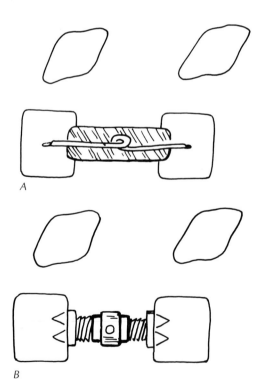

FIGURE 13-2 Adjuncts to abutting implant–bone interface systems in the interbody region include (*A*) a rigid wire stabilizer in acrylic, and (*B*) the Rezaian spinal implant with its terminal spikes. Both adjuncts minimize lateral migration of the implant.

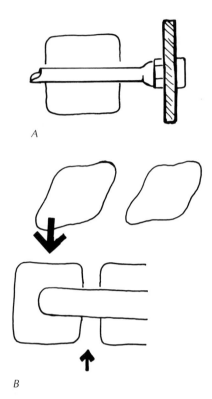

FIGURE 13-3 A penetrating implant without pullout resistance (post type) can function as an implant stabilizer (see Fig. 13-2), as a fixed moment arm cantilever beam (*A*), or as the cantilever component of a terminal three-point bending construct (*B*). In the latter case, an interbody bone graft can resist forces that induce translation *(large arrow)* via a cantilever beam technique *(small arrow)*.

Penetrating Implant-Bone Interfaces with Pullout Resistance—Implants that Change Configuration Following Insertion

Implants that change configuration following insertion into bone have the capacity to resist pullout (Fig. 13-4). They are not commonly used in clinical practice; therefore, little biomechanical information is available.[1]

Penetrating Implant-Bone Interfaces with Pullout Resistance—Screws

Most of the information available on implant-bone interfaces is about screws. This parallels the frequency of their clinical use. In fact, the screw, alone or as a component of a more complex spinal implant, is used clinically with increasing frequency and through increasingly broader applications. A relatively deep knowledge of screw anatomy, screw interactions with bone, and screw biomechanics is mandatory for effective and safe use of screws.[2,3]

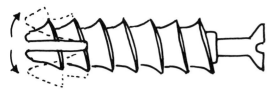

FIGURE 13-4 Implants that change configuration within bone provide an augmentation of pullout resistance.[1] Note splaying of screw tip by a drywall-like screw mechanism *(arrows).*

SCREW ANATOMY

A screw has four basic components: (1) the head, (2) the core, (3) the thread, and (4) the tip (Fig. 13-5). Each component can be altered to achieve a specific desired clinical effect.

Head The head of the screw resists the translational force created by the rotation of the thread through the bone at the termination of screw tightening (Fig. 13-6). The screw head, therefore, should be designed to optimally abut the underlying surface. If this surface is medullary bone, a wide head is necessary to minimize the chance of pull-through. A smaller diameter is required for cortical bone. If the underlying surface is metal, as with a dynamic or semiconstrained screw-plate system, the undersurface of the screw head should conform to the trough in the plate; that is, it should have rounded undersurface. This usually allows toggling. On the other hand, if toggling is not desired, a flat undersurface that abuts the flat surface of the plate may be desirable. Obviously, because of the significant deformation resistance of metal as compared to bone, the head diameter can be smaller with metal-on-metal applications than with metal-on-bone applications (Fig. 13-7).

Once the screw head has come into contact with the underlying surface during tightening, one or a combination of two sequelae will result from further tightening of the screw: (1) screw thread–bone interface failure (stripping, or pullout), and (2) deformation of the underlying surface against the undersurface of the screw head.

Core The core gives the screw most of its fracture resistance, in the form of resistance to cantilever bending and torsion. In clinical practice the torsional strength of the screw

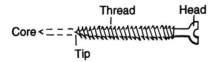

FIGURE 13-5 The important anatomic aspects and characteristics of a screw: the head, the core, the thread, and the tip.

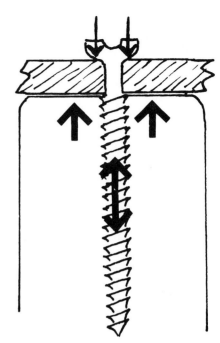

FIGURE 13-6 The head of the screw resists translational forces at the terminus of screw tightening. This causes tensile forces to be applied to the screw and compressive forces to be applied to the bone and plate *(arrows).*

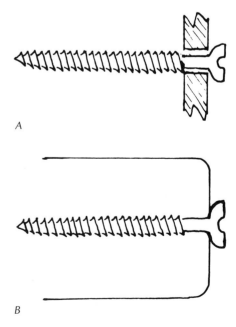

FIGURE 13-7 Screw head diameter can be smaller with metal undersurfaces (*A*) than with bone undersurfaces (*B*).

is relatively insignificant. But screws are frequently to bear substantial cantilevered loads; hence bending strength is of considerable importance. This strength is proportional to the *section modulus* (*Z*) and is defined by the equation already presented in Chap. 2:

$$Z = \frac{\pi D^3}{32}$$

where *D* = core diameter. Therefore, screw (or rod) strength is proportional to the cube of the core diameter. As the core diameter rises, the strength of the screw rises exponentially. This is especially significant for the core diameters commonly used clinically (Table 13-1). Note that the difference in strength between a 5.0-mm and a 6.0-mm core diameter screw is nearly twofold (125 versus 216). Hence the largest screw diameter allowed by the local bony anatomy should be used, so that the likelihood of screw failure (fracture) can be minimized.[4] This principle is difficult to apply in places where the pedicles are narrow, as in the thoracolumbar region. This underscores, in part, the biomechanical and clinical problems associated with pedicle fixation in this region. In view of the simplicity of the mathematical relationship between screw diameter and screw strength, it is not surprising that different systems have similar stabilization attributes.[5]

Stress reduction osteoporosis results from *stress shielding* associated with the use of very rigid implant systems. It is intuitive that the shielding of bone from applied loads may result in demineralization. This indeed occurs, but the stiffness and stability imparted to the spine more than compensate for the phenomenon.[6] With less rigid systems, move-

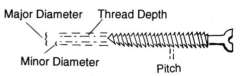

FIGURE 13-8 Screw core (minor) and outside (major) diameters, thread depth, and screw pitch.

ment at the screw-bone interface may occur. Movement at the screw-bone interface causes the screw to become enveloped with fibrous tissue,[7] with weakening of the screw-bone interface.

Thread and tip   Screw *core diameter* (minor diameter) is proportional to strength. *Outside diameter* (major diameter) on the other hand, is more important as a determinant of screw pullout resistance. The depth of the thread may be even more important in this regard (Fig. 13-8).

Three types of screw are used in spinal surgery: machine screws (cortical screws), self-tapping machine screws, and wood screws (cancellous screws). Cortical screws are used in hard, relatively incompressible bone. Their shallow threads minimize the need for bone compression during screw insertion. The problem of pathological bone compression by the screw during insertion is eased by pretapping of the hole for the screw. For a cortical screw to provide maximal pullout resistance, pretapping is optimal. Tapping carves threads into the wall of the screw hole. The cutting edges of the tap screw perform this task. Two characteristics of a screw tap are fundamental to its success: a tapered tip and a full-length flute. The tapered tip helps to align the screw in the desired direction by directing it down the predrilled hole. The full-length flute gathers bone debris carved from the wall of the drill hole by the tap screw (Fig. 13-9*A*). *This is enhanced by periodic loosening of the screw by approximately one-quarter to one-half turn during tightening, which allows the bone debris to collect in the flute.*

Self-tapping screws obviate the need for several steps. A leading-edge flute is built into the tip, allowing debris to accumulate within its confines. The shorter flute of self-tapping screws cannot accommodate all the debris created (Fig. 13-9*B*). Thus the the drill holes should be larger with self-tapping screws (slightly larger than the core diameter of the screw), in order to facilitate debris accumulation around the threads.

Pretapped and self-tapped screws, if used properly, provide similar pullout strengths. Furthermore, the pullout strength of both pretapped and self-tapped screws is not significantly affected by multiple insertions and removals *in cortical bone.*[8]

Cancellous (wood) screws are used in softer material— that is, in cancellous bone. Compression of cancellous bone by the screw during insertion increases its density and, thus, its pullout resistance. (With cortical bone, compression dur-

TABLE 13-1 Relationship of screw strength to core diameter (comparison to a core diameter of 1.0 mm)

Core diameter (mm)	Relative strength (cube of core diameter)
1.0	1.0
1.5	3.4
2.0	8.0
2.5	15.6
3.0	27.0
3.5	42.9
4.0	64.0
4.5	91.1
5.0	125.0
5.5	166.4
6.0	216.0
6.5	274.6
7.0	343.0
7.5	421.9
8.0	512.0
8.5	614.1
9.0	729.0

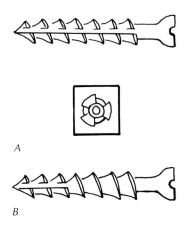

A

B

FIGURE 13-9 *A.* A screw tap. Note the tapered tip and the full-length flute. *B.* A self-tapping screw. Note the leading-edge flute that does not extend the length of the screw. *Inset:* An end-on view of the tip.

ing screw insertion causes microfractures that decrease bone integrity.) Therefore, whereas pretapping is desirable in cortical bone, it is less desirable in cancellous bone. *In fact, in cancellous bone, tapping weakens the implant-bone interface.*

Pedicle screws rarely obtain cortical purchase within the pedicle.[9] Since tapping weakens the implant-bone interface in cancellous bone, the tapping of pedicle screw holes is of questionable value. However, in cortical bone, bone micro-cracking around screw threads is greater with untapped than with tapped screws.[10] Therefore, in cortical bone, untapped screws loosen more frequently than tapped screws.

PULLOUT RESISTANCE

As mentioned above, the main determinants of screw pull-out resistance are major screw diameter[11] and thread depth. Other important facts are extent of cortical purchase, depth of screw penetration, and thread design. The several threads nearest the screw's head bear most of the load transferred from bone during pullout stressing. Therefore, proximal cortical "purchase" is very important to pullout resistance. Of secondary importance is the depth of penetration of the screw within bone.[12] Third, opposite cortical purchase seems to be even less important to pullout resistance.[13,14] This last point is understandable in view of the fact that the greatest load is transferred by the most superficial threads.

Thread design also plays a role in screw pullout resistance. Two factors dominate this aspect of screw mechanics: thread *pitch* and thread *shape*. Thread pitch is the distance from any point on a screw thread to the corresponding point on the next thread. This is essentially equal to the distance a screw advances axially in one turn (the *lead*). A fundamental rule of screw biomechanics is that *pullout resistance is proportional to the volume of bone between threads.* As pre-

viously mentioned, increased thread depth increases pullout resistance. Thread depth is obviously proportional to bone volume between threads. Similarly, the pitch of the thread is proportional to the volume of bone between threads and, thus, to pullout resitance.

Finally, alteration of the shape of the thread can increase or decrease the interthread volume. For example, flattening or reversing the angle of the following edge of the thread will further increase interthread volume (by decreasing metal volume) and result in an even greater increase in pullout resistance. Screw toe-in (triangulation) also contributes to pullout resistance, if the two sides of the construct are rigidly affixed to each other via a crossmember[15] (Fig. 13-10).

Security of the implant-bone interface can be problematic. This commonly occurs in osteoporotic patients. Mineral density of bone has been shown to correlate inversely with pullout resistance.[16] In severely osteopenic patients, screw pullout resistance may be diminished so much that screw fixation may be a suboptimal choice for the implant-bone interface.

In cases where screw hole stripping or cutout has occurred intraoperatively, injection of polymethylmethacrylate into the screw hole prior to screw insertion should be considered. Zindrick and coworkers showed this to be a viable option only when the polymethylmethacrylate is injected under pressure.[17] In this case, the acrylic most likely is forced into the interstices of the medullary bone, thus providing an equivalent, of sorts, of increased thread depth.

Screw-bone interface failure may be minimized by scrupulous attention to screw configuration. Rigidly connected diverging or converging screws have increased pullout resistance. This is optimal with screws placed at approximately a 90-degree angle.[18] Further advantages are gained by elimination of excessive compression stress during tightening. Some compressive stresses are applied to bone by the screw threads, however. They provide adequate fixation, without excessive bone resorption, until bone fusion occurs.[19]

LAG SCREW

Three conditions must obtain for a screw to function as a lag: (1) The near surface of the bone hole must allow the unthreaded screw shaft to glide freely; (2) the far surface of the bone-screw interface must be threaded; and (3) when the screw is tightened, its head must contact the near surface to halt progression of the screw's longitudinal movement.[3] The tension within the screw causes compression between bone fragments (Fig. 13-11).

GRIPPING IMPLANT-BONE INTERFACES

Hooks and wire provide a "grip" of the spine that is not provided by screws, nails, acrylic, or bone. Pullout resistances

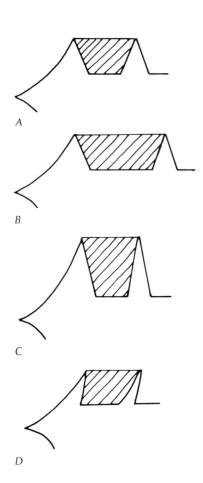

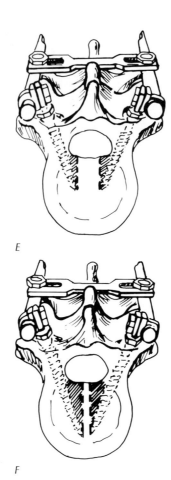

FIGURE 13-10 *A.* Screw pullout resistance is mainly a function of the volume of bone (*hatched area*) between screw threads. *B.* Thread pitch affects this by altering inter-thread distance. *C.* Thread depth affects this by altering thread width. *D.* Thread shape affects this by altering the amount of bone volume directly; if the pitch is unchanged, the only factor affecting bone volume is screw thread volume (metal volume). Decreasing screw thread volume (metal volume) increases bone volume. The triangulation of pedicle screws provides additional resistance to pullout. Pullout resistance is proportional not only to volume of bone between screw threads, but also to the triangular area defined by the screw, the perpendicular, and the posterior vertebral body surface (*shaded area, E*). Whereas screw length does not routinely contribute significantly to pullout resistance, it contributes significantly when screws are triangulated (*F*). Note the increase in the shaded area. Note also that increasing the screw angle also increases the size of the shaded area and, thus, pullout resistance.

for hooks and wire are substantial. Hooks and wire provide particular advantages in osteoporotic bone.[20] This is due to the greater surface of contact and the fact that the contact usually is on cortical bone along the entire contact surface of the hook or wire.

Hooks obviously provide a larger contact surface than wire. Double strands of wire or cable double the contact surface, thus increasing the pullthrough resistance.

Although pullout and pullthrough resistances of hook-bone and wire-bone interfaces are important, equally or more important are the integrity of the bone component through which the interface occurs and the mode of force application to the spine by the implant. For example, a small lamina may fracture if significant stresses are placed on it, regardless of the type of implant-bone interface employed. Similarly, the types of stress placed on the interface may partly determine the likelihood of eventual failure. The pedicle–transverse process claw configuration, as well as the technique of insertion, is pertinent in this regard.

A pedicle hook inserted too deeply may cut into the pedicle, diminishing its integrity. Hook insertion to an insufficient depth results in improper engagement of the pedicle, reducing the interface's ability to augment torsional stabil-

ity. Finally, the addition of a transverse process hook applies a torque to the pedicle that may have the undesirable consequence of failure of the pedicle, the facet, or the transverse process. These mechanisms of failure are illustrated in Fig. 13-12.

Screw pullout resistance may be augmented in the thoracic and lumbar regions by screw-hook claw application. This single-level claw configuration is made possible by the anatomy of the spinal segment—specifically, the relative location of the lamina approximately one-half segment below the centroid of the vertebral body and the pedicle. This leaves room for placement of a hook caudal to the pedicle. This combination increases the implant's pullout resistance while maintaining the rotation-, flexion-, and extension-resisting abilities of the screw (Fig. 13-13). It also takes advantage of the good pullout-resistance attributes of sublaminar hooks.[15,20]

CONFORMING BONE-IMPLANT INTERFACES

Polymethylmethacrylate may be used as an implant material that conforms to the contours of bone. Two common

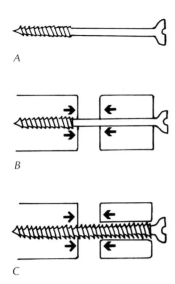

FIGURE 13-11 The lag screw. *A.* The lag screw is threaded only on its leading end. This allows the unthreaded screw shaft to glide freely when the threaded end of the screw pulls the screw through the bone during insertion. *B.* During tightening, the screw threads pull the head onto (and into) the near surface of the bone. The tensile stresses thus created in the screw are translated into compression of the surrounding bone between the screw threads and the screw head. A lag-screw effect can be obtained by drilling the near bone fragment hole to a diameter greater than, or equal to, the outer diameter of a non-lag screw. Arrows depict the compression forces within the bone.

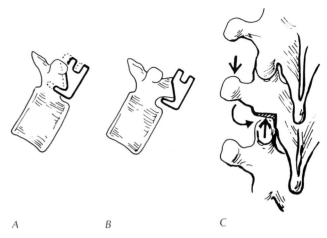

FIGURE 13-12 *A.* Pedicle hooks may fail via excessively deep insertion resulting in a cut-through of the pedicle (*ghosted hook*). *B.* Insufficiently deep insertion results in inadequate pedicle engagement, with consequent loss of torsional stabilizing characteristics. *C.* The addition of a transverse process hook applies a force vector at some distance from the force vector applied by the pedicle hook (*straight arrows*), resulting in the application of a torque to the pedicle (*curved arrow*).

misconceptions about this require clarification. First, the acrylic usually does not conform *precisely* to the bone, because of blood interfacing between the acrylic and bone, and because gravity may cause the acrylic to flow away from important interface points. Second, bone does *not* bond to acrylic; osteointegration between surfaces (see below) does not occur. Therefore, loosening of acrylic-bone interfaces is common. Some authors have found acrylic to be useful in spinal implants,[21,22] but others have found it to have little utility.[23]

OSTEOINTEGRATION

Some implant materials have the capacity for *osteointegration*. This is the bonding or binding of a nonbiological material (e.g., a spinal implant) to bone. Facial and oral applications have dominated this field to date. Titanium has an increased capacity for osteointegration. The phenomenon of osteointegration may be due partly to its matte surface.[24] Peened or matted stainless steel appears to have similar advantages over smooth, non-matte stainless steel surfaces.

When osteointegration occurs, the "attachment" of the implant to the bone over the entire contact surface means that load transfer from implant to bone (and vice versa) is

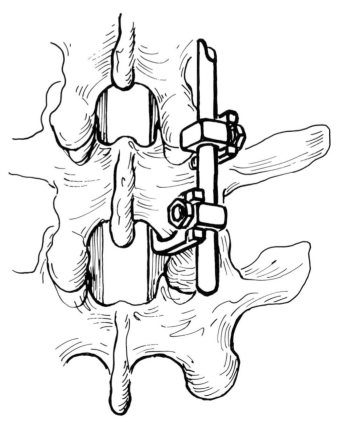

FIGURE 13-13 A caudal sublaminar hook, placed at the same spinal segmental level as a pedicle screw, augments the screw's pullout resistance.

distributed over a much larger surface area than if osteointegration had not occcurred. This reduces focal stress concentration (stress risers). Increased resistance to insertion (torsional resistance) is observed with coarse finishes. This may weaken the bone at the implant-bone interface, negating part of the advantage of osteointegration.

REFERENCES

1. Lesoin F, Jomin M, Viaud C: Expanding bolt for anterior cervical spine osteosynthesis: Technical note. *Neurosurgery* 1983; 12:458–459.
2. Bennett GJ: Materials and material testing, in Benzel EC (ed): *Spinal Instrumentation.* American Association of Neurological Surgeons, 1993.
3. Uhl RL: The biomechanics of screws. *Orthop Rev* 1989; 18:1302–1307.
4. Matsuzaki H, Tokuhashi Y, Matsumoto F, et al: Problems and solutions of pedicle screw plate fixation of the lumbar spine. *Spine* 1990; 15:1159–1165.
5. Ashmann RB, Galpin RD, Corin JD, et al: Biomechanical analysis of pedicle screw instrumentation systems in a corpectomy model. *Spine* 1989; 14:1398–1405.
6. McAfee PC, Farey ID, Sutterlin CE, et al: Device-related osteoporosis with spinal instrumentation. *Spine* 1989; 14:919–926.
7. Schatzker J, Horne JG, Sumner-Smith G: The effect of movement on the holding power of screws in bone. *Clin Orthop Rel Res* 1975; 111:257–262.
8. Foley WL, Frost DE, Tucker MR: The effect of repetitive screw hole use on the retentive strength of pretapped and self-tapped screws. *J Oral Maxillofac Surg* 1990; 48:264–267.
9. Misenhimer GR, Peek RD, Wiltse LL, et al: Anatomic analysis of pedicle cortical and calcellous diameter as related to screw size. *Spine* 1989; 14:367–372.
10. Vangsness CT, Carter DR, Frankel VH: In vitro evaluation of the loosening characteristics of self-tapped and non-self-tapped cortical bone screws. *Clin Orthop Rel Res* 1981; 157:279–286.
11. Skinner R, Maybee J, Transfeldt E, et al: Experimental pullout testing and comparison of variables in transpedicular screw fixation: A biomechanical study. *Spine* 1990; 15:195–201.
12. Krag MH, Beynnon BD, Pope MH, et al: Depth of insertion of transpedicular vertebral screws into human vertebrae: Effect upon screw-vertebra interface strength. *J Spinal Disord* 1989; 1:287–294.
13. Maiman DJ, Pintar FA, Yoganandan N, et al: Pull-out strength of Caspar cervical screws. *Neurosurgery* 1992; 31:1097–1101.
14. Smith SA, Abitbol JJ, Carlson GD, et al: The effects of depth of penetration, screw orientation, and bone density and sacral screw fixation. *Spine* 1993; 18:1006–1010.
15. Ruland CM, McAfee PC, Warden KE, et al: Triangulation of pedicular instrumentation. A biomechanical analysis. *Spine* 1991; 16:S270–S276.
16. Wittenberg RH, Shea M, Swartz DE, et al: Importance of bone mineral density in instrumented spine fusions. *Spine* 1991; 16:647–652.
17. Zindrick MR, Wilstse LL, Eidell EH, et al: A biomechanical study of intrapeduncular screw fixation in the lumbosacral spine. *Clin Orthop Rel Res* 1986; 203:99–112.
18. Benzel EC, Baldwin NG: Crossed screw fixation of the unstable thoracic and lumbar spine. (Submitted.)
19. Schatzker J, Horne JG, Sumner-Smith G: The reaction of cortical bone to compression by screw threads. *Clin Orthop Rel Res* 1975; 111:263–265.
20. Coe JD, Warden KE, Herzig MA, et al: Influence of bone mineral density on the fixation of thoracolumbar implants: A comparative study of transpedicular screws, laminar hooks, and spinous process wires. *Spine* 1990; 15:902–907.
21. Duff TA: Surgical stabilization of traumatic cervical spine dislocation using methylmethacrylate. *J Neurosurg* 1986; 64:39–44.
22. Panjabi MM, Hopper W, White AA, et al: Posterior spine stabilization with methylmethacrylate: biomechanical testing of a surgical specimen. *Spine* 1977; 2:241–247.
23. Whitehill R, Cicoria AD, Hooper WE, et al: Posterior cervical reconstruction with methyl methacrylate cement and wire: A clinical review. *J Neurosurg* 1988; 68:576–584.
24. Cohen J: Tissue reactions to metals: The influence of surface finish. *J Bone Joint Surg* 1961; 43A:687–699.

Chapter *14*

Qualitative Attributes
of Spinal Implants

INTRODUCTION

Spinal implants are either predominantly rigid (constrained) or dynamic (semirigid, or semiconstrained) and impart distractive, compressive, or neutral axial forces to the spine (Table 14-1). Rigid implants are used to achieve rigid fixation of the spine. Dynamic implants allow some intersegmental movement, which eases stresses placed elsewhere in the system (usually at the implant-bone interface). These factors are the determinants of the mode of application.

Most spinal implants apply forces to the spine in a complex manner. The complex nature of their force applications is illustrated by the forces applied by the six construct types discussed in Chap. 15 (simple distraction, three-point bending, tension-band fixation, fixed moment arm cantilever beam fixation, nonfixed moment arm cantilever beam fixation, and applied moment arm cantilever beam fixation). These complex force applications comprise axial, flexion-extension, lateral bending, and translational forces.

It is important to recognize that there is no truly neutral spinal implant. For example, if an implant is placed in a neutral mode at the time of surgery, its characteristics soon change when the spine is loaded (e.g., by the assumption of an upright posture after surgery) (Fig. 14-1).

Thus most spinal implants that are initially placed in a neutral mode eventually bear axial loads. This means that they *function* in a distraction mode. For the purpose of consistency, and with this in mind, *neutral devices* are considered herein as those placed in a neutral mode *at the time of surgery* (i.e., without distraction, compression, bending, or translational force application).

What follows is a discussion of the "desired forces applied" by the spine surgeon via spinal implants. The axial components of these "desired forces" can be broken down into 10 categories. They include both posterior and anterior techniques (5 varieties of each) for spinal instrumentation. The posterior categories are (1) rigid distraction (with or

without three-point bending), (2) rigid neutral, (3) rigid compression (including most tension-band fixation constructs), (4) dynamic neutral fixation (including most cantilever bending constructs with nonfixed moment arms), and (5) dynamic compression (including some tension-band fixation constructs—i.e., springs). The anterior categories are (1) rigid distraction (simple distraction or interbody buttressing), (2) rigid neutral (cantilever bending constructs with fixed and nonfixed moment arms), (3) rigid compression, (4) dynamic neutral fixation (interbody strut placed without distraction), and (5) dynamic compression (Table 14-1). There are no true dynamic distraction devices (anterior or posterior) readily available for clinical use.

Clean separation of these "desired axial force applications" into their respective categories is often impossible. The attempt made here, therefore, is somewhat artificial. This material is presented in order to facilitate understanding of spinal implants and to foster matching of what the surgeon expects from the implant ("desired force application") to what is actually achieved ("achieved force application").

Newton's third law of motion states that interactions between objects result in no net change in momentum; in other words, for every action there is an equal (in magnitude) but opposite (in direction) reaction (see Chap. 2). Spinal instrumentation constructs, as well as all other methods of force application in nature, obey this law. Since spinal instrumentation constructs do not "move" the spine after insertion, we may presume that *all forces applied to the spine are applied in pairs;* that is, since spinal movement does not occur, all forces must be balanced, with a net force of zero (see Chap. 2). Therefore, two equal (but opposite in direction) linear or moment creating forces act on the instantaneous axis of rotation (IAR) of a vertebral spinal segment when a spinal implant either applies a force to the spine or resists spinal movement (Fig. 14-2). The importance of this

TABLE 14-1 Qualitative categorization of spinal implants

Rigid		Dynamic	
Posterior	Anterior	Posterior	Anterior
Distraction	Distraction		
Neutral	Neutral	Neutral	Neutral
Compression	Compression	Compression	Compression

concept cannot be overstated. The various "desired force applications" (modes of application) are presented in the pages that follow.

Specific attention is usually paid to axial force applications (compression and distraction). Flexion-extension, lateral bending, and translational force applications are more complex and less frequently considered than compression and distraction forces. In the spirit of simplicity, the common emphasis of axial force applications is sustained here. Flexion-extension, lateral bending, and translational fixation force applications, however, are discussed where appropriate.

RIGID FIXATION

The goal of rigid spinal instrumentation is absolute immobilization of the spine. Under most circumstances this goal ("desired force application") cannot be completely achieved. Because bone is a biologic material, it deforms and reforms according to the stresses placed on it. Therefore, even the most "rigid" device allows some movement. The range of this movement increases with time, as the implant-bone interface becomes looser. If this movement occurs with enough repetitions and with enough force, it will eventually cause failure at the construct-bone interface, unless at least one of two conditions exists: (1) Either bony fusion occurs (taking over the weight- and stress-bearing burden

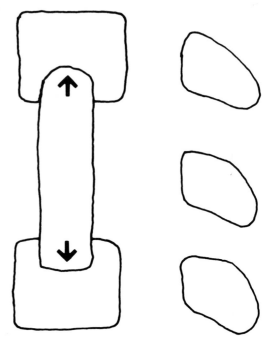

FIGURE 14-2 In this anterior interbody implant, two equal, but directionally opposite, forces (arrows) are applied by an implant placed in distraction or by the assumption of the upright posture (see Fig. 14-1).

from the construct-bone interface), or (2) the instrumentation device itself fails (see Chap. 10). The surgeon's awareness of the "race" between the acquisition of solid bony fusion and eventual instrumentation failure is critical to the clinical decision-making process (see Chap. 10).

When we recognize that even the most rigid of implants eventually allows some spinal movement, the distinctions between the various modes of application of spinal instrumentation again becomes ill-defined. Rigid implants, in a sense, eventually become dynamic, because of the impossibility of permanently rigid fixation to the bones of the spine.

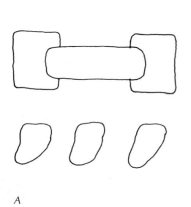

A

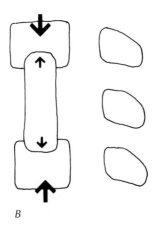

B

FIGURE 14-1 *A*. With the patient in the supine position during surgery, an anterior interbody implant may be placed in a relatively neutral mode; that is, without significant distractive force application to the spine. *B*. When the patient assumes the upright position, axial loads (*large arrows*) are applied to the spine and are resisted by the implant (*small arrows*).

Rigid fixation does not optimize bony fusion acquisition, because of the phenomenon of *stress shielding;* but if it holds rigidly for a sufficient time, bony fusion will eventually be achieved. Unless the fixation devices are removed, however, the ultimately desired fusion strength may not be realized, because of stress shielding and *stress reduction osteoporosis.* Fusion rates, however, have apparently not been adversely affected by the application of rigid instrumentation constructs.[1] These phenomena, therefore, are more theoretical than real.

Rigid Axial Force Applications

POSTERIOR RIGID DISTRACTION FIXATION

Harrington distraction rod (HDR) fixation has been the "gold standard" for thoracic and lumbar stabilization for more than 20 years.[2,3] Its durability as a favored technique is testament to its utility. It uses rigid distraction force application, usually combined with three-point bending forces. It provides an opportunity to reduce kyphoses or retropulsed bone and/or disk fragments. This can be accomplished with or without the use of adjuncts to enhance the kyphosis reduction, such as dorsally positioned sleeves.[4] The latter technique uses distraction and a three-point bending mechanism of load application to achieve its effect (see Chap. 15) (Fig. 14-3). This is a good example of the complex nature of force application by an implant. A spacer, such as a sleeve, can be used to exaggerate the ventrally directed force at the fulcrum (three-point bending) (Fig. 14-3*B*).

Modifications have been made to the Harrington system in order to make it a more stable construct; these include the use of square-ended rods to minimize rotatory instability[5] and the use of Edwards sleeves to minimize kyphotic deformation.[4]

Failure at the hook-bone interface is a common problem associated with HDR application.[6] This is a function of the nature and magnitude of the forces applied at the hook-bone interface.

The rods may also fail (fracture), most commonly at the proximal ratchet of the rod and at sites of rod contouring, due to metal fatigue (stress risers). One may reduce the risk of metal fracture by *not* contouring the rods before placement[7] and by placing the hook as proximal as possible on the rod (i.e., by using the longest rod possible), thus using only a few ratchets. The latter strategy reduces the length of the lever arm (moment arm) between the hook and the first ratchet (the weakest point on the HDR construct).

Posterior spinal distraction has several inherent drawbacks (see Chap. 7). First, *axial ligamentous resistance* is required for the Harrington rods to be effective (Fig. 14-4), since a "claw" configuration (which circumferentially "grips" a lamina) is not used with the standard Harrington system (see Chap. 9).

Another inherent drawback of posterior spinal distraction is its inconsistent ability to reduce retropulsed bone and disk fragments even when applied in combination with a three-point bending force. This may contribute to the observed lack of neurological improvement seen with this technique, as compared with nonoperative approaches.[2] Although an intact anterior longitudinal ligament augments the efficacy, and may be a requirement for the appropriate application, of HDR fixation, it may hinder reduction of retropulsed bone and disk fragments. This technique, there-

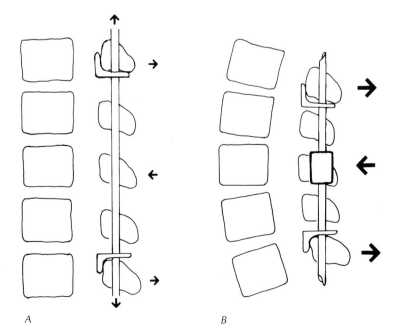

FIGURE 14-3 *A.* The Harrington distraction rod uses rigid distraction *(vertical arrows)* and a three-point bending force application *(horizontal arrows).* Note that the distraction and three-point bending force vectors are oriented at 90° from each other (see Chap. 15). *B.* The use of sleeves about the rods at the level of the fulcrum provides an advantage for reduction of kyphotic deformation by placing a greater ventrally directed force *(ventrally directed horizontal arrow)* at the fulcrum.[4] This, in turn, places a greater dorsally directed force at the termini of the implant *(arrows).*

A   *B*

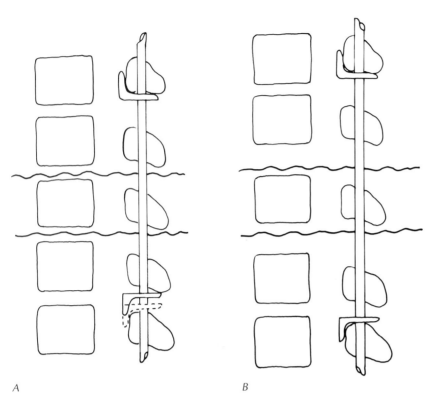

A   *B*

FIGURE 14-4 Axial ligamentous resistance is required if the rods of a posterior distraction system (e.g., Harrington distraction rod) are to be effective. Their distraction force application is nil if intrinsic spinal resistance is not met—as in the case of complete loss of ligamentous integrity at the level of trauma. This results in either an inadequate force application and lack of optimal contact at the hook-bone interface (*A*) or excessive distraction accompanying the force application (*B*). Wavy lines represent soft tissue disruption.

fore, may fail because of one or more of three anatomic and pathological factors: (1) the relative weakness of the posterior longitudinal ligament, (2) the relative strength of the anterior longitudinal ligament, and (3) the frequent occurrence of posterior longitudinal ligament disruption following trauma (see Chap. 7). The anterior longitudinal ligament is often preserved following trauma. Its location allows it to be the distraction-limiting structure (providing axial ligamentous resistance), minimizing the extent of spinal distraction achieved by instrumentation techniques. This is because the ligament itself often prevents the distraction required to reduce these fragments. In addition, spinal cord distraction (especially over a ventral mass) may cause further neural injury via a tethering mechanism.[8,9] Finally, Dickson, Harrington, and Erwin have shown—as mentioned above—that neurological outcome is no better with posterior instrumentation techniques *without* an accompanying anterior neural decompression procedure than with postural nonoperative treatment.[2] The end result "no neurological improvement" may reflect the "averaging" of a neurological improvement associated with neural decompression (associated with the instrumentation technique in some cases) and a worsening of neurological outcome (or lack of achievement of the fullest possible neurological recovery) arising from distraction of neural elements over irreducible retropulsed ventral bony and soft tissues (see Chap. 7).

Elimination of the normal lumbar lordosis with distraction techniques, similarly, may cause adverse sequelae (Fig. 14-5).[7] These complications may be minimized by the use of a spacer or sleeve (Fig. 14-3), or by rod contouring combined with a technique to prevent rod rotation—such as square-ended rods, crossfixation, or intermediate points of segmental fixation with sublaminar wires, hooks, or screws.

Multisegmental fixation can be used to gain the advantage of *load-sharing*. Load-sharing involves the distribution of an applied load between multiple components of an implant system and/or between the implant itself and intrinsic spinal elements. Augmentation of HDR fixation with multiple-level sublaminar wire fixation adjuncts substantially increases stability and decreases the failure rate of HDR fixation.[10–17] However, it carries with it the risks associated with the placement of sublaminar wires.[11,18]

Universal spinal instrumentation (USI) fixation (placed in distraction) can provide multisegmental rigid distraction.[19–23] It often requires complex and time-consuming placement techniques. However, it achieves substantial stability with a minimal chance of instrument failure at the hook-bone interface. Multisegmental fixation that distributes the construct's applied forces over multiple segmental levels allows the realization of these results (see Posterior Rigid Neutral Fixation, and Posterior Rigid Compression Fixation, below).[21] Because of the substantial stability and the minimal chance of instrument failure achieved with

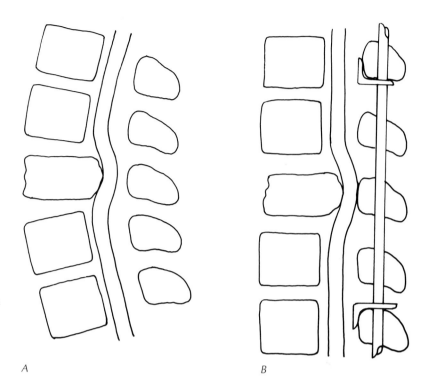

FIGURE 14-5 Distraction of the naturally lordotic spine (*A*) may result in the exaggeration of pathological anatomy (*B*). Note that a three-point bending construct is not achieved in this case, because of the remaining space between the rod and the dorsal elements at the level of the injury.   *A*   *B*

these techniques, USI fixation systems should, perhaps, be considered the new "gold standard" for posttraumatic thoracic and lumbar hook-rod spinal instrumentation.

Jacob's locking-hook spinal rods offer an alternative to simple HDR techniques.[24] Security is provided by locking hooks that help prevent failure at the hook-bone interface by employing a claw configuration at each end of the rod. This claw configuration eliminates the need for intrinsic axial ligamentous resistance. This advantage is also observed with USI systems. The claw configuration allows the use of smaller distractive forces; this, in turn, decreases the chance of failure. One can use smaller distractive forces with locking hooks because distraction in a nonlocking system is the mechanism by which failure is prevented; thus intrinsic axial ligamentous resistance is optimally exploited. The greater the distractive force (up to a point), the lesser the chance of hook dislodgement. If the distractive forces are applied to excess, hook insertion site failure will occur.

In selected cases external skeletal fixation likewise may play a role in spinal trauma management.[25] It can be placed in a distraction posture. However, the risk of infection, the requirement for transpendicular placement, and the less-than-optimal fixation obtained detract substantially from its utility.

POSTERIOR RIGID NEUTRAL FIXATION

There are several types of posterior rigid neutral fixation. They differ widely enough in structural characteristics and

techniques of application that each subset will be discussed independently.

To minimize the chance of failure of rigid fixation devices (either failure at the metal-bone interface or metal fracture), multisegmental fixation has been used. The Luque rod technique is the prototype of posterior rigid neutral rod fixation.[11,17,22,26,27] It provides increased stability by distributing the fixation forces over multiple segmental levels (load-sharing); this increases the cumulative fixation (resistance to movement). This distribution of forces decreases the stresses applied to the metal-bone interface at each individual segmental level. Some posterior rigid neutral rod fixation devices allow for axial growth when applied before the growth potential is acheived (Luque rods). This effect is usually considered a positive attribute of this type of fixation. On the other hand, undesirable settling of the spine may occur occasionally. The settling occurs via the rods' sliding in opposite directions past one another as the spine settles. This can be partly rectified by the crossfixation of the rod on one side to the rod on the other (Fig. 14-6). One must keep in mind, however, that with Luque rod instrumentation, the risks associated with the passage and inadvertent manipulation of sublaminar wires are ever-present.[11,18,28]

USI fixation (neutrally placed) can be used in a posterior rigid neutral mode. Transpedicular instrumentation techniques can also be employed in a rigid neutral mode. Modifications of these techniques for application in the upper cervical spine and the suboccipital region may occasionally be indicated.[29] The risks of transpedicular screw placement

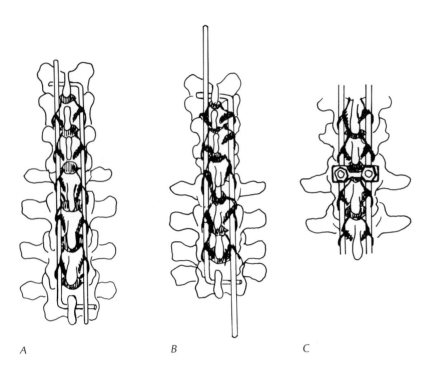

A   *B*   *C*

FIGURE 14-6 Spine settling can occur following insertion of Luque rods. The immediate postoperative configuration (*A*) can settle via the rods' sliding past one another (*B*). This can be partly rectified by rigid fixation of the rods to one another with crossmembers (*C*).

in the cervical region are considered prohibitive by most surgeons, whereas lateral mass plating techniques are common.

Rigid low thoracic and lumbar transpedicular plating and related rodding techniques for spinal instability have been used to provide alternatives to the abovementioned rigid fixation approaches.[21,30,31,32] These alternative techniques use either a rod or a plate as the longitudinal connector between screws. They provide the rigid application of a plate or rod to transpedicular screws. Although these techniques eliminate the well-known risks of sublaminar wiring, they introduce another threat to neural elements and surrounding structures via the inherent difficulty of placing the screws precisely through the pedicle into the vertebral body, particularly in the thoracic region. With good screw fixation, the constructs that provide true rigid fixation may fail at the screw-plate or screw-rod interface. Because the screws are rigidly fixed to the plates or rods, and because the predominant forces applied to these devices are axial, the majority of the stresses are focused at the screw-plate or screw-rod interface (see Chaps. 2 and 15).[33]

A lesser pullout stress is applied at the screw-bone interface because pivoting of the screw at the plate (as occurs with dynamic, semirigid, and semiconstrained devices) cannot occur. (The construct is loaded as with a fixed moment arm cantilever beam; see Chap. 15.) Hence, screw pullout infrequently occurs with this technique. Therefore, the screw pullout characteristics of rigid neutral spine screw fixation techniques are good, but metal failure characteristics at the screw-plate or screw-rod interface are poor (Fig.

14-7). Hence these devices may be more useful where screw pullout is a significant risk, as in patients with osteoporosis. Their applicability in situations where anterior weight-bearing ability is impaired (e.g., following trauma) is also suspect.[33]

Facet wiring and bone grafting techniques use bone graft that is wired to the facet at each involved spinal level.[34] This technique offers acute stability, but may fail on account of wire pullout or fracture of the graft. In addition, remodeling of graft bone at its interface with the wire, resulting in loosening, may occur prior to the acquisition of solid fusion. The technique is most applicable in the cervical region, where stresses placed on the spine are smaller than in the thoracic and lumbar regions. It is inferior to an interspinous wiring technique, because of the shorter length of the fixation lever arm (Fig. 14-8), but is appropriate when posterior elements are not available for applying wires, as after a laminectomy.

POSTERIOR RIGID COMPRESSION FIXATION

The Harrington compression rod was the first posterior rigid compression fixation device to achieve wide clinical use.[35] Harrington compression rods are thinner, and hence weaker, than distraction rods. However, they fracture infrequently, because of the tensile nature of the stresses applied to the rods and the positive tensile stress–resisting characteristics of nearly all materials used as spinal implants. They may occasionally be difficult to apply. Segmental fixation (using multiple hooks) may add to the security of the construct.

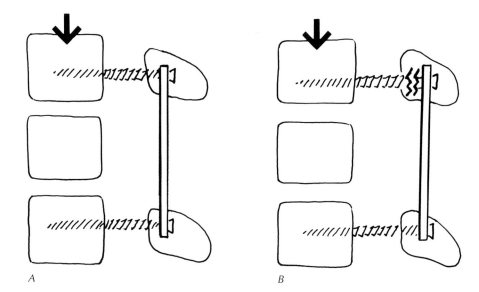

FIGURE 14-7 *A.* Since rigid neutral transpedicular screw fixation constructs are indeed rigid, they make screw pullout under axial loads less likely. *B.* These same loads, however, may result in failure of the construct at the point of the longest moment arm: the screw–longitudinal member junction.

A   *B*

A word of caution: It may be that systems using sublaminar hooks should not be segmentally fixed with sublaminar wires in patients with incomplete myelopathies, because of the possibility of forcing the hooks ventrally into the spinal canal (Fig. 14-9).[35]

USI instrumentation, placed in compression, provides multiple-level fixation, larger rods, and security of placement on account of the use of multiple hooks. The technique is especially useful with thoracic and lumbar fractures.[19–23]

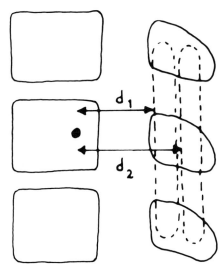

FIGURE 14-8 The fixation lever arm for resistance to flexion with a facet-level tension-band fixation technique (rigid or dynamic) is shorter than that with a spinous process–level fixation technique (rigid or dynamic). Arrows depict tension-band fixation forces; d_1 and d_2 represent the length of the tension-band fixation moment arms; dots represent IARs.

The Halifax clamp may provide an advantage in the upper thoracic and cervical regions, where larger devices are not necessary.[36,37] A clamp designed specifically for atlantoaxial fusions likewise has been employed.[38] Its bulkiness, however, renders it cumbersome and potentially dangerous. In situations where translational instability exists, a posteriorly applied clamp, or any posterior tension-band fixation implant, may not prevent a parallelogram-like translational deformation (Fig. 14-10A). However, if natural anatomic constraints on translation exist, a clamp may be all that is needed to secure stability (Fig. 14-10B).

Knodt rods[39,40] (applied in compression) may provide rigid compression in selected situations (absence of translational instability) in the mid- to low lumbar region, where the normal lumbar lordosis complicates the placement of more complex compression devices. Excessive multilevel compression may exaggerate the normal lordotic posture of the lumbar spine; therefore, single-level immobilization is especially desirable in this region. Figure 14-11A illustrates the use of Knodt rods in a patient with an L4 flexion-distraction fracture (Chance fracture). Because of the rod's small diameter and short length, the use of Knodt rods in extension should rarely be considered in patients with spine trauma. Although Harrington compression rods may also be used under these circumstances, application over only two lumbar segments may prove difficult. The ease of placement of Knodt rods, on the other hand, is facilitated by the use of the turnbuckle effect. (The threads on the two ends of the rod face in opposite directions.) This allows for a much simpler application procedure than that required for Harrington compression rods. The Jacob's system may also be applied in compression.[24]

Interspinous wiring techniques are used almost exclusively in the cervical region, because of the lesser stresses

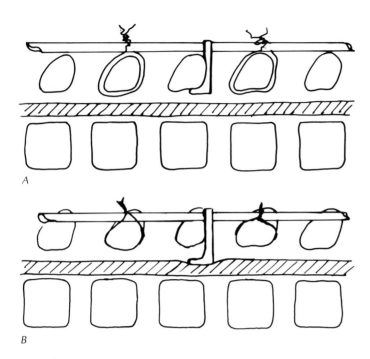

A

B

FIGURE 14-9 If sublaminar hooks are placed (*A*), forcible approximation of the rod to the lamina by sublaminar wiring may result in dural sac impingement (*B*).

placed on the construct in this region (compared to the thoracic and lumbar regions).[41–43] These techniques have been used occasionally with accompanying HDRs in the thoracic and lumbar spine.[44] Interspinous wiring techniques provide tension-band fixation (in flexion) over two or more spinal segments (see "Anterior Rigid Neutral Fixation, below). In the cervical region, the fusion of only two vertebrae may decrease the incidence of flexible kyphosis.[45,46] It also may decrease the incidence of accelerated segmental degenerative disease of the spine.[47] Lumbar facet wiring and facet screw fixation techniques[48–50] provide a lesser degree of immediate stability, because of the inherent weakness of the facet joints and the short length of the fixation lever arm (Fig. 14-8).

The interspinous compression wiring and fusion technique encourages bone healing by enhancing the forces of compression at the bone graft–spinous process junction while increasing acute stability (Fig. 14-11*B*).[41] Bone graft remodeling (and thus loosening) at the wire-bone interface is a theoretical, but infrequently encountered, problem. This and related techniques are recommended for use solely in the cervical region.

ANTERIOR RIGID DISTRACTION FIXATION

Anterior cervical plates, anterior thoracic and lumbar devices,[51] and acrylic or bone graft struts (either acrylic or bone, placed after corpectomy) can be placed in a distraction mode or into a distracted spine, thus providing distraction of the spine in a rigid or semirigid manner. However, neither bone nor acrylic alone can provide acute stability, except via a contribution to axial load support. If significant acute stability is absolutely necessary other approaches may be preferable. Because acrylic does not incorporate into bone, it never offers a truly solid fusion. It does not bond with bone. Therefore, it should be reserved for selected cases, such as stabilization following the resection of neoplasms, usually in conjunction with a metal reinforcer/stabilizer.[52] *In order to attain long-term stability, bony fusion must be obtained.*

The technique of placing an anterior interbody fusion in a distraction mode may reduce translational deformities and provide significant stabilizing characteristics. This is especially so if the anterior longitudinal ligament is not injured (see Chap. 10). (The anterior longitudinal ligament is a particularly strong spinal ligament; see Chap. 1.) The posterior

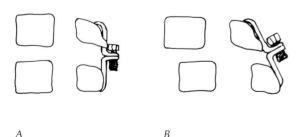

A

B

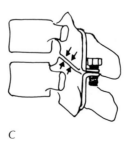

C

FIGURE 14-10 *A* and *B*. Translational deformation may follow the application of a tension-band fixation "clamp." *C*. However, if there is an anatomic constraint to translation—such as intact facet joints—then tension-band fixation can prevent translation.

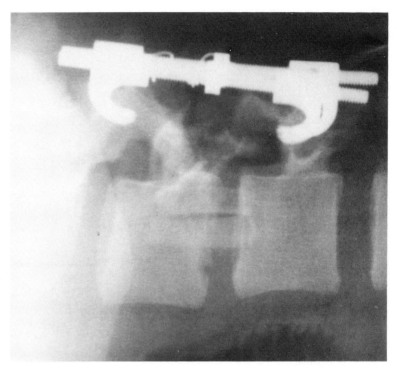

A

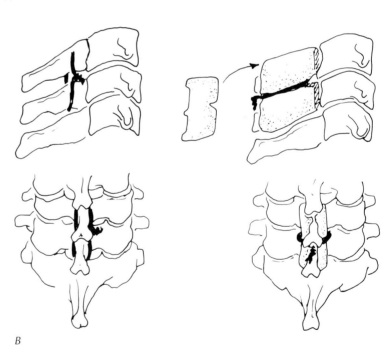

FIGURE 14-11 *A.* Knodt rods placed in a compression mode for the fixation of a flexion-distraction deformity. *B.* Another application of the tension-band fixation technique is that associated with the interspinous compression wire fixation technique.[41] This technique provides both tension-band fixation, via the cerclage wire, and compression of the bone graft to the spinous processes, via a dorsal "pull" on the cerclage wire by the compression wire.

B

lumbar interbody fusion (PLIF) technique also takes advantage of this concept.

The Kostuik-Harrington device,[53] the Kaneda device,[51] and other screw-rod techniques are true anterior rigid distraction devices that can be applied to the thoracic and lumbar regions. The risk of soft tissue erosion as a complication with these devices must be considered before application.

ANTERIOR RIGID NEUTRAL FIXATION

Anterior vertebral body plating can provide substantial acute stability while allowing bony fusion to progress.[51,54–59] This technique is used mainly in the cervical region. Visceral soft tissue erosion in the cervical region, as observed with the Dunn apparatus in the thoracic and lumbar regions, is a potential problem. Following extension, failure at the

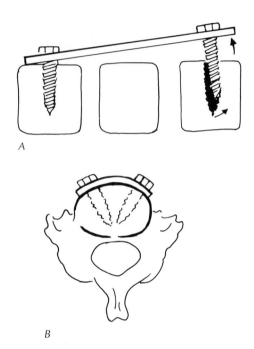

FIGURE 14-12 Rigid anterior neutral fixation techniques may fail by screw cutout (*A*). Toeing-in of the screws minimizes the chance of screw pullout (but not cutout) by requiring a volume of bone between the screws to be dislodged in order for pullout to occur. This obviously requires that the screws be attached via a rigid plate, or be connected via a crossmember (*B*). Anterior plate implants function as tension-band fixation constructs in extension. However, they provide limited resistance to flexion in this regard. In order to provide maximal stability, a posterior tension-band fixation construct may be used in conjunction. This complex construct provides tension-band fixation attributes in both flexion and extension.

screw-bone interface may occur. Screw cutout, rather than pullout, occurs most commonly in this situation (Fig. 14-12*A*). The Synthes locking screw-plate system uses a toed-in screw configuration in which the screw is locked to the plate.[58] The toed-in mechanism compensates, at least in part, for the screw pullout (but not cutout) tendencies of this construct (Fig. 14-12*B*).

Anterior rigid devices for application in the thoracic and lumbar regions must be used with great caution.[60] The Zielke technique, although previously used for scoliosis, may occasionally be applicable to trauma with scoliotic deformities[61] Other devices and techniques may be used too.[53,62]

These devices provide significant immediate stability in extension, because of their excellent tension-band fixation characteristics. In flexion, however, the failure of a less-than-substantial construct may occur if posterior instability coexists. This is due to the inherent weakness of this type of construct in flexion, either at the plate or at the screw-plate or screw-bone interface (Fig. 14-12*D*).

In order to provide maximal stability, a posterior compressive force (as from an interspinous cerclage wire) may be applied. This posterior compressive force provides tension-band fixation in flexion that complements a similar fixation in extension, provided by the anterior plating technique (Fig. 14-12*E*). A very stable construct is thus achieved. Obviously, if tension-band fixation in extension is adequate following the placement of an anterior fusion and posterior cerclage wiring (which provides secure tension-band fixation in flexion), the placement of an anterior plate is inappropriate. *Clinically adequate degrees of stability are usually realized with lesser operations.* The question of whether the degree of stability achieved with anterior plating techniques is worth the risk of both short- and long-term complications is yet to be answered.

ANTERIOR RIGID COMPRESSION FIXATION

Anterior compression fixation can be rigidly applied in the thoracic and lumbar regions by a variety of techniques. The application of compression forces to the spine provides an element of stability not offered by neutral or dynamic techniques. This application takes advantage of the intrinsic ability of the spine to participate in load-sharing. The forcing of the spine into compression causes the spine to assume a greater percentage of axial load-bearing (i.e., it increases load-sharing). This is in contrast to the construct itself bearing the majority of the load (Fig. 14-13). Anterior longitudinal ligament integrity and ventral spinal canal decompression are necessary for optimal efficacy and safety of this technique.

Rigid Device–Related Flexion-Extension Force Application

Anterior, posterior, or lateral points of force application may be used for the acquisition of flexion and extension. This may be achieved by an applied moment arm cantilever beam, simple distraction, tension-band fixation, or a three-point bending fixation technique (see Chap. 15).

Rigid Device–Related Lateral Bending Force Application

Reduction of a scoliotic curvature may be accomplished by the application of either rigid distraction on the convex side of the curve or rigid or dynamic compression on the concave side of the curve. Rigid distraction may be applied on the concave side of the curve. Rigid or dynamic compression must be applied lateral to the IAR, on the convex side of the curve. If it is not applied in this manner, the exaggeration of the scoliotic curvature will result (Fig. 14-14). The principles of these techniques have been addressed under Rigid Axial Force Applications, above.

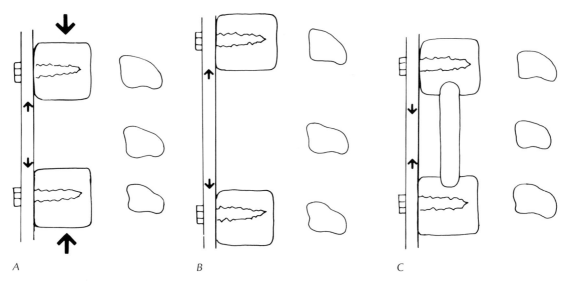

A   B   C

FIGURE 14-13 Rigid distraction fixation forces *(short arrows)* cause the implant to *bear* the majority of the axial load *(long arrows)* during assumption of the upright posture *(A)*. This may cause failure of the construct, either at the construct-bone interface or via construct fracture. If the construct is first distracted (following spinal canal decompression) *(B)* and then compressed *(short arrows)* on an inserted interbody bone graft, the bone graft and intrinsic spinal elements will bear a substantial portion of the axial load during assumption of the upright posture *(C)*.

Rigid Device–Related Translational Force Application

Translational deformities may be reduced by the application of rigid forces to the spine via a *longitudinal member* (rod or plate) anchored by screws, wires, or hooks. These force applications are often complex. Often, simple distraction can be used to reduce translational deformities. These techniques take advantage of the existing ligamentous stability and tethering abilities of the intact spinal ligaments (Fig. 14-4). Three-point bending constructs may also be used for translational deformity reduction (Fig. 14-15).

DYNAMIC FIXATION

Dynamic spinal instrumentation allows varying degrees of intersegmental movement. Although excessive movement suppresses bony fusion, minimal intersegmental movement increases the chance for bone healing via the augmentation of bone healing–enhancing forces. The major advantage of this type of fixation, however, is that the minimal intersegmental movement allowed by the device absorbs some of the movement that would normally be absorbed at the hook-bone interface of the screw-plate interface. This markedly decreases the chance of failure at the metal-bone inter-

FIGURE 14-14 *A.* A scoliotic curvature can be corrected by applying rigid distraction on the concave side of the curve, or by applying rigid or dynamic compression on the convex side of the curve. *B.* A Dwyer device may be used in the latter case. *C.* If a compression force is applied on the convex side of the curve, but medial to the IAR at any level, an exaggeration of the curvature will become manifest.

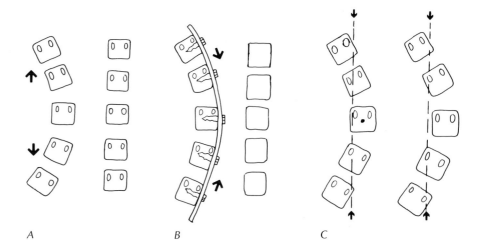

A   B   C

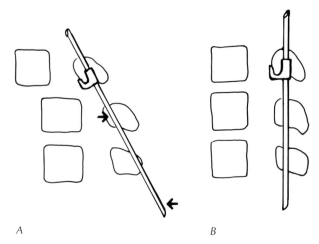

A   B

FIGURE 14-15 A translation deformation (A) can be corrected by a three-point bending force application (B).

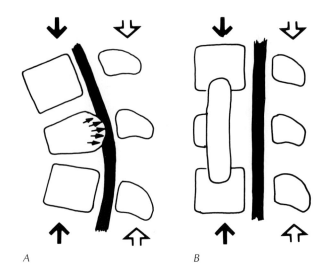

A   B

FIGURE 14-16 *A. Posterior dynamic compression (hollow arrows)* should be applied only in the presence of adequate anterior axial load-bearing capabilities or following interbody weight-bearing fusion. If this cardinal rule is not obeyed, the bearing of an axial load *(solid arrows)* will result in deformation and, in this case, spinal canal encroachment *(horizontal arrows)*. *B.* If ventral spinal decompression is performed, and followed by placement of an anterior interbody weight-bearing strut, these complications rarely occur.

face. However, *posterior dynamic fixation devices must be applied in conjunction with a solid anterior intervertebral strut or in the presence of existing ventral stability with respect to axial loading.*[6,45] Following axial loading, excessive flexion will result if this cardinal rule is violated (Fig. 14-16).

Dynamic Axial Force Applications

POSTERIOR DYNAMIC NEUTRAL FIXATION

The Roy-Camille plate, the Luque plate, the semi-contrained screws of the Dynalok (Danek) system, the lateral mass cervical plates, and related devices are available for posterior dynamic neutral fixation.[63,64] They allow some movement between screw and plate (toggling). These techniques use a screw with a rounded hub that pivots in a concave bed on the plate. This allows movement (rocking) of the screw on the plate (hence the dynamic nature of the device—Fig. 14-17) and minimizes the chance of metal failure at the screw-plate interface. However, it places greater stress at the screw-bone interface. Attempted spine flexion or axial loading may result in screw pullout (Fig. 14-18). Hence the weak link in this type of construct is at the screw-bone interface. With rigid techniques, the weakest point of the system is at the screw-plate or screw-rod interface (Fig. 14-7). If the screws have a good purchase in bone, the device is a strong dynamic neutral spine stabilization construct.

The injection of pressurized polymethylmethacrylate into the screw hole may help to prevent screw pullout.[65] This, however, can set up an oxygen deprivation anode at the acrylic end of the screw, which may result in metal corrosion. *The use of dynamic neutral plating techniques in patients with osteoporotic bone may be fraught with difficulty.* This is due to the poor screw-pullout resistance of osteoporotic bone (see Chap. 13) and the construct's dynamic nature.

Posterior dynamic neutral plates, similarly, must be used in the presence of a significant anterior interbody (axial load–resisting) support. This type of construct is stable in flexion (in the presence of adequate anterior support), because of its tension-band-fixation–in–flexion character-

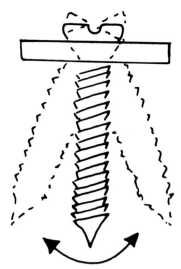

FIGURE 14-17 Most dynamic or semiconstrained screw-plate fixation constructs use a screw with a rounded hub that fits into a rounded slot in the plate. This allows toggling and gives the construct its dynamic or semiconstrained nature.

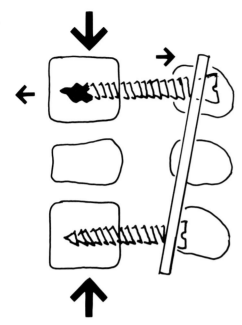

FIGURE 14-18 Dynamic or semiconstrained screw-plate fixation constructs may fail via screw pullout, because of their allowance of toggling. The bearing of an axial load (*vertical arrows*) can cause screw pullout (*horizontal arrows*).

istics. Excessive flexion, however, may result in construct failure if an anterior interbody support is not present or if intrinsic axial load–resisting abilities are inadequate (Fig. 14-16). This support may be lent by an interbody strut graft or by existing anterior axial load–resisting abilities of the spine.

Posterior interspinous compression wiring and posterior acrylic fixation techniques provide a modified type of dynamic neutral fixation of the spine. Interspinous compression wiring with fusion gives a very stable construct and should be considered a rigid stabilization technique (Fig. 14-11). The submaximal tension applied by the cerclage wire, however, allows some movement. This provides stabilization in a manner akin to the rod within the spring of the modified Weiss spring system; it creates a dynamic, but somewhat rigid, fixation.[41]

Although most surgeons do not routinely use acrylic for dorsal application in spine trauma, its occasional use may be appropriate. Panjabi and coworkers demonstrated that wire-and-methylmethacrylate stabilization provides significant acute stability.[66] Other authors, however, have demonstrated the theoretical and clinical problems associated with this construct.[67,68] The poor fit often achieved between bone and acrylic is explained by "wear and tear" on the adjacent bone in response to the stress of the interface with the acrylic and to the often-poor contact between the bone and the acrylic achieved during hardening. Blood often intervenes between the bone and the acrylic at this time, decreasing the integrity of the interface.

POSTERIOR DYNAMIC COMPRESSION FIXATION

The Weiss spring, with or without modifications, has been the only true posterior dynamic compression device clinically available.[6,69,70] It is no longer available for clinical use.

ANTERIOR DYNAMIC NEUTRAL FIXATION

Semirigid (dynamic) anterior fixation of the spine can be performed with any system that uses an interbody axial load–resisting structural support of the spine. This type of support can be provided by acrylic placed in an interbody location. The semirigid, or dynamic, nature of the technique is magnified by the ultimate absence of bony fusion. Some movement is allowed at the application site. This movement allows the development of a pseudoarthrosis-like fibrous tissue union at the margin of the acrylic (which provides a significiant portion of the stability of the construct). As in the application of acrylic to posterior spine fixation techniques, problems occur with regard to long-term stability when acrylic is placed anteriorly. The technique has been used with efficacy, however, especially with metastatic spine cancer applications. In this situation, bone grafting offers little chance of fusion and long-term stability.[52]

An anterior interbody bone graft, until fusion is acquired, also functions as a dynamic instrumentation construct. This dynamic construct gradually merges into a solid, or rigid, construct as fusion is achieved.

The Caspar anterior cervical spine plating technique[71] and equivalent techniques applied in the thoracic and lumbar spine[72] should also be considered anterior dynamic neutral fixation devices, because they allow some movement at the screw-plate interface. The advantage of this type of construct include the augmentation of bone healing–enhancing forces, the application of tension-band fixation forces (in extension) to the spine, and the intrinsic additional advantages of dynamic fixation.

Anterior (Lateral Bending) Dynamic Compression Fixation

Dynamic compression force application on the convex side of a scoliotic curvature uses forces similar to those used by its rigid counterpart (Fig. 14-14). The Dwyer apparatus is the prototype device in this category.[72] It applies its intended force at a point lateral to the IAR. With this device, however, there is a loss of biomechanical advantage proportional to the extent of the curvature present (Fig. 14-14).

Dynamic Device–Related Translational Force Application

In general, translational deformation is difficult to reduce with dynamic (semirigid or semiconstrained) constructs. Implant rigidity, to one degree or another, is nearly always required for this purpose. Hence there are no specific applications that warrant discussion here.

SPECIAL CONSIDERATIONS

Knowledge of the mechanism of a given spinal injury may help one to determine the most appropriate construct-induced force vector application technique. For example, a hangman's fracture (which usually results from excessive capital extention) requires a capital flexion vector, with accompanying distraction and true neck extension to assist with this reduction; the force application is akin to that used for reduction of a Colles fracture of the wrist. Similarly, for a Chance fracture, a ventral neural decompression, followed by the application of dorsal compression instrumentation, is an appropriate treatment plan (Fig. 14-11). The stabilization techniques in these two examples use forces that are opposite in orientation to those that caused the injuries.

The fracture type and location obviously dictate, to a significant degree, the type of reduction and fixation technique to be used. Substantial translational injuries may be best reduced and fixated with rigid distraction techniques. In these cases, segmental sublaminar wiring or pedicle fixation may substantially augment stability (Fig. 14-19). Other complex fractures may require long posterior rigid neutral rod fixation techniques with multiple-level fixation. Rigid distraction techniques, when combined with three-point bending force application, should at least partly correct scoliotic deformities; and they should provide stable constructs for kyphotic deformities when applied with multiple segmental fixation. Rigid distraction, using accompanying multiple segmental fixation and crossfixation, may provide a strong construct for complex fractures in the low lumbar region. This provides an alternative to pedicle fixation techniques (Fig. 14-19).

The extent of neurological injury obviously plays a major role in operation selection. There are two indications for surgery after spine trauma: (1) neural element decompression, and (2) spine stabilization. Either may stand alone as an indication for surgery.[6,73–75] Obviously, a more "cavalier"' approach to spine reduction and fixation may be undertaken when the patient manifests a complete myelopathic injury. Only minimal hope for neurological recovery, other than nerve root function, exists in these patients, even following dural sac decompression.[73–75]

Conversely, if any neurological function distal to the injury is present preoperatively, a chance for neurological recovery exists.[73,74] Therefore, great care should be taken to prevent neurological deterioration and to promote neurological recovery. Aggressive surgery for spinal canal decompression should be considered, where appropriate.

EFFECTIVE USE OF INTRINSIC SPINAL ANATOMY

Several anatomic features of the spine can be effectively used by the spine surgeon during the application of instrumentation. The orientation of the facet joints may provide a substantial biomechanical advantage in the application of tension-band fixation constructs in the cervical region. The orientation of the cervical facet joints is essentially in a coronal plane (see Chap. 1). This orientation does not lend itself well to resistance of rotation, flexion, or dorsal translation. Ventral translation without flexion is resisted well, provided there is an intact facet joint complex (Fig. 14-10). If an element of cervical instability in flexion is present, with an accompanying disruption of the disk space, the facet joint cannot function in this capacity as a resister of ventral translational deformation. This is seen in situations where posterior interspinous ligamentous instability has been incurred, the mechanism being a distraction injury (usually with accompany flexion). The correction of an interspinous ligament disruption injury by the application of a tension-band fixation construct allows reduction of the deformity and the prevention of further ventral translation via the "locking" of the intact facet joints against each other. Longer constructs may occasionally be required (Fig. 24-10).

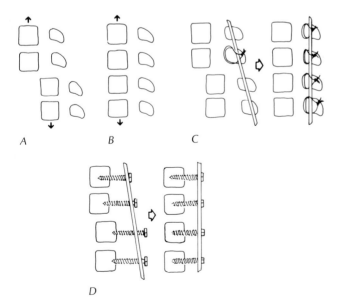

FIGURE 14-19 *A* and *B*. Translational deformations may be reducible by the simple application of distraction forces to the spine. This maneuver, however, may prove to be inadequate. *C*. Sublaminar wiring may be used to pull the translated segments back toward the rod and into proper alignment. *D*. Pedicle screws may also be used for this purpose.

REFERENCES

1. McAfee PC, Farey ID, Sutterlin CE, et al: Device-related osteoporosis with spinal instrumentation. *Spine* 1989; 14:919–926.
2. Dickson JH, Harrington, PR, Erwin WD: Results of reduction and

stabilization of the severely fractured thoracic and lumbar spine. *J Bone Joint Surg* 1978; 60A:799–805.

3. Flesch JR, Leider LL, Erickson DL, et al: Harrington instrumentation and spine fusion for unstable fractures and fracture-dislocations of the thoracic and lumbar spine. *J Bone Joint Surg* 1977; 59A:143–153.

4. Edwards CC, Levine AM: Early rod-sleeve stabilization of the injured thoracic and lumbar spine. *Orthop Clin North Am* 1986; 17:121–145.

5. Denis F, Ruiz H, Searls K: Comparison between square-ended distraction rods and standard round-ended distraction rods in the treatment of thoracolumbar spinal injuries. *Clin Orthop Rel Res* 1984; 189:162–167.

6. Benzel EC, Larson SJ: Operative stabilization of the post-traumatic thoracic and lumbar spine: A comparative analysis of the Harrington distraction rod and the modified Weiss spring. *Neurosurgery* 1986; 19:379–385.

7. Johnston CE, Ashman RB, Sherman MC, et al: Mechanical consequences of rod contouring and residual scoliosis in sublaminar segmental instrumentation. *J Orthop Res* 1987; 5:206–216.

8. Cusick JF, Mykelbust J, Zyvoloski M, et al: Effects of vertebral column distraction in the monkey. *J Neurosurg* 1982; 57:651–659.

9. Dolan EJ, Transfeldt EE, Tator CH, et al: The effect of spinal distraction on regional spinal cord blood flow in cats. *J Neurosurg* 1980; 53:756–764.

10. Anden U, Lake A, Nordwall A: The role of the anterior longitudinal ligament in Harrington rod fixation of unstable thoracolumbar spinal fractures. *Spine* 1980; 5:23–25.

11. Akbarnia BA, Fogarty JP, Smith KR: New trends in surgical stabilization of thoraco-lumbar spinal fractures with emphasis for sublaminar wiring. *Paraplegia* 1985; 23:27–33.

12. Akbarnia BA, Fogarty, JP, Tayob AA: Contoured Harrington instrumentation in the treatment of unstable spinal fractures: The effect of supplementary sublaminar wires. *Clin Orthop Rel Res* 1984; 189:186–194.

13. Bryant CE, Sullivan JA: Management of thoracic and lumbar spine fractures with Harrington distraction rods supplemented with segmental wiring. *Spine* 1983; 8:532–537.

14. Gaines RW, Breedlove RF, Munson G: Stabilization of thoracic and thoracolumbar fracture-dislocations with Harrington rods and sublaminar wires. *Clin Orthop Rel Res* 1984; 189:195–203.

15. Munson G, Satterlee C, Hammond S, et al: Experimental evaluation of Harrington rod fixation supplemented with sublaminar wires in stabilizing thoracolumbar fracture-dislocations. *Clin Orthop Rel Res* 1984; 189:97–102.

16. Sullivan JA: Sublaminar wiring of Harrington distraction rods for unstable thoracolumbar spine fractures. *Clin Orthop Rel Res* 1984; 189:178–185.

17. Yngve DA, Burke SW, Price CT, et al: Sublaminar wiring. *J Pediatr Orthop* 1986; 6:605–608.

18. Johnston CE, Happel LT, Norris R, et al: Delayed paraplegia complicating sublaminar segmental spinal instrumentation. *J Bone Joint Surg* 1986; 68A:556–563.

19. Benzel EC, Kesterson L, Marchand EP: Texas Scottish Rite Hospital rod instrumentation for thoracic and lumbar spine trauma. *J Neurosurg* 1991; 75:382–387.

20. Birch JG, Herring JA, Roach JW, et al: Cotrel-Dubousset instrumentation in idiopathic scoliosis. *Clin Orthop Rel Res* 1988; 227:24–29.

21. Cotrel Y, Dubousset J: Nouvelle technique d'osteosynthèse rachidian segmentaire par voie posterieure. *Rev Chir Orthop* 1984; 70:489–494.

22. Farcy JP, Weidenbaum M, Michelsen CB, et al: A comparative biomechancial study of spinal fixation using Cotrel-Dubousset instrumentation. *Spine* 1987; 12:877–881.

23. Herring JA, Wenger DR: Segmental spinal instrumentation. *Spine* 1982; 7:285–298.

24. Jacobs RR, Schlaepfer F, Mathys R, et al: A locking hook spinal rod system for stabilization of fracture-dislocations and correction of deformities of the dorsolumbar spine. *Clin Orthop Rel Res* 1984; 189:168–177.

25. Magerl FP: Stabilization of the lower thoracic and lumbar spine with external skeletal fixation. *Clin Orthop Rel Res* 1984; 189:125–141.

26. Cybulski GR, Von Roenn KA, D'Angelo CM, et al: Luque rod stabilization for metastatic disease of the spine. *Surg Neurol* 1987; 28:277–283.

27. Luque ER: Segmental spinal instrumentation of the lumbar spine. *Clin Orthop Rel Res* 1986; 203:126–134.

28. Benzel EC: Luque rod segmental spinal instrumentation, in Wilkins R, Rengachary S (eds): *Neurosurgical Operative Atlas.* 1992:433–438.

29. Flint GA, Hockley AD, McMillan JJ, et al: A new method of occipitocervical fusion using internal fixation. *Neurosurgery* 1987; 21:947–950.

30. Dick W: The "fixatuer interne" as a versatile implant for spine surgery. *Spine* 1987; 13:882–900.

32. Steffee AD, Biscup RS, Sitkowski DJ: Segmental spine plates with pedicle screw fixation: A new internal fixation device for disorders of the lumbar and thoracolumbar spine. *Clin Orthop Rel Res* 1986; 203:45–53.

33. Yoganandan N, Larson SJ, Pintar F, et al: Biomechanics of lumbar pedicle screw/plate fixation in trauma. *Neurosurgery* 1990; 27:873–880.

34. Callahan RA, Hohnson RM, Margolis RN, et al: Cervical facet fusion for control of instability following laminectomy. *J Bone Joint Surg* 1977; 59A:991–1002.

35. Ferguson RL, Allen BL: An algorithm for the treatment of unstable thoracolumbar fractures. *Orthop Clin North Am* 1986; 17:105–112.

36. Cybulski GR, Stone JL, Crowell RM, et al: Use of Halifax interlaminar clamps for posterior C1-C2 arthrodesis. *Neurosurgery* 1988; 22:429–431.

37. Holness RO, Huestis WS, Howes WJ, et al: Posterior stabilization with an interlaminar clamp in cervical injuries: Technical note and review of the long term experience with the method. *Neurosurgery* 1984; 14:318–322.

38. Mill KLG, Scotland TR, Wardlow D, et al: An implant clamp for atlanto-axial fusion. *J Neurol Neurosurg Psychiatry* 1988; 51:450–451.

39. Benzel EC: Biomechanics of lumbar and lumbosacral fractures, in Rea GL, Miller CA (ed): *Spinal Trauma: Current Evaluation and Management.* American Association of Neurological Surgeons, 2d ed. Philadelphia, Lippincott, 1993:1–105.

40. Selby D: Internal fixation with Knodt's rods. *Clin Orthop Rel Res* 1986; 203:179–184.

41. Benzel EC, Kesterson L: Posterior cervical interspinous compression wiring and fusion for mid to low cervical spinal injuries. *J Neurosurg* 1989; 70:893–899.

42. Robinson RA, Southwick WO: Indications and technics for early stabilization of the neck in some fracture dislocations of the cervical spine. *South Med J* 1960; 53:565–579.

43. Rogers WA: Treatment of fracture-dislocation of the cervical spine. *J Bone Joint Surg* 1942; 24:245–258.

44. Floman Y, Fast A, Pollack D, et al: The simultaneous application of an interspinous compressive wire and Harrington distraction rods in the treatment of fracture-dislocation of the thoracic and lumbar spine. *Clin Orthop Rel Res* 1986; 205:207–215.

45. Benzel EC: Short segment compression instrumentation for selected thoracic and lumbar spine fractures: The short rod–two claw technique. *J Neurosurg* 1993; 79:335–340.

46. Whitehill R, Schmidt R: The posterior interspinous fusion in the treatment of quadriplegia. *Spine* 1983; 8:733–740.

47. Hunter LY, Braunstein EM, Bailey RW: Radiographic changes following anterior cervical fusion. *Spine* 1980; 5:399–411.

48. Andrew TA, Brooks S, Piggott H: Long-term follow-up evaluation of screw-and-graft fusion of the lumbar spine. *Clin Orthop Rel Res* 1986; 203:113–119.

49. Jacobs RR, Montesano PX, Jackson RP: Enhancement of lumbar spine fusion by use of translaminar facet joint screws. *Spine* 1989; 14:12–15.

50. Kornblatt MD, Casey MP, Jacobs RR: Internal fixation in lumbosacral spine fusion: A biomechanical and clinical sutdy. *Clin Orthop Rel Res* 1986; 203:141–150.

51. Kaneda K: Kaneda anterior spinal instrumentation for the thoracic and lumbar spine, in An HS, Cotler JM (eds): *Spinal Instrumentation*. Baltimore: Williams and Wilkins, 1992:413–433.

52. Lozes G, Fawaz A, Devos P, et al: Operative treatment of thoracolumbar metastases, using methylmethacrylate and Kempf's rods for vertebral replacement and stabilization; Report of 15 cases. *Acta Neurochir (Wien)* 1987; 84:118–123.

53. Kostuik JP: Anterior fixation for fractures of the thoracic and lumbar spine with or without neurological involvement. *Clin Orthop Rel Res* 1984; 189:103–115.

54. Bremer AM, Nguyen TQ: Internal metal plate fixation combined with anterior interbody fusion in cases of cervical spine injury. *Neurosurgery* 1983; 12:649–653.

55. Brown JA, Havel P, Ebraheim N, et al: Cervical stabilization by plate and bone fusion. *Spine* 1988; 13:236–240.

56. Dunn HK: Anterior stabilization of thoracolumbar injuries. *Clin Rel Res* 1984; 189:116–124.

57. Dunn HK: Anterior spine stabilization and decompression for thoracolumbar injuries. *Orthop Clin North Am* 1986; 17:113–119.

58. Morscher E, Sutter F, Jenny H, et al: Die vorder Verplattung der Halswirbelsaule mit dem Holschrauben-Plattensystem aus Titanium. *Chirurgia* 1986; 57:702–707.

59. Yuan HA, Mann KA, Found EM, et al: Early clinical experience with the Syracuse I-plate: An anterior spinal fixation device. *Spine* 1988; 3:278–285.

60. Woolsey RM: Aortic laceration after anterior spinal fusion. *Surg Neurol* 1986; 25:267–268.

61. Kaneda K, Fujiya N, Satoh S: Results with Zielke instrumentation for idiopathic thoracolumbar and lumbar scoliosis. *Clin Orthop Rel Res* 1986; 205:195–203.

62. Ryan MD, Taylor TK, Sherwood AA: Bolt-plate fixation for anterior spinal fusion. *Clin Orthop Rel Res* 1986; 203:196–202.

63. Luque ER: Interpeduncular segmental fixation. *Clin Orthop Rel Res* 1986; 203:54–57.

64. Roy-Camille R, Saillant G, Mazel C: Internal fixation of the lumbar spine with pedicle screw plating. *Clin Orthop Rel Res* 1986; 203:7–17.

65. Zindrick MR, Wiltse LL, Widell EH, et al: A biomechanical study of interpeduncular screw fixation in the lumbosacral spine. *Clin Orthop Rel Res* 1986; 203:99–112.

66. Panjabi MM, Hopper W, White AA, et al: Posterior spine stabilization with methylmethacrylate: Biomechanical testing of a surgical specimen. *Spine* 1977; 2:241–247.

67. Eismont FJ, Bohlman HH: Posterior methylmethacrylate fixation for cervical trauma. *Spine* 1981; 6:347–353.

68. Whitehill R, Cicoria AD, Hooper WE, et al: Posterior cervical reconstruction with methylmethacrylate cement and wire: A clinical review. *J Neurosurg* 1988; 68:576–584.

69. Weiss M: Dynamic spine alloplasty (spring-loading corrective devices) after fracture and spinal cord injury. *Clin Orthop Rel Res* 1975; 112:150–157.

70. Weiss M, Bentkowski Z: Biomechanical study in dynamic spondylosis of the spine. *Clin Orthop Rel Res* 1974; 103:199–203.

71. Tippets RH, Apfelbaum RI: Anterior cervical fusion with the Caspar instrumentation system. *Neurosurgery* 1988; 22:1008–1013.

72. Black RC, Eng P, Gardner VO, et al: A contoured anterior spinal fixation plate. *Clin Orthop* 1988; 227:135–142.

72. Dwyer AF, Schafer MF: Anterior approach to scoliosis. *J Bone Joint Surg* 1974; 56B:218–224.

73. Benzel EC, Larson SJ: Functional recovery after decompressive operation for thoracic and lumbar spine fractures. *Neurosurgery* 1986; 19:772–777.

74. Benzel EC, Larson SJ: Functional recovery after decompressive spinal operation for cervical spine fractures. *Neurosurgery* 1987; 20:742–746.

75. Benzel EC, Larson SJ: Recovery of nerve root function after complete quadriplegia from cervical spine fractures. *Neurosurgery* 1986; 19:809–811.

Chapter 15

Mechanical (Quantitative) Attributes of Spinal Implants: Construct Types

INTRODUCTION

A thorough understanding of the forces applied to the spine by spinal implants is mandatory. These applied forces are often extremely complex. However, if these applied forces are broken down into components, the component force vectors may be quantitated.

The force vector of a simple compression instrumentation construct is usually applied at a finite distance from the instantaneous axis of rotation (IAR) and perpendicular to the long axis of the spine, thus creating a bending moment that is proportional to the perpendicular distance from the point of application of that force to the IAR (i.e., proportional to the lever arm, or moment arm; see below and Chap. 2).

Application of distraction as an isolated force to the posterior aspect of the spine is uncommon. Ventrally or dorsally, however, distraction may be applied in the form of true distraction, or as a buttress that resists axial loading (by applying a distraction force when an axial load is borne). Usually this is placed in an interbody location and so is "in line" with the IAR along the neutral axis. A distraction force applied "in line" with the IAR does not result in a bending moment, whereas a distraction force placed at a perpendicular distance from the IAR applies a bending moment proportional to the length of the lever arm (Fig. 15-1).

Of course, most spinal implants may be placed in a neutral mode; that is, applying no forces of any type to the spinal column at the time of surgery (see Chap. 14). However, the application of an implant device so that it never applies (or bears) a force is impossible. Even if the device is placed in a neutral mode at the time of surgery, any movement or change in body position after surgery presents stresses to the construct that alter its neutral-mode characteristic. Hence an implant placed in a neutral mode resists compression when the patient assumes an upright posture. Thus this

implant, in a sense, is placed in a distraction mode (see Chap. 14) (Fig. 15-2A). Conversely, a spinal implant placed in a compression mode may be used to "share" the load with an accompanying interbody strut implant (Fig. 15-2B). *If a cantilever beam is placed in a distraction mode, it bears all of the load. If placed in a compression mode, it shares the load with intrinsic vertebral components or interbody struts. Such an implant placed in compression might become non-weight-bearing in the upright position ("zero weight-bearing").* These points must always be considered during the clinical decision-making process.

All spinal instrumentation techniques apply forces to the spine via one or a combination of six basic mechanisms: (1) simple distraction, (2) three-point bending, (3) tension-band fixation, (4) fixed moment arm cantilever beam fixation, (5) nonfixed moment arm cantilever beam fixation, and (6) applied moment arm cantilever beam fixation. The biomechanical principles of these techniques will be discussed separately. Each of these techniques may be applied from either an anterior, a lateral, or a posterior spinal approach.

SIMPLE DISTRACTION FIXATION

Simple distraction fixation can be applied from either an anterior interbody or a posterior position. Anterior distraction constructs generally apply forces that are in line with the IAR; that is, in the interbody region. This allows the anterior distraction implant to effectively resist axial loads without employing a bending moment (Fig. 15-1). Anterior interbody distraction can cause extension of the spine if the distraction forces are applied ventral to the IAR (ventral to the neutral axis) (Fig. 15-3A). Application of posterior distraction force as an isolated entity is uncommon. This is so because of its propensity to pathologically encourage exag-

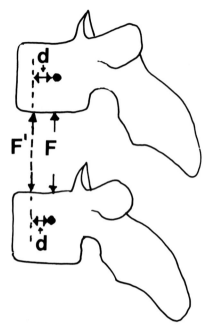

FIGURE 15-1 A distraction force (*F*) that is applied "in line" with the IAR (in the neutral axis) does not result in bending moment application. A distraction force (*F′*) that is applied at some distance from the neutral axis causes a bending moment, the magnitude of which is dictated by the perpendicular distance (*d*) from the IAR (center of the neutral axis).

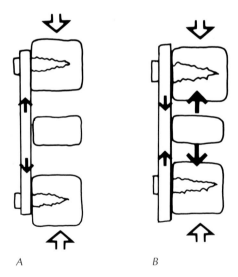

FIGURE 15-2 A. A spinal implant placed in distraction (*thin arrows*) bears most of the axial load (*hollow arrows*). B. A spinal implant placed in compression (*thin arrows*) shares the axial load (*hollow arrows*) with intrinsic spinal elements (*solid arrows*). The spinal implant is thus unloaded during weight-bearing. If enough compression were applied, the spinal implant might conceivably bear no load during the assumption of the upright position. This would be the case if the compression force applied by the implant were equal to the weight of the torso above the implant itself; that is, in the case of zero weight-bearing.

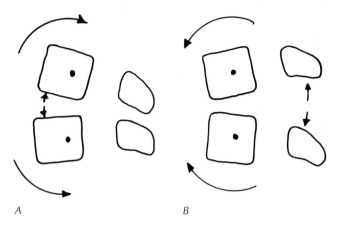

    A   *B*

FIGURE 15-3 A. Anterior spinal distraction (*straight arrows*) can cause spinal extension (*curved arrows*) if the distraction forces are applied ventral to the IAR (neutral axis). B. Conversely, the application of distraction forces (*straight arrows*) dorsal to the IAR (neutral axis) results in spinal flexion (*curved arrows*) (i.e., in tension-band distraction).

geration of a kyphotic deformity. The location of force application dorsal to the IAR causes a bending moment that results in flexion (Fig. 15-3*B*). The combination of distraction and three-point bending instrumentation application eliminates this pathological situation by applying a ventrally directed force at the fulcrum (Fig. 15-4).

Distraction applied to the spine at a finite perpendicular distance from the IAR causes a bending moment to be applied to the spine. This results in a force application similar (but opposite in direction) to that achieved with tension-band (compression) fixation. This distraction force application might be called *tension-band (distraction) fixation* (Fig. 15-3*B*).

THREE-POINT BENDING FIXATION

A springboard in action is a common example of a three-point bending force application. It consists of a fulcrum that directs a force vector opposite the direction of the terminal force vectors (Fig. 15-4*A*). Three-point bending spinal instrumentation constructs apply similar force vectors (Fig. 15-4*B*). They are usually applied with an accompanying distraction force application; for example, by Harrington distraction rods, or by universal spinal instrumentation techniques applied in a distraction mode (Fig. 15-4*C*). Three-point bending constructs usually involve instrumentation application over multiple spinal segments (five or more spinal segments), with accompany dorsally directed forces at the upper and lower construct-bone interfaces and a ventrally directed force at the fulcrum that is equal to the sum of the two dorsally directed forces (Fig. 15-4*B*). This technique is often used to accomplish ventral decompres-

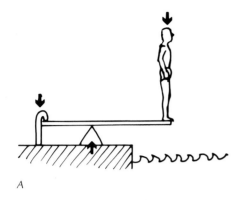

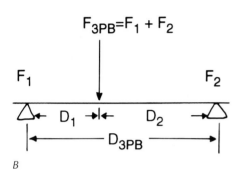

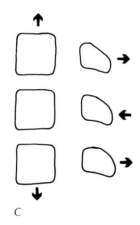

FIGURE 15-4 The force vectors at work when a person is standing on the end of a springboard (*A*). These 3-point bending forces are defined by the equation ($M = D_1 D_2 F_{3pb}/D_{3pb}$) where D_1 and D_2 are the distances from the fulcrum to the terminal hook-bone interfaces, D_{3pb} is the sum of D_1 and D_2, and F_{3pb} is the ventrally directed force applied at the fulcrum (*B*). Spinal three-point bending constructs (the forces of which are depicted as horizontal arrows) are usually applied in combination with another force vector complex; usually distraction (*vertical arrows, C*).

sion of the dural sac by distracting the posterior longitudinal ligament (*ligamentotaxis*). The desired resultant force should push the offending fragments ventrally and away from the dural sac (see Chap. 7).[1,2] Because of the relative

weakness of the posterior longitudinal ligament and/or the fixed nature of the retropulsed fragments, however, this technique may not always succeed (Chap. 7).

Posterior distraction force vector application is rarely "pure." It is frequently associated with the application of a three-point bending force to the spine. The application of sufficient posterior distraction will result in enough spinal flexion (since posterior spinal distraction force vectors are applied dorsal to the IAR, causing a flexion bending moment) that the construct will make contact with the spine at the level of the fracture site at an intermediate point along the construct (i.e., at a fulcrum).[1,3] The application of a distraction force between two adjacent spinal levels where a fulcrum is not present is an exception; for example, the application of a Knodt rod in distraction that spans only one motion segment. Prior to engagement of the fulcrum, flexion occurs because of the application of the distraction force at points dorsal to the IAR. This is most common in the lumbar region, where a lordotic posture is present (Fig. 15-5).

The bending moment at the fracture site resulting from a three-point fixation construct is defined mathematically by the equation

$$M = \frac{D_1 \times D_2 \times F_{3pb}}{D_{3pb}}$$

where *M* is the bending moment, D_1 and D_2 are the distances from the fulcrum to the terminal hook-bone inter-

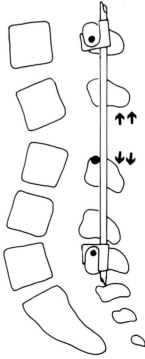

FIGURE 15-5 The application of posterior distraction forces to a lordotic spine may result in inadvertent flexion.

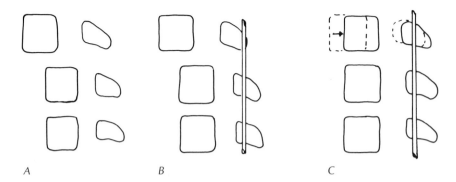

A   *B*   *C*

FIGURE 15-6 Terminal three-point bending. A ventral translational deformation relative to the next most caudal segment (*A*) can be corrected by the application of three-point bending forces to each of the three segments depicted (*B*). This results in translational deformation reduction (*C*).

faces, D_{3pb} is the sum of D_1 and D_2, and F_{3pb} is the ventrally directed force applied at the fulcrum by the three-point bending technique (Fig. 15-4).[1,4]

Terminal Three-Point Bending Fixation

Three-point bending fixation should not be considered as applying only to mid-construct deformation reduction. A three-point bending construct can also be used to correct a deformity at either of the termini of a construct (Fig. 15-6). Usually the construct is positioned so that the sagittal deformation is at its rostral end of the construct. This is so because sagittal plane deformations usually occur with the more rostral segment translating in a ventral direction with respect to the more caudal segment (Fig. 15-6).

In reality, terminal three-point bending fixation is simply a three-point bending construct in which the fulcrum is situated near one end of the construct; that is, D_1 is short and D_2 is relatively long. In light of this, the springboard discussed above is more appropriately considered a terminal three-point bending structure.

TENSION-BAND (COMPRESSION) FIXATION

Posterior spinal compression (tension-band fixation) is usually applied by wires, clamps, springs, or rigid constructs, such as Knodt rods in compression, Harrington compression rods, or universal spinal instrumentation techniques applied in compression. These techniques apply spinal compression forces at their dorsal application sites (Fig. 15-7*A*). Ventral tension-band fixation constructs, however, may also be applied (Fig. 15-7*B*).

By the nature of the tension-band fixation construct, extension (dorsal bending moment) or flexion (ventral bending moment) is applied to the spinal segments that are "compressed." For tension-band fixation techniques, the bending moment applied at the fracture site by the tension-band fixation technique is defined mathematically by the equation

$$M_{tbf} = F_{tbf} \times D_{iar\text{-}tbf}$$

where M_{tbf} is the bending moment, F_{tbf} is the compression force applied at the upper and lower termini of the construct at the instrument-bone interface, and $D_{iar\text{-}tbf}$ is the perpendicular distance from the IAR to the applied force (Fig. 15-8).[1] Generally, only a few segments can be fixated with this technique.

Ventrally positioned extradural masses (bone and/or disk fragments) might be thrust dorsally into the spinal canal during instrumentation application. Therefore, decompression procedures may be appropriate prior to the application of the instrumentation construct (see Chap. 14).[3]

COMPARING RIGID OR SEMIRIGID DISTRACTION AND COMPRESSION

The concepts of *load-bearing* and *load-sharing* should be considered whenever a spinal implant is used. Neutral implants, in the truest sense, do not exist. When weight is borne by the torso, the implant is exposed to myriad forces (load-bearing). This occurs inevitably, even in cases where an implant is initially placed in a neutral mode (Fig. 15-9).

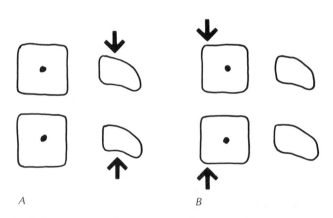

A   *B*

FIGURE 15-7 *A.* Posterior spinal tension-band fixation. *B.* Anterior spinal tension-band fixation.

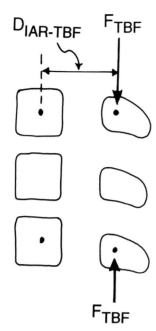

FIGURE 15-8 The forces applied by a tension-band fixation construct are described by the equation ($M_{tbf} = F_{tbf} D_{iar=tbf}$) where M_{tbf} is the bending moment, F_{tbf} is the compression force applied at the upper and lower termini of the construct at the instrument-bone interface, and $D_{iar=tbf}$ is the perpendicular distance from the IAR to the tension-band fixation applied-force vector.

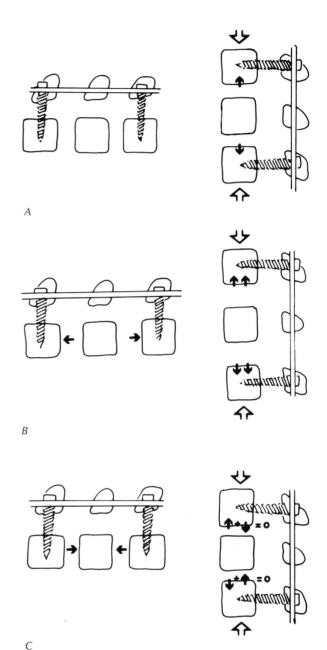

FIGURE 15-9 Changes in position alter the load borne by an implant. *A.* If an implant is placed in a neutral mode (zero surgical load, *left*), then when an upright posture is assumed the axial load applied to the implant (*hollow arrows*) is approximately equal to the weight of the torso positioned above the implant (*right, solid arrows*). *B.* If the implant is placed in a distraction mode (*left, solid arrows*), then when an upright posture is assumed the implant bears the surgical load plus the weight of the torso above the spinal implant (*hollow arrows*). Thus the implant bears a greater load (*paired solid arrows*). *C.* If the implant is placed in compression (negative surgical load, *solid arrows*), then assumption of the upright posture results in the implant's bearing an axial load that is less than the weight of the torso positioned above the implant. In fact, if the negative surgical load is equal to the weight of the torso positioned above the implant, the load borne by the implant during the assumption of an upright posture is zero; that is, the surgical load is equal, and opposite in direction, to the weight of the torso positioned above the implant (*solid arrows*).

For the purposes of this discussion we have considered isolated axial loads and force applications. The clinical situation, however, is quite different; myriad forces are applied by the torso to the implant, and by the implant to the torso. The bearing of a load by the torso during the assumption of an upright posture causes a spinal implant to absorb an axial load. If the implant was placed in a neutral mode, the axial load borne changes from zero (the load borne by the implant at the time of surgery) to roughly the weight of the torso positioned above the implant (Fig. 15-9A). If the implant was placed in a distraction mode, the additional axial load borne by the implant with the patient assuming the upright posture is the sum of the load borne at the time of surgery (surgical load-bearing) and the weight of the torso above the implant (Fig. 15-9B).

The placement of an implant in a compression mode alters the forces considerably. In the hypothetical situation where only axial forces are considered, the placement of an implant in a compression mode results in negative surgical load-bearing. If an axial load is subsequently borne by a patient assuming an upright posture, the surgical compression load is effectively diminished, and the net load approaches, or passes, zero (Fig. 15-9C). Thus a spinal implant placed in a compression mode can share the load applied by the torso with the spine proper, by leaving some of the load to be borne by existing spinal axial load-bearing capabilities or by an interbody strut graft.

COMPARING THREE-POINT BENDING AND TENSION-BAND FIXATION

Three-point bending and tension-band fixation constructs differ considerably. Three-point bending fixation techniques require the use of long constructs to optimize efficacy of the construct; the bending moment applied by a three-point bending construct is proportional the length of the construct. The bending moment applied by a tension-band fixation construct is independent of construct length. Therefore, three-point bending constructs are usually employed over more spinal segments than tension-band fixation constructs.

The bending moment applied at the fracture site by three-point bending fixation techniques is defined mathematically by the equation[1,4]

$$M_{3pb} = \frac{D_1 \times D_2 \times F_{3pb}}{D_{3pb}}$$

whereas the bending moment applied by tension-band fixation techniques is defined mathematically by the equation[1]

$$M_{3pb} = F_{3pb} \times D_{iar\text{-}3pb}$$

If D_1 is equal to D_2 (as it usually is), then both D_1 and D_2 are equal to $\frac{1}{2}D_{3pb}$. Solving the equation thus yields the following

$$M_{3pb} = \frac{[(\frac{1}{2})D_{3pb}]^2 \times F_{3pb}}{D_{3pb}} = \frac{0.25D_{3pb}^2 \times F_{3pb}}{D_{3pb}}$$
$$= 0.25D_{3pb} \times F_{3pb}$$

where M_{3pb} is the bending moment at the fracture site, F_{3pb} is the ventrally directed force applied at the fulcrum, and D_{3pb} is the length of the construct (Fig. 15-10).[1]

Since the two bending moments from the two forces applied to a structure by the construct are equal (because the net bending of a structure in equilibrium is zero), the situation observed in the case of a tension-band fixation construct (Fig. 15-11A) is defined by the equation

$$M_{tbf} = F_{tbf} \times D_{iar\text{-}tbf} = F_{e\text{-}tbf} \times \frac{1}{2} \times D_{tbf}$$
$$F_{e\text{-}tbf} = \frac{2 \times F_{tbf} \times D_{iar\text{-}tbf}}{D_{tbf}}$$

$F_{e\text{-}tbf}$ is the "effective" ventrally directed force created by the torque associated with the force (F_{tbf}) and lever arm ($D_{iar\text{-}tbf}$). Since the product of F_{tbf} and $D_{iar\text{-}tbf}$ is fixed by the characteristics of the construct, increasing construct length (D_{tbf}) decreases the effective ventrally directed force applied

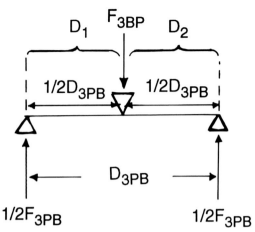

FIGURE 15-10 If a three-point bending construct is symmetrically placed—that is, if the length of the construct above the fulcrum is equal to that below the fulcrum—then D_1 is equal to D_2, both of these are equal to $\frac{1}{2}D_{3pb}$, and the situation is described by the equation $[M_{3pb} = (\frac{1}{2}D_{3pb})^2 F_{3pb}/D_{3pb} = 0.25\,D_{3pb} F_{3pb}/D_{3pb} = 0.25\,D_{3pb} \times F_{3pb}]$ where M_{3pb} is the bending moment at the fracture site, F_{3pb} is the ventrally directed force applied at the fulcrum, and D_{3pb} is the length of the construct.

at the fulcrum ($F_{e\text{-}tbf}$). Therefore, since a ventrally directed force at the fulcrum ($F_{e\text{-}tbf}$) is usually a desirable force, the use of a long tension-band fixation construct may often *not* be desirable. A long tension-band fixation construct, in fact, may be associated with an exaggerated extension of the spine via the application of widely separated bending moments, in spite of the lesser $F_{e\text{-}tbf}$ (Fig. 15-11B). Long constructs allow the application of two widely-spaced bending moments (at the termini of the construct). This encourages the development of an exaggerated extension–buckling type of deformity.

If the bending moment applied at the fracture site is the same for three-point bending and tension-band fixation techniques, the two equations may be simultaneously solved:

$$M = D_{iar\text{-}tbf} \times F_{tbf} = 0.25D_{3pb} \times F_{3pb}$$

This implies that in order to achieve an equal bending moment, the two instrumentation constructs use moment arm lengths that differ by a factor of 4:

$$D_{iar\text{-}tbf} = 0.25D_{3pb}, \text{ or } D_{3pb} = 4\,D_{iar\text{-}3pb}$$

These moment arms are not equivalent with regard to orientation (Fig. 15-12). The $D_{iar\text{-}tbf}$ refers to a lever arm that is perpendicular to the long axis of the spine (and the instrumentation construct), whereas the D_{3pb} refers to a lever arm that is parallel to the long axis of the spine (and the instru-

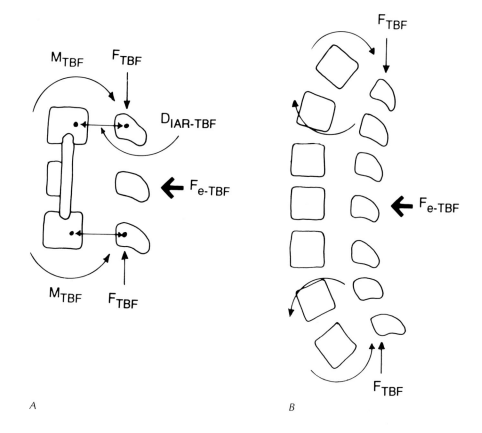

FIGURE 15-11 Tension-band fixation constructs (*A*) may not be desirable, because of the following relationships ($M_{tbf} = F_{tbf} D_{iar=tbf} = F_{e=tbf} \frac{1}{2} D_{tbf}$) and ($F_{e=tbf} = 2 F_{tbf} D_{iar=tbf}/D_{tbf}$). $F_{e=tbf}$ is the "effective ventrally directed force created by the torque associated with the force (F_{tbf}) and lever arm ($D_{iar=tbf}$). Since the product of F_{tbf} and $D_{iar=tbf}$ is fixed by the characteristics of the construct, increasing the construct length (D_{tbf}) decreases the effective ventrally directed force applied at the fulcrum ($F_{e=tbf}$). In addition, this may cause hyperextension of the spine by creating terminal bending moments (*B*).

A   *B*

mentation construct) (Fig. 15-12). Nevertheless, a three-point bending technique requires a longer construct than does the tension-band fixation technique in order to achieve the same bending moment at the fracture site with similar applied forces. Since the bending moment at the fracture site is unchanged by the length of a tension-band fixation construct, and since the ventrally directed effective force $F_{e\text{-}tbf}$ diminishes as the construct length is increased, short tension-band constructs may often be more desirable. Conversely, longer three-point bending constructs offer greater stability (i.e., better biomechanical advantages for deformity progression prevention and deformity correction). Therefore, if substantial axial loading–, rotation-, and/or translation-resisting characteristics are desired, long three-point bending constructs (spanning more than five spinal segments) may be most appropriate.

Three-point bending fixation techniques use additional superimposed forces applied in distraction at the terminal (and intermediate) construct-bone interfaces. These add to the stresses applied to the bone (by adding a distraction component). However, they do not alter the bending moment if the ventrally directed force at the fulcrum (F_d) is not changed (Fig. 15-13). Some authors have advocated the exaggeration of such forces in order to accomplish spinal column reduction and spinal canal decompression (see Chap. 7)[2]; this has not always met with success.

The use of terminology associated with biomechanics and physics in the literature of spine surgery has often been confusing. Much of the confusion has had to do with the biomechanics of injury and instrumentation. The concept of the bending moment has been misrepresented and poorly understood.

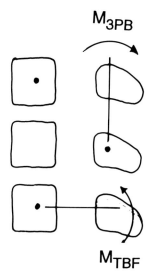

FIGURE 15-12 The moment arm applied by three-point bending constructs (M_{3pb}) is parallel to the long axis of the spine, whereas that applied by tension-band fixation constructs (M_{tbf}) is perpendicular to the long axis of the spine.

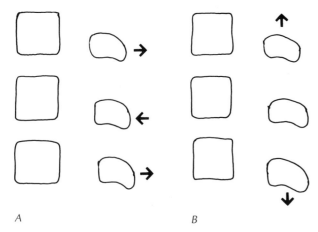

A   *B*

FIGURE 15-13 Three-point bending constructs nearly always are applied in combination with distraction (see Fig. 15-4*A*). These two components, three-point bending (*A*) and distraction (*B*), are independent of each other with respect to the forces they apply to the spine.

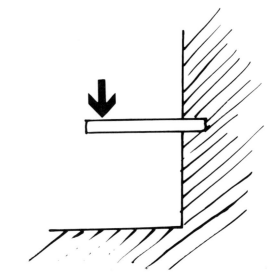

FIGURE 15-14 A fixed moment arm cantilever beam. In this case the cantilever beam is rigidly fixed to the wall. Note the lack of need for an accompanying applied-force vector during the bearing of a load (*arrow*).

The bending moment associated with instrumentation application is often greatest at the level of the deformity (particularly with three-point bending techniques).[4] This is fortuitous for deformity reduction, because of the requirement for torque application at the deformity site in order to achieve spinal deformity reduction. The maximum bending moment applied at the deformity site is located at the center of the circle defined by the arc of the force causing the bending moment.[1] However, this has not always been so depicted in the literature; the nomenclature currently used is inconsistent.[2] One should consider the bending moment as the *torque* applied to the spine by the instrumentation construct. This allows a better understanding of its true nature.

FIXED MOMENT ARM CANTILEVER BEAM FIXATION

A *cantilever* is a large projecting bracket or beam supported at one end only. A cantilever is usually designed to bear a weight or structure over a space where support cannot be placed or is not desired. There are three types of cantilever beams: those with fixed moment arms, those with nonfixed moment arms, and those that apply moment arms. A fixed moment arm cantilever beam is illustrated in Fig. 15-14. The most common example of this type of structure among spinal instrumentation constructs is the rigid pedicle fixator. Rigid pedicle fixation techniques (such as rigid plate or screw-rod combinations) may compensate for a short moment arm by providing a fixed moment arm cantilever beam configuration for structural support. Although the initial application of such a construct may be in a neutral mode

(no distraction, rotation, compression, or translational forces applied to the spine at the time of surgery), when an axial load is applied (e.g., during the assumption of an erect posture), the construct must resist the axial load by virtue of its intrinsic cantilever beam with fixed moment arm characteristics; that is, by rigidly buttressing the spine. Worthy of note is its lack of need for a ventrally directed force at the fulcrum. This is compensated for by the inherent buttressing effect. This places a significant stress at the point of maximum bending moment; that is, at the screw-plate or screw-rod interface (Fig. 15-15). This stress may be excessive, resulting in screw fracture (an infrequently observed phenomenon with modern construct designs). Biomechanical studies have confirmed this.[5]

NONFIXED MOMENT ARM CANTILEVER BEAM FIXATION

A nonfixed moment arm cantilever beam does not effectively bear an axial load without the assistance of other structures (e.g., vertebral body, bone graft, etc.). However, it helps the already-present axial load–supporting structures to do so (Fig. 15-16). Nonfixed moment arm cantilever beam constructs do not apply substantial axial load–resisting forces to the spine. The toggling of the screw on the plate allowed by this technique dictates that little, if any, bending moment is applied to the spine. These techniques are appropriately used only when axial load–resisting capabilities of

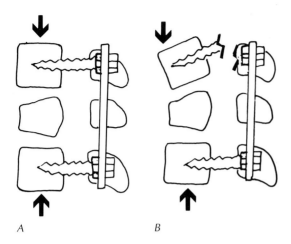

FIGURE 15-15 *A.* The bending moment realized by a fixed moment arm cantilever beam during load bearing is maximal at the screw-plate or screw-rod interface. *B.* This may result in construct failure at this location following the bearing of an axial load *(arrows)*.

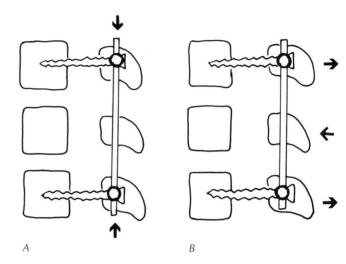

FIGURE 15-17 Nonfixed moment arm cantilever beam constructs can function in a tension-band fixation mode *(A)* or in a three-point bending mode *(B)*.

the spine are present. Because of their biomechanical characteristics, their ability to resist screw pullout is diminished (Fig. 15-16*B*) (see Chap. 14).

The application of these constructs in the cervical spine, via lateral mass screw-plate systems, or in the lumbar spine, via transpedicular screw-plate or screw-rod systems, may create situations where they function, at least in part, as tension-band fixation constructs in flexion (see Chap. 14) (Fig. 15-17*A*). They can also function as three-point bending con-

structs (Fig. 15-17*B*), especially if used in predominantly cortical bone, with its relatively good screw-pullout resistance. Finally, they augment stability by pulling the bone to the underside of the plate (see below). In light of all this, the construct-type categories cannot be completely separated in the end.

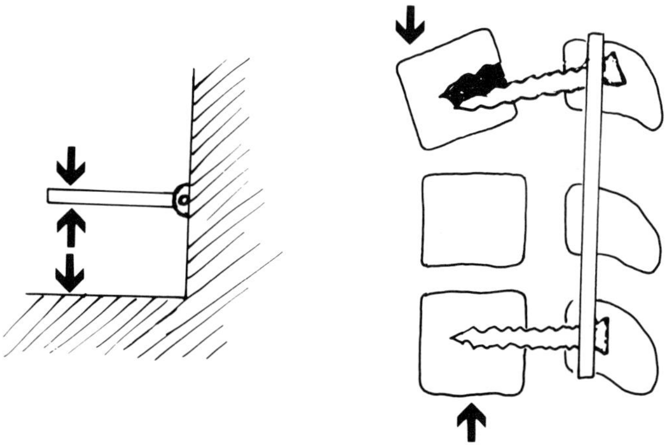

APPLIED MOMENT ARM CANTILEVER BEAM FIXATION

Finally, cantilever beam fixation can be applied with either a flexion component (Fig. 15-18*A*) or an extension component (Fig. 15-18*B*) to the applied moment arm. These constructs usually are rigid and are used to reduce deformities. Extension moment arm application is their most common clinical use at present.

COMMENTS

Although a fixed moment arm cantilever beam can be applied in a distraction mode, the buttressing effect of this construct clearly separates it biomechanically from a simple distraction construct. Simple distraction can apply a torque to the IAR if it is applied at a perpendicular distance from the IAR, whereas the cantilever beam technique applies no effective torque unless an applied moment is used.

Pedicle fixation devices may fail to bear axial loads effectively, because of a lateral parallelogram-like translational deformition. A simple toeing-in of the screws should prevent this mechanism of construct failure.[1,6] Rigid crossfixation of

FIGURE 15-16 *A.* A nonfixed moment arm cantilever beam. In this case the cantilever beam is fixed by a hinge to the wall. Note the requirement for an accompanying applied force vector *(double-headed arrow)* during the bearing of a load *(single-headed arrow)*. *B.* Nonfixed moment arm cantilever beam constructs may fail via screw pullout.

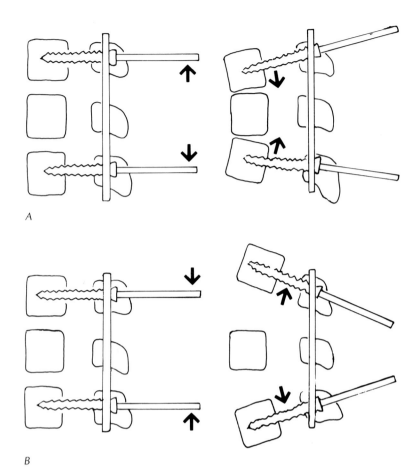

A

B

FIGURE 15-18 *A.* Applied moment arm cantilever beam construct employing a flexion moment. *B.* Applied moment arm cantilever beam construct employing an extension moment.

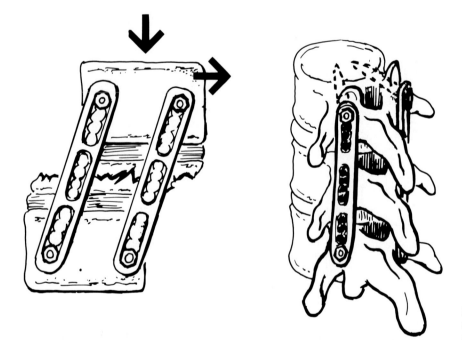

A

B

FIGURE 15-19 The parallelogram-like effect of lateral translational deformation (*A*) can be prevented by the toeing-in of the screws of the construct (*B*).

FIGURE 15-20 A parallelogram-like translational deformation of the spine in the sagittal plane can occur with nonfixed moment arm cantilever beam constructs (*A*). This untoward occurrence can be minimized by the use of more rigid constructs or the employment of a nonfixed moment arm construct over additional caudal segment(s) (*B*). This is similar in principle to the strategy shown in Fig. 15-6 for three-point bending constructs.

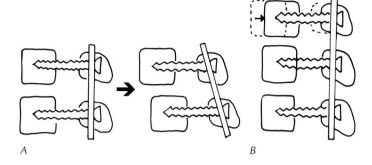

the rod on each side to its counterpart would also prevent this complication (Fig. 15-19).

The ability of a cantilever beam construct to resist translation may be limited (especially a construct with a nonfixed moment arm). In this situation a parallelogram-like effect may occur in the sagittal plane, particularly if only one motion segment is encompassed by the construct (Fig. 15-20*A*). If a more rigid construct is used (e.g., a fixed moment arm cantilever beam construct) (Fig. 15-20*B*), or if a longer construct (e.g., a nonfixed moment arm cantilever beam construct) is used over more motion segments, sagittal

translational deformation is more effectively resisted. In the former case the rigidity of the construct does not allow translation unless screw pullout occurs. In the latter, the increased length of the lever arm with at least three points of attachment to the spine creates a substantial biomechanical advantage. Note that the extra level encompassed by the construct should optimally be caudal to the unstable motion segment if the translational deformity of the upper segment is ventral in direction and cephalad to the unstable motion segment of the translational deformity is dorsal in direction (Fig. 15-21).

Similarly, nonfixed moment arm cantilever beam constructs may achieve some of the rigidity characteristics of their fixed moment arm counterparts via the "pulling" of the spine to the construct. This restricts vertebral bending and increases axial load–resisting abilities (Fig. 15-22). The

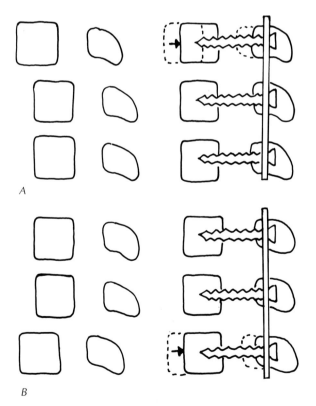

FIGURE 15-21 A terminal three-point bending construct may have a nonfixed moment arm. The long arm of the construct is situated caudally if a ventral translational deformity is to be resisted (*A*), and rostrally if a dorsal translational deformity is to be resisted (*B*).

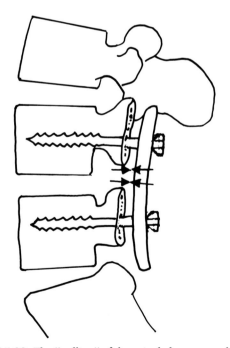

FIGURE 15-22 The "pulling" of the spinal elements to the plate of a nonfixed moment arm cantilever beam construct may lend a considerable degree of stability to the construct.

extent of the contribution of this factor varies and is not readily measurable. This attribute of the nonfixed moment arm cantilever beam construct is augmented by increased construct length.

REFERENCES

1. Benzel EC: Biomechanics of lumbar and lumbosacral spine fractures, in Rea GL (ed): *Spinal Trauma: Current Evaluation and Management.* American Association of Neurological Surgeons, 1993.
2. Edwards CC, Levine AM: Early rod-sleeve stabilization of the injured thoracic and lumbar spine. *Orthop Clin North Am* 1986; 17:121–145.
3. Benzel EC, Larson SJ: Operative stabilization of the posttraumatic thoracic and lumbar spine: A comparative analysis of the Harrington distraction rod and the modified Weiss spring. *Neurosurgery* 1986; 19:378–385.
4. White AA, Panjabi MM: *Clinical Biomechanics of the Spine* (2d ed). Philadelphia: Lippincott, 1990, 1–125.
5. Yoganandan N, Larson SJ, Pintar F, et al: Biomechanics of lumbar pedicle screw/plate fixation in trauma. *Neurosurgery* 1990; 27:873–881.
6. Carson WL, Duffield RC, Arendt M, et al: Internal forces and moments in transpedicular spine instrumentation. *Spine* 1990; 15:893–901.

Chapter 16

Construct Design

For the purposes of this discussion, *construct design* is defined as *the act of laying out an operative instrumentation plan for a case-specific instability problem that includes formulating both a blueprint for the instrumentation construct to be placed and a strategy for the implementation of the blueprint.*[1] Meticulous preoperative strategy definition is vital to a successful outcome.

FUNDAMENTAL CONCEPTS

The nomenclature of spinal instrumentation is both complex and, by definition, confusing. The wide variety of implant and implant-component choices, of modes of application, and of construct purchase-site choices contributes to this comlexity and confusion. The determinants of the spinal construct of choice in each clinical situation must be carefully addressed by the surgeon. They include the indication for instrumentation, the fundamental type of instrumentation to be used, the mode of application of the implant, and the complexity of the construct to be implanted.

Indications for Spinal Instrumentation

Indications for surgery depend on the extent and type of spinal instability present. The quest to quantitate the extent of spinal instability in order to optimize its management should lead the surgeon to the following questions: What is expected from the implant? And is this expectation reasonable? If these questions are appropriately answered, the foundation of the construct design process has been properly established.[1]

Implant Construct Choices

The employment of a spinal implant involves the making of several choices: the choice of the longitudinal member (rod or plate), the choice of the implant component of the implant-bone interface (wire, hook, or screw), and the choice of crossfixation mechanism.

Mode of Application of the Implant

The mode of application of the implant is a critical element in the construct design process. The surgical placement of the implant in a distraction, compression, neutral, translation, flexion, extension, or lateral-bending mode affects the extent of load-bearing and load-sharing by the implant, the extent of deformity exaggeration or correction, and the exaggeration or relief of neural compression.[1]

Mechanism of Load-Bearing

As was outlined in Chap. 15, there are six fundamental construct types. This implies that there are six fundamental mechanisms of load-bearing. These are associated, respectively, with corresponding construct types:(1) simple distraction, (2) three-point bending, (3) tension-band fixation, (4) fixed moment arm cantilever beam fixation, (5) nonfixed moment arm cantilever beam fixation, and (6) applied moment arm cantilever beam fixation.

NOMENCLATURE OF CONSTRUCT DESIGN

Methodical and prospective (preoperative) construction of a "blueprint" for implant placement helps the surgeon plan the operation. It also facilitates communication between the surgeon, his or her assistants, the nurses, and the implant vendors.

A simple scheme has previously been presented,[1] and will be outlined here, that provides information regarding (1) the level of the lesion or of the unstable segment(s), (2) the most advantageous type of implant (which includes the implant component of the implant-bone interface, the longitudinal member, and the crossmember), (3) the mode of application at each segmental level, (4) the method of load-

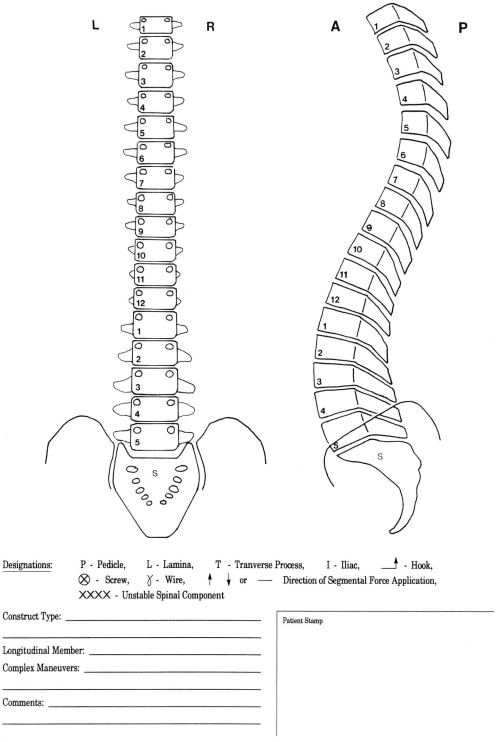

Designations: P - Pedicle,   L - Lamina,   T - Tranverse Process,   I - Iliac,   ⊥ - Hook,
⊗ - Screw,   ᛉ - Wire,   ↑ ↓ or — Direction of Segmental Force Application,
XXXX - Unstable Spinal Component

Construct Type: _____

Longitudinal Member: _____

Complex Maneuvers: _____

Comments: _____

Patient Stamp

FIGURE 16-1 A blueprint format for the planning of a construct-design strategy. A posterior-anterior view is shown on the left, and a lateral view on the right. Note that the diagram does not include the cervical spine. If instrumentation is planned in this region, the line drawing can be extended or the spinal segments relabeled to conform to the extent of operative plan. Room at the bottom of the page allows for other vital information, such as the patient's demographic data (bottom right) and information on (1) the method of load bearing (distraction, three-point bending, tension-band fixation, cantilever beam with a fixed moment arm, cantilever beam with a nonfixed moment arm, or cantilever beam with an applied moment arm); (2) the longitudinal member type (rod or plate); and (3) a description of planned complex maneuvers (i.e., derotation maneuvers). (*From E.C. Benzel.*[4])

bearing by the construct, and (5) a clear definition of the complexity of the construct. This scheme "forces" the surgeon to select the appropriate implant components in advance, so that intraoperative communication between the surgeon and his or her assistants is facilitated and the likelihood of a well-conceived operation and a satisfactory outcome is maximized.

Although the principles that govern decision-making in construct design are common to all aspects of spinal instrumentation surgery in all regions of the spine, they are more graphically and clinically obvious in the thoracic and lumbar regions than in the cervical region. In the cervical region implant choices seem to be simpler conceptually, and fewer implant choices are available. For example, a dislocated cervical facet may be surgically managed by open reduction, fusion, and spinal instrumentation. The spinal instrumentation, be it a spinous process wiring or facet screw-plating technique, usually is applied in a standard way; that is, the spinous process wiring construct is placed in a tension-band fixation mode and the screw-plate construct is placed in a neutral mode. Either of these can be readily visualized by the surgeon.

A thoracolumbar fracture, on the other hand, may be managed by a variety of techniques, including short segment fixation techniques, long rod–short fusion techniques, long rod–long fusion techniques, ventral fixation techniques, combination techniques, and so on. Each of these techniques can be applied in a variety of modes of application—compression, distraction, neutral, distraction followed by compression, or distraction and compression at differing segmental levels of the spine. It is in consideration of these clinical dilemmas that this chapter focuses on thoracic and lumbar fixation design strategies. The information gleaned from these considerations can then easily be applied to the cervical spine.

Line Drawing Framework

A simple posterior-anterior and lateral line drawing of the spine provides a framework for the clear definition of the operative plan (Fig. 16-1). Often only a posterior-anterior drawing is necessary, unless the operative plan includes the reduction of a deformity in the sagittal plane (e.g., a kyphotic deformity). Redundant information should not be depicted on the lateral view. The line drawing provides the blueprint for surgery.

The convention for the posterior-anterior line drawing is that the left side of the drawing portrays the left side of the patient; that is, the drawing portrays the patient as viewed from behind. This is in accordance with the most common surgical approach and so reduces the chance of confusion.

Level of Pathology and Level of Fusion

The designation of the level of pathology or spinal instability, the levels to be fused, and the type of fusion should next be placed on the line drawing. The level(s) of instability or pathology are designated by Xs and the fusion by a hatched outline of an anatomically correct depiction of the fusion (Fig. 16-2).

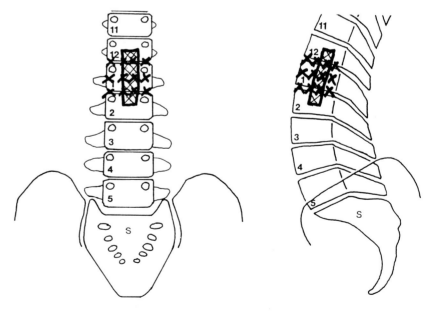

FIGURE 16-2 The level of instability has been designated by Xs in both of the disrupted disk interspaces and the injured vertebral body in this case of unstable L1 compression fracture. An anterior interbody fusion is planned and is depicted by the hatched area. *(From E.C. Benzel.⁴)*

Designations: P - Pedicle, L - Lamina, T - Tranverse Process, I - Iliac, — Hook, ⊗ - Screw, γ - Wire, ↑ ↓ or — Direction of Segmental Force Application, XXXX - Unstable Spinal Component

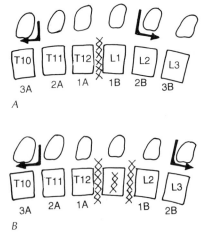

A

B

FIGURE 16-3 An illustration of the changes in instrumentation length caused by changes in the definition of the specific location of the area(s) of instability. *A.* A T12-L1 translational deformity, with the T11-T12 and L1-L2 disk interspaces and endplates left unharmed. A 3A-2B construct extends from T10 to L2. T10 is 3 segments above the T12-L1 interspace, and L2 is 2 segments below this interspace. *B.* An unstable L1 compression fracture. Both the T12-L1 and L1-L2 disk interspaces have been violated. A 3A-2B construct, in this situation, extends from T10 above to L3 below. This construct is one segment longer than that shown in *A.* The difference resides in the definition of the lower extent of the instability; in *A* it is at T12-L1, whereas in *B* it is at L1-L2. *(From E.C. Benzel.[4])*

Accurate delineation of the unstable motion segment(s) is important to the definition of the number of spinal levels to be spanned, both above and below the level of pathology. For example, the instability consists only of a loss of integrity of the T12-L1 motion segment, the instrumentation of three levels *above* places the upper end of the implant at T10, and the instrumentation of two levels *below* places the lower end of the implant at L2 (Fig. 16-3A). This is designated by the nomenclature *3A-2B,* which describes an implant extending from three spinal levels above to two levels below the pathology.

If, however, the L1 vertebral body is fractured and its juxtaposed disk interspaces disrupted, the T12-L1 and L1-L2 motion segments are structurally disrupted. In this case the same implant-design designation described above (3A-2B) gives an implant extending from T10 (three levels above the upper extent of the pathology) to L3 (two levels below the lower extent of the pathology) (Fig. 16-3B). In the former case the implant extends from T10 to L2 (the lower extent of the pathology being the upper aspect of T12); in the latter it extends from T10 to L3 (the lower extent of the pathology being the lower aspect of L1).

The mechanical effect of immobilizing any motion segment unnecessarily may be significant. Therefore, the definition of the level of instability is critical in the surgical decision-making process.

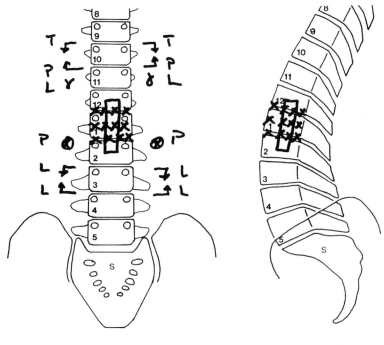

FIGURE 16-4 The types of implant components, their purchase sites, and their locations are illustrated in this hypothetical and somewhat unconventional 3A-2B construct using hooks, sublaminar wire, and pedicle screws attached to a rod. Many fixation modalities are depicted for illustrative purposes. Hooks are designated by right-angled arrows (with arrowheads pointing in the direction of the orientation of the hook—i.e., the side of the hook-bone interface). Screws are designated by circled *X*s, and wires by loops. The location of each is defined by *P* for pedicle, *L* for laminar or sublaminar, *T* for transverse process, or *I* for iliac. *(From E.C. Benzel.[4])*

Designations: P - Pedicle,   L - Lamina,   T - Tranverse Process,   I - Iliac,   — Hook,
⊗ - Screw,   γ - Wire,   ↑ ↓ or — Direction of Segmental Force Application,
XXXX - Unstable Spinal Component

Type of Implant Components

The type of implant components used in the instrumentation construct should be delineated clearly on the blueprint. The implant component at each implant-bone interface is a wire, hook, or screw. The convention used here is to designate hooks by a right-angle arrow, with the arrowhead pointing in the direction of the orientation of the hook—that is, toward the bone-purchase side of the hook. Each screw is designated by an *X* surrounded by a circle. Wire is depicted as a loop.[1]

The insertion sites of these components are indicated by placement of the above-described symbols at the appropriate levels of the spine on the line drawing, with accompanying designations to specify anatomic sites of purchase: *P* for pedicle, *L* for laminar or sublaminar, *T* for transverse process, and *I* for iliac (Fig. 16-4).[1]

Mode of Application at Each Segmental Level

The mode of axial load application (distraction, compression, or neutral) at each implant-bone interface is indicated by an arrow pointing in the direction of force application, for distraction and compression, or by a horizontal line, for neutral.

Bending moments are difficult to depict accurately on the line drawing; hence they are described. For example, a derotation maneuver may be described by the notation, "The rods are placed in a concave left configuration, which is then followed by a 90-degree counterclockwise rotation to convert the scoliotic deformity to a kyphotic deformity."

The modes of application at each segmental level are depicted with the arrows and lines, as described above. These are drawn laterally to the implant-type designations (Fig. 16-5A). If sagittal plane forces are planned, they are depicted on the lateral line drawing (Fig. 16-5B). Finally, crossmember location can be designated by elongated rectangles with circles (Fig. 16-5A).

Mechanical Attributes of Spinal Implants: Construct Type

The mechanism by which the construct will bear loads is also specified. There are six methods of load-bearing asso-

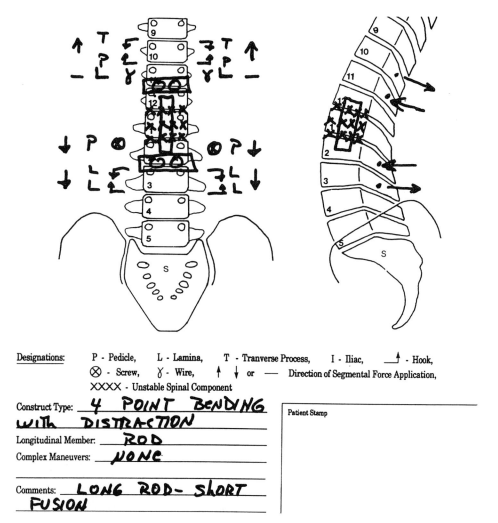

FIGURE 16-5 The totality of forces applied to the spine by the implant (i.e., the mode of application) is depicted. This force distribution can be created by distraction and compression maneuvers performed intraoperatively. The axial forces thus attained are supplemented by deformity correction via the application of four-point bending forces to the spine *(right)*. The placement of a crossmember is designated by elongated rectangles with open circles *(left)*. *(From E.C. Benzel.[4])*

Designations: P - Pedicle,   L - Lamina,   T - Tranverse Process,   I - Iliac,   ⌐↑ - Hook,
⊗ - Screw,   γ - Wire,   ↑ ↓ or —   Direction of Segmental Force Application,
XXXX - Unstable Spinal Component

Construct Type: **4 POINT BENDING WITH DISTRACTION**
Longitudinal Member: **ROD**
Complex Maneuvers: **NONE**

Comments: **LONG ROD- SHORT FUSION**

Patient Stamp

ciated with the six construct types (see Chap. 15): (1) distraction, (2) three-point bending, (3) tension-band fixation, (4) fixed moment arm cantilever beam, (5) nonfixed moment arm cantilever beam, and (6) applied moment arm cantilever beam. Since this information is difficult to depict on the line drawing, it is simply recorded in the space provided at the bottom of the page.

CONSTRUCT DESIGN STRATEGIES

There are many factors in the design of a spinal instrumentation construct. Attention should be paid specifically to bony integrity, the location of the unstable spinal segment, implant length, the need for crossfixation, the axial load-bearing capacity of the instrumented spine, the orientation of the instability, the need for dural sac decompression, and the armamentarium of the surgeon. Each of these factors must be adequately addressed if the outcome is to be optimal.

Bony Integrity

Osteoporosis creates a surgical dilemma in the form of reduced integrity of the implant-bone interface. Hooks and sublaminar wires resist pullout better than screws and therefore are advantageous in the osteoporotic patient. Hooks and sublaminar wires apply forces to the spine at a considerable perpendicular distance from the instantaneous axis of rotation (IAR). The pivoting moment created by these constructs is exaggerated when shorter constructs are employed. Short constructs, therefore, are more prone to the ill effects of this pivoting movement than longer constructs. Thus, longer constructs using hooks or wires are more efficacious than shorter ones using hooks or wires. This is particularly so in osteoporotic patients. This difference may be minimized by the placement of shorter constructs in a compression mode[2] (Fig. 16-6).

Location of the Unstable Spinal Segment

The nearer the pathological process or unstable spinal segment to the occiput or sacrum, the less leverage is applied by the terminal end of the implant (i.e., the shorter the lever arm). Therefore, rigid implant-bone interfaces are often desirable at the terminal end of the construct.

Implant Length

The degree of the instability largely dictates the extent of instrumentation used. Longer constructs are more effective at maintaining alignment—all other factors being equal—than shorter ones. They achieve this by employing longer lever arms (moment arms).

An *instrumentation-fusion mismatch* is a discrepancy

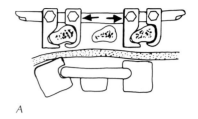

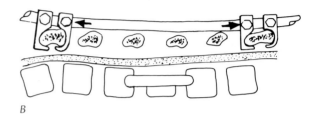

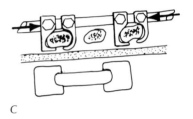

FIGURE 16-6 *A.* The placement of a short construct in a distraction mode causes an excessive pivoting moment to be placed at the implant-bone interfaces. *B.* Although a similar pivoting moment is applied at the terminal implant-bone interfaces of longer constructs, the resulting pivoting motion has less effect on the unstable spinal segment. *C.* The placement of the construct in a compression mode allows the "sharing" of the axial load between the spine and the construct.

between the number of spinal levels incorporated within an instrumentation construct and the number of spinal levels fused [i.e., between the number of fused segments and the (greater) number of instrumented segments]. Long spinal fusions often immobilize an excessive length of the spine. This reduces the chance for the acquisition of spinal fusion. On the other hand, the fusion of only the unstable spinal segments, with a long instrumentation construct used to gain the leverage needed for a solid fusion (instrumentation-fusion mismatch), creates the potential for the implant eventually to "work out" of the unfused, but instrumented, segments.

For these reasons, rigid shorter implants that incorporate only the segmental levels fused are optimal. The use of such short implants is called *short segment fixation*.[2,3]

In cases where instrumentation-fusion mismatch exists, some tolerance for movement at the unfused implant/bone interfaces is mandatory. Hooks and wires allow some movement at this interface; screws do not. The fact that screws do not allow movement without becoming overtly incompetent (at least in a screw-pullout sense) implies that *if an instrumentation-fusion mismatch is planned, screws should not be used as the implant-bone interface in the unfused segments.*

As a general rule of thumb, when long constructs are employed (usually three-point bending constructs or universal spinal instrumentation systems), an additional spinal level above the unstable spinal segment should be incorporated by the instrumentation construct. This allows the use of similar lengths of instrumentation construct above and below the unstable spinal segment. The points of attachment for hooks or wires are at the lower extent of the vertebral body (i.e., about one-half of a spinal segment *lower* than the middle of the vertebral body). This is illustrated in Fig. 16-7*A*. When failure of a long instrumentation system occurs, the upper rostral fixation points most commonly fail. This is often due to a lever arm of inadequate length and to the relatively poor fixation achieved. This may be the case when a 2A-2B construct (2 segments above and 2 segments below the unstable segment) is employed. Therefore, the extension of the construct rostrally by one segment (3A-

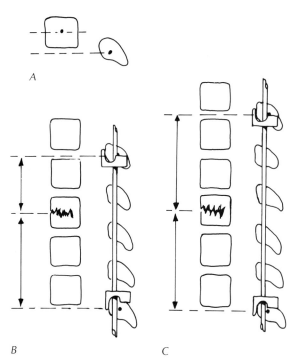

FIGURE 16-7 *A.* The points of attachment on the spinal segment of hooks or wires are at the caudal portion of the spinal segment. This is about one-half of a spinal segment *below* the centroid of the spinal segment. This discrepancy becomes clinically manifest in the definition of the length of the moment arm applied by the construct. *B.* A 2A-2B (2 above and 2 below the unstable segment) three-point bending hook/rod construct. The lever arm (moment arm) rostral to the unstable segment is shorter than the caudal moment arm. *C.* Extending the construct rostrally another level causes the rostral and caudal moment arms to be of roughly equal lengths.

2B) provides a longer and more efficient moment arm, which strengthens this weaker link (Fig. 16-7*B* and *C*).[2]

The 3A-2B configuration is a logical compromise between the problems associated with longer constructs and the shorter moment arm achieved with shorter ones. This is especially so when universal spinal instrumentation constructs are used, with their inherent multisegmental points of secure fixation.

In cases of extreme or multilevel instability, longer constructs may be appropriate. A 4A-3B construct is an example of such an approach (Fig. 16-8). Short segment fixation provides an increasingly popular alternative, especially when applied in a compressive, load-sharing manner (Fig. 16-9).[2,3]

Crossfixation

Crossfixation usually is not necessary for short segment fixation unless it helps reduce the deformity. For longer constructs—especially hook-rod systems—crossfixation most certainly assists in the stabilization process. It creates a quadrilateral frame construct. This resists torsional deformation of the rods about each other (Fig. 16-10*A* and *B*) and helps to minimize the chance of hook-bone interface failure. The latter benefit is acheived via the minimization of the chance that hook-bone interfaces will fail one at a time. Since all hooks are rigidly interconnected by the crossmember(s), several hooks would have to fail simultaneously in order for the system to fail at the implant-bone interface. The likelihood of this is small (Fig. 16-10*C*).

With long constructs, two crossmembers are better than one. Three or more crossmembers offer no significant advantage over two. Terminal crossmembers are not as efficient as more centrally placed crossmembers. In general, the two crossmembers should be placed roughly at the junctions of the middle third of the construct with the two terminal thirds of the construct.

Axial Load-Bearing Capacity of the Instrumented Spine

The need for surgical reconstitution of spinal integrity is an extremely important consideration in the choice of instrumentation constructs. Of prime importance in this regard is the ability of the spine to bear axial loads. If adequate axial load-bearing capacity already exists or has been surgically recreated, the load-bearing responsibilities of the spinal implant are less than if adequate axial load-bearing capacity does not exist or cannot be restored.

In cases where axial load-bearing capacity exists, as in that of a grade 1 degenerative L4-L5 spondylolisthesis (glacial instability), the role, and thus the design requirements, of the spinal implant are much different from those in an overtly unstable spine. In the former case the spinal implant serves two main purposes. First, it theoretically increases the rate of fusion. Second, it theoretically minimizes the

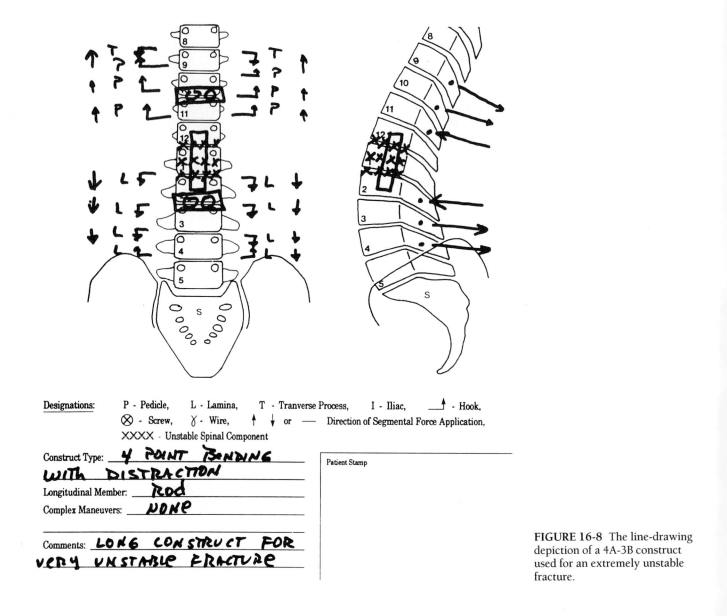

Designations: P - Pedicle, L - Lamina, T - Tranverse Process, I - Iliac, ⌐↑ - Hook,
⊗ - Screw, γ - Wire, ↑ ↓ or — Direction of Segmental Force Application,
XXXX - Unstable Spinal Component

Construct Type: __4 POINT BENDING WITH DISTRACTION__

Longitudinal Member: __Rod__

Complex Maneuvers: __NONE__

Comments: __LONG CONSTRUCT FOR VERY UNSTABLE FRACTURE__

Patient Stamp

FIGURE 16-8 The line-drawing depiction of a 4A-3B construct used for an extremely unstable fracture.

chance of translational deformation. In the latter case, besides serving these two purposes, it also assists in the bearing of the axial load.

If axial load-bearing capacity is inadequate, the instrumentation construct must both prevent translational deformation and provide axial load support. The provision of axial load support by the spinal implant dictates that the construct do some or all of the load-bearing for the unstable spinal segment during the acquisition of solid fusion. Long distraction or three-point bending constructs and short fixed or applied moment arm cantilever beam constructs are suitable to this task.

If adequate axial load-bearing capacity exists, a substantial portion of the axial load may be borne by the remaining intrinsic strength of the spine. The surgeon may take advan-

tage of this. By definition, in this situation the instrumentation construct need not bear all of the axial load. Therefore, it need not apply an excessively long lever arm to the spine in order to achieve stability. In other words, in this situation a shorter construct may be as effective as a longer one. Furthermore, the instrumentation construct may be placed in a compression mode, which causes the load to be shared between the spine itself and the instrumentation construct.[2,3] As has been said elsewhere, *the placement of a spinal implant in a compression mode requires that the dural sac be adequately decompressed and that any existing neural impingement be immune to exaggeration by the application of compression forces to the spine.*[2,4] Cantilever beam and tension-band fixation constructs can be used for this purpose.

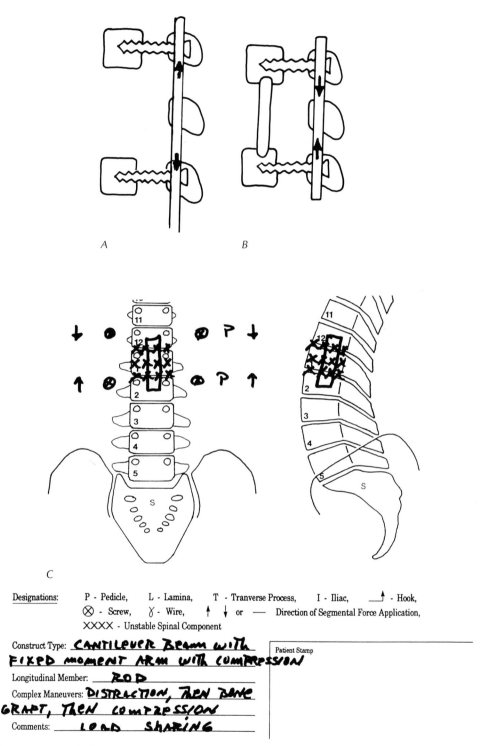

A

B

C

Designations: P - Pedicle,   L - Lamina,   T - Tranverse Process,   I - Iliac,   ⌐̶ - Hook,

$\otimes$ - Screw,   ɣ - Wire,   ↑ ↓ or ── Direction of Segmental Force Application,

XXXX - Unstable Spinal Component

Construct Type: **CANTILEVER BEAM WITH FIXED MOMENT ARM WITH COMPRESSION**

Longitudinal Member: **ROD**

Complex Maneuvers: **DISTRACTION, THEN BONE GRAFT, THEN COMPRESSION**

Comments: **LOAD SHARING**

Patient Stamp

FIGURE 16-9 A short segment pedicle screw fixation construct used for an unstable fracture. *A.* The device was initially placed in a distraction mode during ventral interbody bone graft placement, to provide room for the bone graft. *B.* It was then placed in a compression mode, to secure the bone graft and to cause sharing of the axial load between the bone graft and intrinsic vertebral axial load-resisting capacity and the instrumentation construct. Failure of the construct will occur less often if the spine and bone graft are "asked" to assume a portion of the axial load-bearing responsibilities (see Chap. 7). *C.* The line drawing of such a construct.

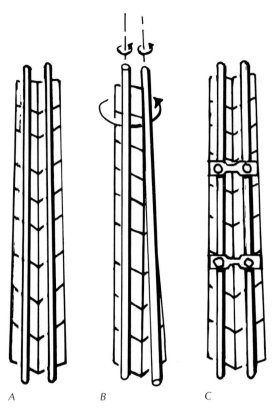

FIGURE 16-10 The effects of crossfixation. Torsional stresses that result in rotation of one rod about the other (*A* and *B*) are effectively resisted by rigid crosslinking of one rod to the other (*C*). When hook-bone interfaces fail, they usually fail one at a time. The rigid crosslinking of one rod to the other minimizes the chance of failure by requiring multiple hook-bone interfaces to fail simultaneously, which is much less likely. With long rod systems, the two crosslinks should be placed approximately at the junctions of the terminal thirds of the construct with the middle third.

Orientation of the Instability

The orientation of the instability largely dictates the choice of construct type. Translational instability in the sagittal plane often dictates that a three-point bending component of the construct be employed to reduce the deformity or "hold" spinal alignment. Screws, sublaminar wires, or hooks may be used.

The use of pedicle screws to reduce or "hold" a translational deformity in the sagittal plane requires that the screw-bone interface resist pullout. Screw-bone interfaces are notoriously weak in this sense. Furthermore, bicortical screw purchase may *not* provide a significant advantage in this regard (see Chap. 13).[5] Hooks and sublaminar wires more effectively resist pullout.

Flexion (kyphotic), extension (lordotic), or lateral-bending (scoliotic) deformities often require complex instrumentation techniques, such as the use of compression fixation (tension-band fixation) on the convex side and/or distraction fixation on the convex side of the deformation. Alternatively, spinal derotation maneuvers may be most appropriate.

True axial-load injuries (burst fractures) may be treated with any of the construct types, given appropriate application. The surgeon's preference and armamentarium dictates which is used.

The Need for Dural Sac Decompression

As a rule, adequate dural sac decompression prior to the placement of a compress construct is mandatory (see Chap. 15). Both anterior and posterior decompressive operations, however, are performed at the expense of structural stability.

The Armamentarium of the Surgeon

The armamentarium of the surgeon may be a major factor in implant selection and in the implementation process. For example, the inability to decompress ventral compressive lesions rules out the use of a dorsal compression construct. The inability to place pedicle screws dictates that hooks or wires be used. Limitations like these are obviously liabilities. Thus the surgeon is rewarded for his or her surgical and clinical acumen.

REFERENCES

1. Benzel EC: Construct design, in Benzel EC (ed): *Spinal Instrumentation.* AANS Publications, 1994.
2. Benzel EC: Short segment compression instrumentation for selected thoracic and lumbar spine fractures: The short rod–two claw (SRTC) technique. *J Neurosurg* 79:335–340, 1993.
3. Benzel EC: Short segment fixation, in Benzel EC (ed): *Spinal Instrumentation.* AANS Publications, 1994.
4. Benzel EC: Biomechanics of lumbar and lumbosacral spine fractures, in Rea GL, Miller CA (eds): *Spine Trauma: Current Evaluation and Management.* AANS Publications, 1993, 165–195.
5. Maiman DJ, Pintar FA, Yoganandan N, et al: Pull-out strength of Caspar cervical screws. *Neurosurgery* 1992;31:1097–1101.

Part V

Anterior Spinal Instrumentation Constructs

Historical and Anatomic Perspective of Anterior Spinal Instrumentation Constructs

It is, indeed, desirable to place an instrumentation construct in a ventral location on the spine if a ventral spinal decompression and fusion operation is performed simultaneously. Attempts at a clinical application of anterior spinal instrumentation, however, have met with varying degress of success.[1,2] One of the first attempts at anterior spinal instrumentation was made by Milgram in 1953. This was unsuccessful.[3] Humphries and coworkers also reported an unsuccessful use of an anterior interbody fusion clamp.[4]

Dwyer was among the first to achieve successful surgical insertion of an instrumentation construct in the anterior thoracic and lumbar spine.[5-7] The Zielke technique, developed subsequently, was usually used for the fixation of fewer spinal segments.[8] Harrington then reported the use of Knodt rods or Harrington distraction rods, combined with acrylic augmentation for ventral spinal use.[9] This was followed by the development of the Kostuik-Harrington distraction system.[3]

Kaneda and coworkers developed a technique of spiked vertebral plates attached to the vertebral bodies via screws interconnected by rigid rods.[10,11] A wide variety of techniques have subsequently been employed clinically.[3,12-17]

The Rezaian device was developed for interbody distraction fixation.[18] It provides a ventral spinal distraction, as do the Kaneda, Kostuik, and Amset devices. The Rezaian device provides simple distraction only, whereas the Kaneda device, for example, provides the option of applying compression or distraction and a method of applying a cantilever beam fixation force to the spine. Other types of system may also be employed ventrally—for example, acrylic or bone.

The Texas Scottish Rite Hospital rod system has been applied as one might use a Kaneda device. It appears to be equally versatile; in addition, the screws are rigidly attached to the rod (cantilever bending with a fixed moment arm). This lessens the need for bicortical screw purchase.

Only recently have anterior instrumentation constructs been applied to the cervical region of the spine. Caspar developed a semiconstrained (semirigid or dynamic) plate system that uses a screw purchase on the posterior vertebral body cortex,[19] and Morcher developed a constrained (rigid) plate system that uses a screw-plate locking mechanism.[20]

Ventral spine approaches for the application of instrumentation are the same as those used routinely for any ventral spinal surgery (see Chap. 8). In the cervical region, if extensive longitudinal exposure is required, a diagonal, rather than horizontal, skin crease incision helps to increase the length of exposure. Ventral exposure for the cervicothoracic region may be gained through the thoracic inlet, via a manubrium-splitting approach, or via the lateral extracavitary or transcavitary approach. In the midthoracic region the ventral spine may be approached via the anterior transthoracic approach or the lateral extracavitary or transcavitary approach.

The thoracolumbar region presents significant anatomic barriers on account of the confines of the diaphragm and associated structures. Nevertheless, via appropriate dissection and appropriate consideration of anatomy, this region can be exposed ventrally. It can also be approached via the lateral extracavitary approach. From L2 inferiorly, the ventral lumbar spine can be approached through the anterolateral extracavitary or lateral extracavitary approach, or even via the transperitoneal approach. The lumbosacral region can be approached via the transperitoneal approach for low (sacral) lesions, the Pfannenstiel extraperitoneal approach, the anterolateral extraperitoneal approach, or the lateral extracavitary approach. The latter requires substantial iliac crest removal to gain access to the sacrum.

Spinal instrumentation constructs are discussed from a biomechanical viewpoint in the several chapters that follow. Although much information is provided about clinically used spinal implants, this information is most certainly not complete, nor is it intended to be so. It is designed to place the final touches on a clinically practical understanding of spinal biomechanics as applied to spinal instrumentation.

REFERENCES

1. Benzel EC: Short segment fixation of the thoracic and lumbar spine, in Benzel EC (ed): *Spinal Instrumentation*. AANS Publications, 1994.
2. Benzel EC, Ball PA: History of spinal instrumentation, in Benzel EC (ed):*Spinal Instrumentation*. AANS Publications, 1993:3–10.
3. Kostuik JP: Anterior fixation for burst fractures of the thoracic and lumbar spine with or without neurologic involvement. *Spine* 1988;13:286–293.
4. Humphries AW, Hawk WA, Berndt AL: Anterior interbody fusion of lumbar vertebrae: A surgical technique. *Surg Clin North Am* 1961;41:1685–1700.
5. Dwyer AF, Newton NC, Sherwood AA: An anterior approach to scoliosis: A preliminary report. *Clin Orthop* 1969;62:192–202.
6. Dwyer AF, Schafer MF: Anterior approach to scoliosis. *J Bone Joint Surg* 1974;56B:218–224.
7. Hall JE: Dwyer instrumentation in anterior fusion of the spine—Current concepts and review. *J Bone Joint Surg* 1981;63A:1188–1190.
8. Kaneda K, Fujiya N, Satoh S: Results with Zielke instrumentation for idiopathic thoracolumbar and lumbar scoliosis. *Clin Orthop* 1986;205:195–203.
9. Harrington KD: The use of methylmethacrylate for vertebral body replacement and anterior stabilization of pathological fracture dislocations of the spine due to metastatic malignant disease. *J Bone Joint Surg* 1981;63A:36–46.
10. Kaneda K: Kaneda anterior spinal instrumentation for the thoracic and lumbar spine, in An HS, Cotler JM (eds): *Spinal Instrumentation*. Baltimore: Williams and Wilkins, 1992:413–433.
11. Kaneda K, Abumi K, Fujiya M: Burst fractures with neurologic deficits of the thoracolumbar-lumbar spine. *Spine* 1984;9:788–795.
12. Black RC, Gardner VO, Armstrong GWD, et al: A contoured anterior spinal fixation plate. *Clin Orthop* 1988;227:135–142.
13. Bone LB, Ashman RB, Roach JW, Johnston CE: Mechanical comparison of anterior spine instrumentation in a burst fracture model. *Orthop Trans* 1987;11:87.
14. Chang KW: Late anterior decompression for incomplete neural deficit secondary to thoracolumbar fractures. *J Surg Assoc ROC* 1989;22:407–414.
15. Dunn HK: Anterior stabilization of thoracolumbar injuries. *Clin Orthop* 1984;189:116–124.
16. Dunn HK: Anterior spine stabilization and decompression for thoracolumbar injuries. *Orthop Clin North Am* 1986;17:113–119.
17. Yuan HA, Mann KA, Found EM, et al: Early clinical experience with the Syracuse I-plate: An anterior spinal fixation device. *Spine* 1988;13:278–285.
18. Dombrowski ET: Rezaian fixator in the anterior stabilization of unstable spine. *Orthop Rev* 1986;15:66–69.
19. Caspar W, Barbier DD, Klara PM: Anterior cervical fusion and Caspar plate stabilization for cervical trauma. *Neurosurgery* 1989;25:491–502.
20. Johnsson H, Cesarini K, Petren-Mallmin M, Raushning W. Locking screw-plate fixation of cervical fractures with and without ancillary posterior plating. *Arch Orthop Trauma Surg* 1991;111:1–12.

Chapter 18

Anterior Spinal Neutral and Distraction Fixation

Anterior interbody spinal distraction may result either from the placement of distraction at the time of surgery or from the placement of a neutral construct in an interbody position at the time of surgery, with the expectation that the construct will subsequently bear an axial load—effectively distracting the spine by applying a resistance to compression (see Chap. 15). Therefore, for the purposes of this chapter, the term *anterior distraction fixation* applies to distraction *and* neutral fixation, unless otherwise specified.

Spinal distraction is similar, but opposite in direction, to force application through tension-band fixation (compression). A comparison of these two techniques, however, is much more complex than simply contrasting them in this manner. For example, the application of distraction force to the spine does not always result in the same type of force application (see Chap. 15). The location of the instantaneous axis of rotation (IAR) in relation to the points of instrumentation-related force application is critical to the definition of the types of forces applied. If the point of application of the force by the construct is ventral to the IAR, forces opposite in orientation, but similar in nature, to tension-band fixation are applied (Fig. 18-1*A*). These are cantilever beam constructs (see Chap. 15).

However, if the point of application of the force by the construct is in line with with the IAR, tension-band-like forces are not applied to the spine (Fig. 18-1*B*). These are simple distraction (buttress) constructs (see Chap. 15). Tension-band forces require a moment arm in order to achieve their desired result. This moment arm is the perpendicular distance from the point of application of the forces (by the construct) to the IAR. If this type of force is applied in the opposite direction (i.e., in a distraction mode), either distraction with extension (Fig. 18-2*A*) or a three-point bending type of fixation is achieved (Fig. 18-2*B*). The former could be considered tension-band distraction fixation (see Chap. 15).

For anterior interbody neutral or distraction fixation to be effective as a technique, intrinsic or surgically created resistance to distraction and/or spinal bracing is required. For example, ligamentous resistance to distraction causes an intrinsic compression of the bone graft into both ends of the strut (see Chaps. 9 and 10), thus providing greater security to the strut graft–mortise relationship.

Similarly, distraction as applied by a semiconstrained (semirigid or dynamic) screw-plate device requires that adequate posterior spinal stability be present. A screw-plate construct, regardless of the mode of application, is effective in resisting axial loads and spinal extension but not in resisting flexion. In this situation, plate bending or screw cut-out may occur following flexion. If posterior spinal stability is present or created, these complications are less likely (Fig. 18-3).

TECHNIQUES

The two fundamental types of anterior distraction spinal implant are (1) an interbody strut that buttresses the spine (Fig. 18-4) and (2) a cantilever beam that uses screws, hooks, or staples in either a fixed moment arm, a nonfixed moment arm, or an applied moment arm configuration (Fig. 18-5). Bone, acrylic, or metal implants (such as the Rezaian device) can be used for the first type; each form of the second can be applied by by a variety of systems.

CLINICAL APPLICATIONS

The decision to use an interbody buttress or a cantilever beam technique with either a fixed moment arm, a nonfixed moment arm, or an applied moment arm is of critical importance. *All too often instrumentation techniques are chosen in*

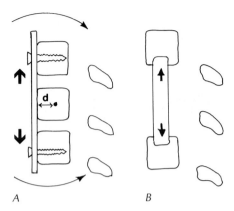

A   B

FIGURE 18-1 *A.* The application of a distraction force to the anterior aspect of the vertebral body (ventral to the neutral axis) results in a construct configured like a cantilever, with the application of a moment arm. *B.* The application of a distraction force to the mid–vertebral body region (in the region of the neutral axis) results in buttressing of the spine, without the application of a moment arm. *d* = moment arm; straight arrows depict implant force applications; curved arrows depict bending moments.

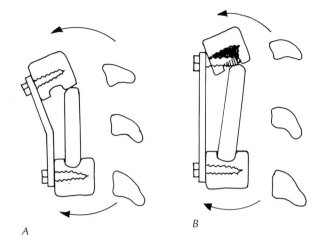

A   B

FIGURE 18-3 Plant bending (*A*) or screw cutout (*B*) may occur if posterior spinal stability is not adequate. The ventral spinal implant can function adequately as a buttress, but not as an effective limiter or flexion deformation.

a cavalier manner, with too little attention to biomechanics. Questions that should be asked prior to the application of instrumentation include the following: Is a spinal implant indicated? Is a rigid or dynamic implant desired or required? Is deformity reduction required, or simply deformity prevention? These questions are not easily answered. Their routine preoperative consideration ensures that the surgeon is

at least placing physical and biomechanical principles in their rightful place—high on the list of preoperative considerations.

Cervical Spine

In the cervical spine, interbody strut buttressing and fixed and nonfixed cantilever beam fixation techniques are

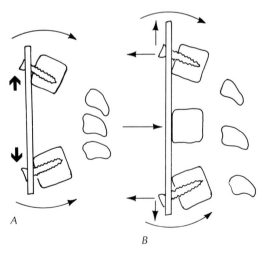

A   B

FIGURE 18-2 *A.* The application of an anterior screw-plate construct in a distraction and extension. The latter occurs because the point of force application by the construct is ventral to the neutral axis. *B.* If a fulcrum intervenes between the termini of the construct, the attainment of security of the construct results in less spinal extension via three-point bending force application. Straight arrows depict implant force applications; curved arrows depict resulting bending moment.

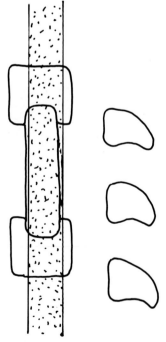

FIGURE 18-4 An interbody strut buttresses the spine by being aligned with the neutral axis. The neutral axis is depicted by the stippled area.

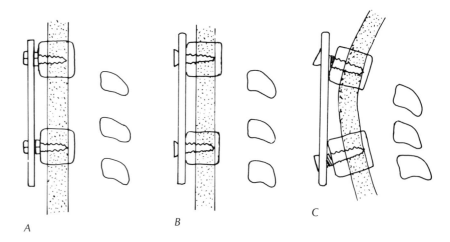

FIGURE 18-5 Cantilever beam fixation stabilizes the spine via the use of a fixed or applied moment arm (*A*) or a nonfixed moment arm (*B*). The fixed or applied moment arm construct functions, in a sense, as a buttress, by "encompassing" the neutral axis. The nonfixed moment arm construct distracts and extends the spine if applied in a distraction mode (see Fig. 18-2*A*). Axial load-bearing may result in spinal extension, because the implant is placed ventral to the neutral axis, and toggling of the screw on the plate is not restricted by this implant (*C*). The neutral axis is depicted by the stippled area.

used—frequently in combination with each other (e.g., simultaneous use of a cantilever beam construct with an interbody bone graft). One must consider preoperatively which technique, if any, is most appropriate to the situation at hand. Is posterior stability adequate? Are the stresses that the construct will be expected to withstand, such that a buttress alone will suffice, reasonable? If greater stability is required from the implant, is a rigid rather than a more dynamic construct more appopriate (Fig. 18-6)?

Since the techniques discussed in this chapter are often used on a distracted spine at the time of surgery and subsequently expected to withstand additional axial loads during the assumption of the upright posture, they are distraction implants. However, because of their obvious cantilever beam configuration, they are additionally discussed in Chap. 20.

Thoracic and Lumbar Spine

Thoracic and lumbar anterior spinal distraction fixation techniques have biomechanical attributes like those of their cervical counterparts. Slight differences, however, do exist—such as the use of ventral rod-screw systems and the need for more substantial constructs on account of the greater stresses applied to them.

MULTISEGMENTAL FIXATION

Multisegmental fixation is not routinely used in the ventral spine—especially not for distraction purposes. Limiting factors include the often-inadequate ventral spinal longitudinal exposure as well as the relatively weak implant–vertebral body interface. The vertebral body is predominantly medullary (cancellous) bone. Its noncompact makeup makes implant purchase sites relatively weak. Attempts to obviate this problem, such as bicortical screw purchase, are potentially dangerous and may not be biomechanically sound (see Chap. 13).

COMPLICATIONS

The impaction of the graft into the vertebral body as a toothpick might penetrate styrofoam must be recognized as a possibility. This may be compensated for, in part, by use of the endplates of the vertebral bodies as barriers to this type of penetration. The creation of a deep mortise may have sig-

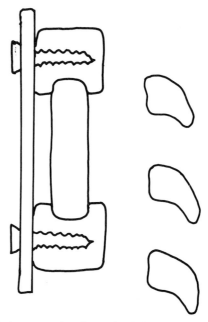

FIGURE 18-6 As an isolated spinal stabilizer, a rigid construct (e.g., a fixed moment arm cantilever beam construct) provides greater stability than a semirigid one (e.g., a nonfixed moment arm cantilever beam construct). The nonfixed moment arm construct allows movement that a rigid construct does not (see Fig. 18-5). However, the nonfixed moment arm construct, if applied appropriately with an accompanying interbody buttress (e.g., an interbody bone graft), may be desirable, as depicted. This is especially so if the spine is distracted, the buttress inserted securely into its interbody position, and the construct then compressed (see Chap. 16).

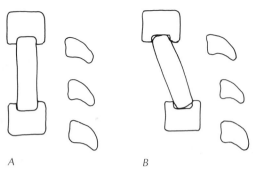

A   B

FIGURE 18-7 "Pole vaulting" of the spine (translational deformation, with the bone graft functioning as the "vaulting pole") may follow anterior interbody buttress placement without adequate accompanying posterior stabilization.

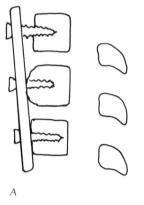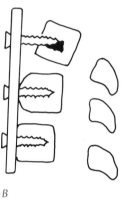

A   B

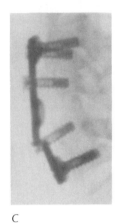

C

FIGURE 18-8 The inadvertent application of a three-point bending force complex to the spine may result in excessive force application unbeknownst to the surgeon (A). Screw pullout or cutout (B) or plate fracture (C) may occur.

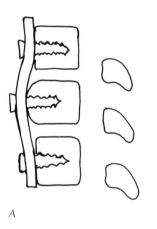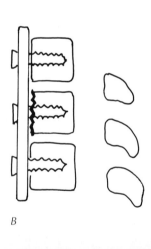

A   B

FIGURE 18-9 The complications shown in Fig. 18-8 may be prevented by adequate plate contouring (A) or ventral spinal surface fashioning (B) so that no three-point bending forces are applied to the spine or plate.

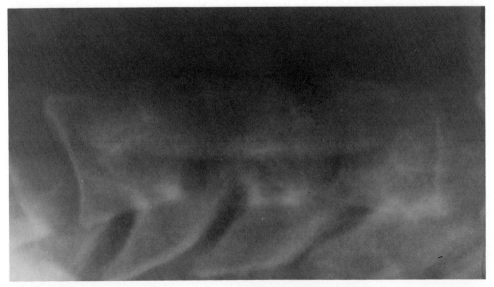

FIGURE 18-10 The creation of deep mortises with an accompanying well-fitted bone graft provides a snug fit, as depicted. Additional instrumentation may not be necessary.

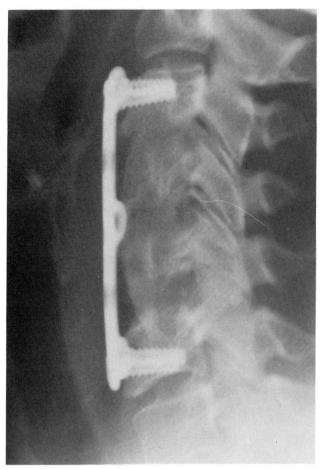

FIGURE 18-11 Security may be enhanced in some cases by the addition of a cantilever beam construct to an anterior interbody fusion. This is depicted in the form of a fixed moment arm cantilever beam construct. In some cases this may obviate the need for placement of a posterior construct.

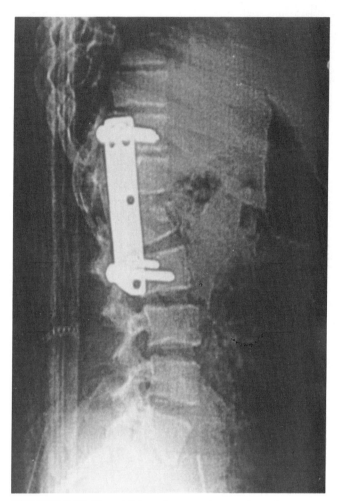

FIGURE 18-12 The addition of an anterior cantilever beam construct to an anterior interbody fusion in the thoracic or lumbar region may also be beneficial. In some cases this may obviate the need for the placement of a posterior construct.

nificant advantages for such a construct. It may help prevent one of the most common complications of this type of fixation: the "pole vaulting" of adjacent vertebral bodies past each other, with the distraction fixation construct serving as the pole (see Chap. 10 and Fig. 18-7). This may be prevented by the use of a different construct altogether, by the creation of a deeper and more appropriate mortise for the distraction construct, or by the use of an accompanying posterior construct.

Although an anterior three-point bending construct may be desirable in some circumstances, it is most often applied inadvertently. The planned or inadvertent application of an anterior screw-plate construct in a three-point bending mode can be used to reduce spinal deformation (Fig. 18-2*B*

and *C*). However, it may result in screw pullout or cutout, or in plate fracture (Fig. 18-8). The contouring of the plate or the bone may minimize the occurrence of this complication (Fig. 18-9).

CLINICAL EXAMPLES

Anterior cervical fusion without instrumentation exemplifies the interbody strut that applies either a neutral or a distractive force at the time of surgery (Fig. 18-10). The addition of an anterior cervical plate may add to the security of fixation (Fig. 18-11). Anterior cantilever beams may be applied in the thoracic or lumbar spine as well (Fig. 18-12).

Chapter 19

Anterior Spinal Compression (Tension-Band) Fixation

INTRODUCTION

Anterior cantilever beam constructs (with or without a non-fixed moment arm) are considered anterior compression fixation *(tension-band fixation)* devices if they resist distraction of the spine. This concept is similar, but opposite in orientation, to those forces and mechanisms associated with non-interbody anterior distraction fixation (Fig. 19-1). These constructs, however, may fail in flexion, much as their distraction counterparts may (see Chap. 18). This has to do mainly with their inherent inability to compensate for absent or lost intrinsic posterior tension-band (compression) characteristics. It should be evident that interbody compression fixation devices are impractical; and they are not used clinically.

Cantilever beam constructs and true tension-band fixation devices, such as the Dwyer apparatus, resist distraction better than flexion (the Dwyer apparatus much more so than cantilever beam constructs). They resist bending in the plane of their application and in an orientation *opposite* the side of their application (Fig. 19-2).

TECHNIQUES

Unlike anterior distraction techniques, anterior compression techniques cannot use an interbody strut to apply forces to the spine. Therefore, fixation techniques that employ hook-bone, screw-bone, staple-bone fixation, and so on, are used. These include the same screw-plate techniques described in Chap. 18. As with anterior distraction techniques, a fundamental difference between cervical, thoracic, and lumbar techniques is the relative inability to use rods in the cervical region; thus, significant compression or distraction cannot be accomplished there.

CLINICAL APPLICATION

Spinal compression allows the surgeon to allow the instrumentation construct to share the bearing of axial loads with the spine. The load is shared either by spinal elements, with their intrinsic spinal integrity, or by interbody strut graft placement (see Chaps. 10, 15, and 18).

The rationale for the use of compression techniques in this regard was briefly outlined in Chap. 15. Suffice it to say that the compression applied by the spinal implant neutralizes the axial forces subsequently accepted by the spine-implant combination. This concept is applicable, however, only if the spine, with or without the interbody strut graft, is capable of accepting its share of the load (Fig. 19-3).

Cervical Spine

Since systems that incorporate rods have not, to date, been used in the anterior cervical spine, screw-plate systems predominate in this region. Therefore, tension-band fixation in compression and cantilever beam fixation are the only biomechanical advantages that can be achieved by these techniques. Both essentially resist extension; both are, therefore, in addition to their cantilever beam properties, tension-band fixators.

Thoracic and Lumbar Spine

The ability to use a rod-screw or equivalent construct (such as the Kaneda device) in the thoracic and lumbar spine provides an additional dimension to anterior compression fixation in this region. As mentioned above, compression force application by the construct allows the sharing of the load with the spine or interbody strut. This can be enhanced by

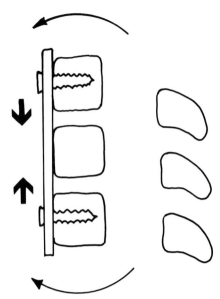

FIGURE 19-1 The forces applied by screw-plate anterior compression fixation. Straight arrows depict implant force applications; curved arrows depict bending moments.

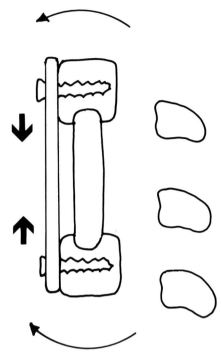

FIGURE 19-3 Tension-band fixation is applicable only in situations where axial load-bearing abilities (either instrinsic or surgically created, as depicted) are present. In such cases the tension-band fixation construct is able to form a load-sharing construct in which the spinal elements share the load with the construct. Straight arrows depict implant force applications; curved arrows depict resulting bending moments.

distraction of the spine with subsequent placement of the interbody graft. (Not all techniques allow this, because of physical limitations of the implant and anatomic limitations of the spine.) The construct may then be compressed onto the previously placed interbody strut graft. This allows (1) increased security of the interbody strut graft–mortise interface, (2) sharing of the load between the implant and the

strut graft, and (3) augmentation of bone-healing-enhancing forces (compression) (see Chap. 10).

MULTISEGMENTAL FIXATION

As with anterior distraction fixation (see Chap. 18), significant longitudinal anterior spinal exposure is often difficult to achieve, and implant-bone fixation points are relatively weak (compared to their dorsal counterparts, such as sublaminar hooks or screws that pass through the pedicle and the vertebral body). Therefore, multisegmental compression fixation is not often employed in its purest sense.

With long anterior compression fixation techniques, care must be taken to minimize the chance of the application of terminal bending moments, as can occur with posterior techniques (see Chap. 15) (Fig. 19-4).

The Dwyer device, or a modification of it made by replacing the cable by a rod (Zielke apparatus), is an exception to this. This technique has been used to achieve deformity correction by the application of compression forces on the convex side of the curvature, via multisegmental points of fixation (Fig. 19-5).

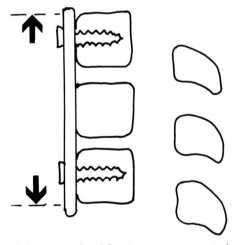

FIGURE 19-2 Tension-band fixation constructs resist bending in the plane of their application and in an orientation opposite the side of their location. In this case the implant resists spinal extension because it is in a ventral location.

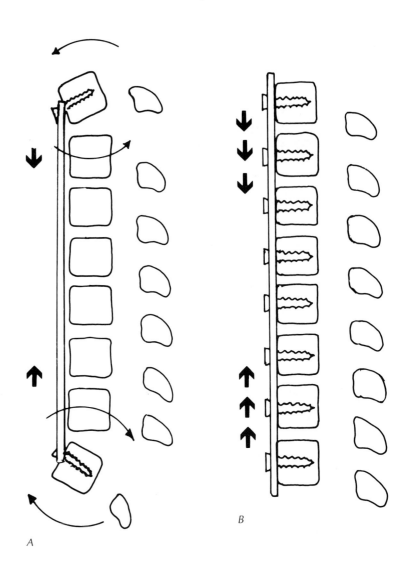

FIGURE 19-4 *A.* Terminal bending moments (*curved arrows*) may become manifest in situations where excessively long tension-band fixation forces (*straight arrows*) are applied to the spine. *B.* Fixating the spine at multiple intervening locations, and thus spreading the load borne by the implant over multiple spinal levels (multisegmental fixation) may eliminate this phenomenon.

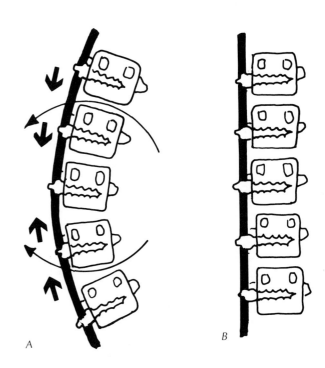

FIGURE 19-5 *A.* The Dwyer and Zielke devices apply compression fixation (tension-band fixation) at multiple segmental levels of the spine. *B.* They are usually applied on the convex side of a scoliotic curvature in order to achieve reduction of the deformity. Straight arrows depict implant force applications; curved arrows depict resulting bending moments.

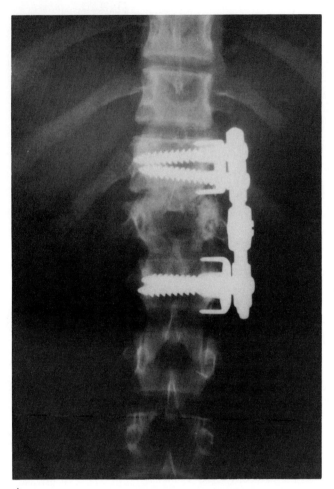

A

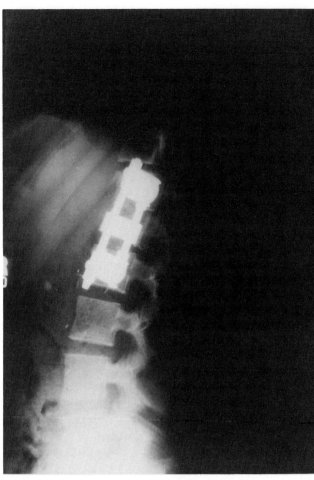

B

FIGURE 19-6 Some ventral devices can be placed in either a distraction or a compresssion mode. In the case depicted, the distraction and subsequent compression of the spine on an interbody bone graft is facilitated by the threaded-bolt-and-nut method of force application. *(Photograph courtesy of L.V. Ansel.)*

COMPLICATIONS

The complications of anterior spinal compression are similar to those of all ventral fixation techniques. The most common ones arise from inappropriate use of the technique. *One must not have unreasonable expectations of any implant.* Complications like those experienced with neutral or distraction fixation constructs may be experienced with common fixation (see Chap. 18).

CLINICAL EXAMPLES

There are few anterior compression techniques currently available. Many techniques perhaps could be applied in a compression mode, but are not designed for such application. Some, however, facilitate such use by providing a user-friendly method of applying compression intraoperatively (Fig. 19-6).

Chapter *20*

Anterior Cantilever Beam Fixation and Related Techniques

INTRODUCTION

Cantilever beam fixation constructs come in three fundamental types: fixed, nonfixed, and applied moment arm (see Chap. 15). Fixed and applied moment arm constructs provide what has been called *constrained* or *rigid* spinal fixation, whereas nonfixed moment arm fixation provides what has been called *semiconstrained, dynamic,* or *semirigid* fixation.

TECHNIQUES

These constructs may be applied from any orientation allowed by the anatomic restrictions of a given spinal segment. This means that these construct types can be placed in a direct anterior position (in the cervical, thoracic, and lumbar spine), as well as in a lateral position (in the thoracic and lumbar spine) (Fig. 20-1). For the constrained (rigid) constructs, the orientation of placement should matter little to spinal stability, unless the anatomic characteristics of the spine dictate length-of-moment-arm differences or the use of especially short, long, narrow, or wide screws (Fig. 20-2).

CLINICAL APPLICATIONS AND COMPLICATIONS

These techniques apply complex forces to the spine. Vertebral body or segmental rotation in the sagittal or coronal plane can be created by application of the devices in parallel with each other or by the use of specially designed constructs, such as the Kaneda device. The application of forces

in opposite directions achieves a rotatory force application. An *intrinsic implant bending moment* is achieved. In most circumstances previously described, implant-derived bending moments resulted from implant-derived force application to the spine through a moment arm [defined as the perpendicular distance from the instantaneous axis of rotation (IAR) to the point of application of the force]. With an intrinsic implant bending moment, the forces are applied by the implant, but the moment arm is also provided by the implant (Fig. 20-3). For optimal force application, the parallel rods should be placed far apart, thus lengthening the moment arm.

These deformity reduction techniques usually are applied to the lateral aspect of the spine (rather than the anterior aspect) in the thoracic and lumbar regions. Cross-fixation of the two segments minimizes the chance of subsequent parallelogram deformation (Fig. 20-4).

Other fixation applications may be used that are similar, if not identical, to those described in Chaps. 18 and 19. As with anterior distraction fixation, three-point bending-like forces may be simultaneously applied to the spine (see Chap. 18). These forces, too, are usually undesirable.

Finally, care must be taken to leave enough room on the surface, and within the vertebral body, for screw insertion. The creation of a deep mortise "takes up" a significant amount of room that could otherwise be used for screw insertion. Conversely, the placement of a ventral spinal plate "takes up" room that might be better used for the creation of a deep mortise. One must continuously assess and reassess the need for screw-plate insertion, especially if it would be done at the expense of interbody strut–vertebral body integrity (Fig. 20-5).

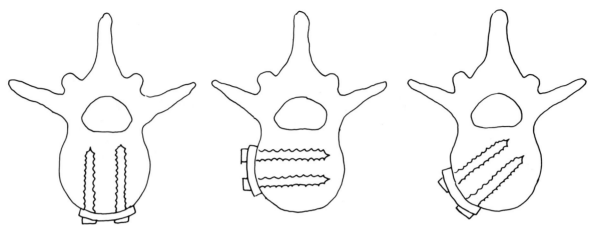

FIGURE 20-1 An anterior cantilever beam implant can be placed in a true anterior, lateral, or intermediate location.

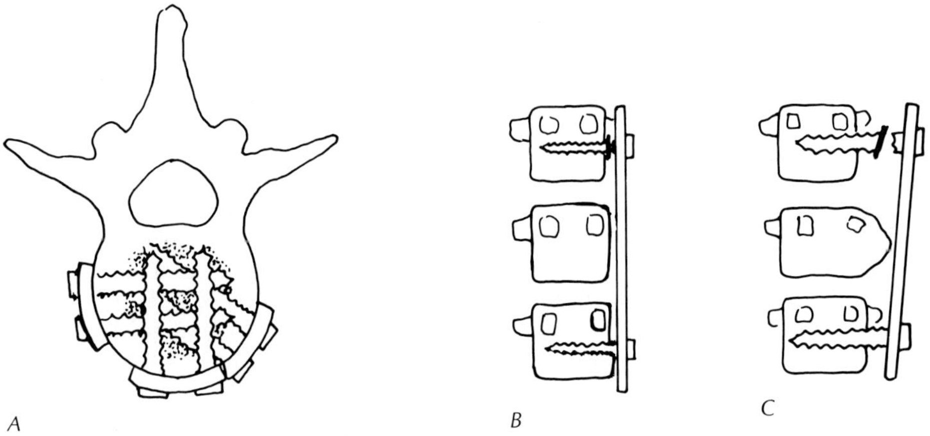

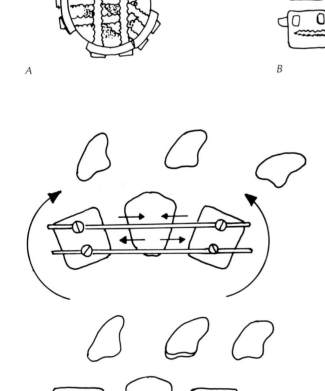

A *B* *C*

FIGURE 20-2 As long as the screws cross the neutral axis (*stippled area*), the orientation of constrained (rigid) implant application should not affect the construct's efficacy (*A*). The use of small diameter (*B*) or long (*C*) screws either of which may be dictated by the confines of the regional anatomy, may result in screw fracture.

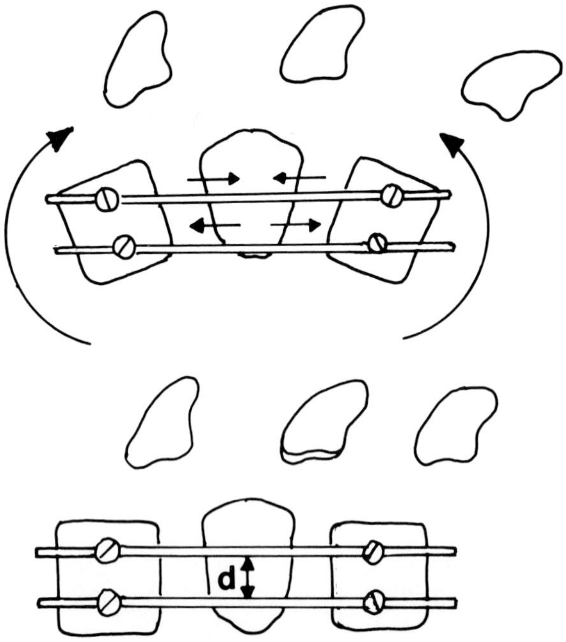

FIGURE 20-3 Intrinsic implant bending moment. Straight arrows depict the forces applied; curved arrows depict the resulting bending moment—in this case, the intrinsic implant bending moment. The greater the distance between the rods, the greater the efficacy achieved (via a greater applied bending moment). The bending moment is proportional to the length of the moment arm, *d*.

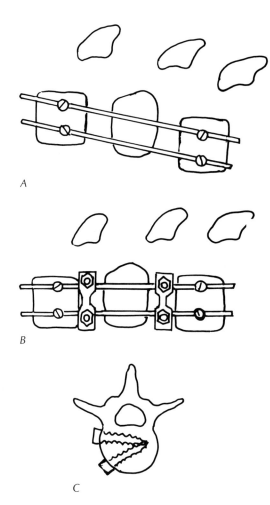

FIGURE 20-4 *A* and *B.* Rigidly crosslinking the two rods depicted in Fig. 20-3 minimizes the chance of parallelogram deformation. *C.* "Toeing-in" of the screws assists in this.

CLINICAL EXAMPLES

Many ventral instrumentation techniques are of a cantilever beam type. There is considerable overlap between those discussed in this chapter and those discussed in Chaps. 18 and

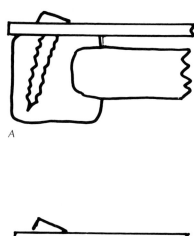

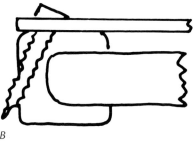

FIGURE 20-5 The dilemma associated with anterior screw-plate construct insertion. *A.* The use of a screw-plate construct somewhat compromises the insertion of a solid interbody strut graft. A shallower mortise is obligatory, so that screw trajectory will not be disturbed. *B.* If, on the other hand, a deep mortise is created and a solid bone graft–mortise relationship thus achieved, the insertion of screws is compromised by the relative spatial constraints at the vertebral body insertion site.

19. Both fixed and nonfixed moment arm cantilever beam constructs, as described in Chaps. 18 and 19, are cantilever beams and apply distraction, neutral, or compression forces to the spine. As shown in Fig. 20-5, great care must be taken to avoid inappropriate application of an implant, especially when it would interfere with bone graft security. Although the techniques may be identical, separate consideration of the principles involved is warranted.

Part VI

Posterior Spinal Instrumentation Constructs

Chapter 21

Historical and Anatomic Perspective of Posterior Instrumentation Constructs

Wire and/or screw fixation of the unstable spine was first reported around the turn of the century. In the United States these techniques remained quietly in vogue until the pre–World War II years.[1-4] During the same time, in Europe, Lange described the use of steel rods to stabilize the spine.[5] In this ill-conceived but innovative approach to spinal stabilization, the rods had no solid bony purchase. Success, therefore, was limited.

In the 20 years after World War II there were two breakthroughs in spinal surgery: the interspinous wiring technique of Rogers, and the Harrington system for spinal stabilization and deformity correction. Rogers described the technique of cervical interspinous wiring in the early 1940s.[6,7] Harrington introduced his instrumentation system in 1962.[8,9]

Since then, modifications of both the Rogers technique and the Harrington system were devised in order to increase the security of fixation. These included a variety of interspinous wiring modifications and the use of sleeves and square-ended modifications of Harrington rods.

The next significant advance in posterior spinal stabilization was the development of multisegmental spinal instrumentation. Multisegmental instrumentation allowed the sharing of the load applied to the instrumentation construct by multiple vertebrae, thus substantially decreasing the chance of failure at the metal-bone interface.

The Luque segmental wiring system, developed in the early 1970s, was the first of this class of implants to achieve wide clinical application.[10] Subsequent modifications have been employed. These include closed loops instead of rods, and techniques for anchoring the rods to the sacrum.[11,12]

Deformity correction is achieved by the sequential tightening of the wires.[13]

Sublaminar wires were used to augment the efficacy of Harrington rod fixation by reducing the chance of hook dislodgment.[14] This combination allowed the surgeon to apply distraction and simultaneously enhance the correction of the spinal deformity. Further modifications were the forerunners of more complex, currently used systems of universal spinal instrumentation (USI).[11,12,15-17]

Harrington was the first to report the use of the pedicle as a fixation site.[18] He abandoned this concept on account of problems with component-component (screw–longitudinal member) integrity. Roy-Camille was principally responsible for the refinement and institution of the common clinical application of pedicle fixation.[19]

The Luque sublaminar wiring technique waned in popularity, mainly because of the associated risk of neurological injury and the lack of ability to exert distractive or compressive forces on the spine. Cotrel and Dubousset developed an instrumentation system that addressed these issues and more.[20,21] The Cotrel-Dobousset (CD) instrumentation system consists of rods and multiple hooks (that can be affixed to the lamina, pedicle, or transverse process) and screws. This provides a reliable segmental fixation of the spine, plus the option to use posterior rotational forces to correct scoliotic deformities. These and other advantages allow safe and efficacious segmental fixation of the spine and the introduction of several additional manufacturer-specific, but similar, implant systems.[22,23]

Roy-Camille pioneered the development of lateral mass plates and screws; these were introduced in the United

States in 1988.[24] They have overtaken cervical wiring techniques in popularity with surgeons.

REFERENCES

1. Albee FH: Transplantation of a portion of the tibia into the spine for Pott's disease. *JAMA* 1911;57:885–886.
2. Hadra BE: The classic: Wiring of the vertebrae as a means of immobilization in fracture and Pott's disease (reprint). *Clin Orthop* 1975;112:4–8.
3. Hibbs RA: An operation for progressive spinal deformities. *NY Med J* 1911;93:1013–1016.
4. Hibbs RA: A report of fifty-nine cases of scoliosis treated by fusion operation. *J Bone Joint Surg* 1924;6:3–37.
5. Lange F: The classic: Support for the spondylitic spine by means of buried steel bars attached to the vertebrae (reprint). *Clin Orthop* 1986;203:3–6.
6. Rogers WA: Fractures and dislocations of the cervical spine. *J Bone Joint Surg* 1957;39A:341–376.
7. Rogers WA: Treatment of fracture-dislocation of the cervical spine. *J Bone Joint Surg* 1942;24:245–258.
8. Harrington PR: The history and development of Harrington instrumentation. *Clin Orthop* 1973;93:110–112.
9. Harrington PR: Treatment of scoliosis: Correction and internal fixation by spine instrumentation. *J Bone Joint Surg* 1962;44:591–610.
10. Luque ER: The anatomic basis and development of segmental spinal instrumentation. *Spine* 1982;7:256–259.
11. Flatley TJ, Derderian H: Closed loop instrumentation of the lumbar spine. *Clin Orthop* 1984;196:273–278.
12. Luque ER: Segmental spinal instrumentation of the lumbar spine. *Clin Orthop* 1986;203:126–135.
13. Luque ER, Cassis N, Ramirez-Wiella G: Segmental spinal instrumentation in the treatment of fractures of the thoracolumbar spine. *Spine* 1982;7:312–317.
14. Bryant CE, Sullivan JA: Management of thoracic and lumbar spine fractures with Harrington distraction rods supplemented with sublaminar wiring. *Spine* 1983;8:532–537.
15. Akbarnia VA, Fogarty JP, Smith KR: New trends in surgical stabilization of thoraco-lumbar spinal fractures with emphasis for sublaminar wiring. *Paraplegia* 1985;23:27–33.
16. Cybulski GR, Von Roenn KA, D'Angelo CM, et al: Luque rod stabilization for metastatic disease of the spine. *Surg Neurol* 1987;28:277–283.
17. Farcy JP, Weidenbaum, Michelsen CB, et al: A comparative biomechanical study of spinal fixation using Cotrel-Dubousset instrumentation. *Spine* 1987;12:877–881.
18. Harrington PR, Tullos HS: Reduction of severe spondylolisthesis in children. *South Med J* 1969;62:1–7.
19. Roy-Camille R, Saillant G, Mazel C: Internal fixation of the lumbar spine with pedicle screw plating. *Clin Orthop* 1986;203:7–17.
20. Birch JG, Herring JA, Roach JW, et al: Cotrel-Dubousset instrumentation in idiopathic scoliosis. *Clin Orthop* 1988;227:24–29.
21. Cotrel Y, Dubousset J, Guillaumat M: New universal instrumentation in spinal surgery. *Clin Orthop* 1988;227:10–23.
22. Dickman CA, Fessler RG, MacMillan M, et al: Transpedicular screw-rod fixation of the lumbar spine: Operative technique and outcome in 104 cases. *J Neurosurg* 1992;77:860–870.
23. Moreland DB, Egnatchik JG, Bennett GJ: Cotrel-Dubousset instrumentation for the treatment of thoracolumbar fractures. *Neurosurg* 1990;27:69–73.
24. Cooper PR, Cohen A, Rosiello A, et al: Posterior stabilization of cervical spine fractures and subluxations using plates and screws. *Neurosurg* 1988;23:300–306.

Chapter 22

Posterior Distraction Fixation

INTRODUCTION

The use of a spinal implant to apply a posterior distraction force alone is uncommon. Usually there is an accompanying three-point bending or cantilever beam force application. The rarity of any need for an implant-derived posterior distraction force application and the possibility of exaggerating spinal deformation tend to discourage the clinical use of such an implant-derived force application.

TECHNIQUES AND CLINICAL APPLICATION

Short-segment applications are the most common. The use of the Knodt rod (via sublaminar hooks) at a single motion segment is an example of such an application (Fig. 22-1). A desired result may be the opening of the neuroforamina.

Rarely, posterior spinal distraction for the reduction of a spinal deformity may be indicated (Fig. 22-2).

COMPLICATIONS

The application of isolated posterior spinal distraction forces may cause exaggeration of a kyphotic deformity. This most often occurs when a segmental kyphotic deformity is superimposed on a normal lordotic curvature. It is due to the moment arm through which the distraction forces act, and to the inability to achieve a three-point bending force application that results from the lack of contact between the rod and the fulcrum (Fig. 22-3).

This type of force application may flatten the normal lordotic curvature (Fig. 22-4). This is sometimes associated with a clinical-anatomic back pain syndrome called the *flat back syndrome*.

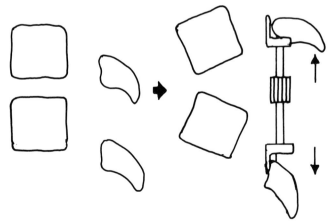

FIGURE 22-1 Knodt rod application over a single motion segment. Note the opening of the neuroforamina. Straight arrows depict the forces applied by the implant.

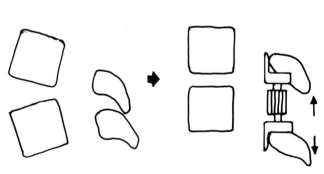

FIGURE 22-2 Isolated posterior spinal distraction forces may be used to reduce the rare extension injury of the spine. Straight arrows depict the forces applied by the implant.

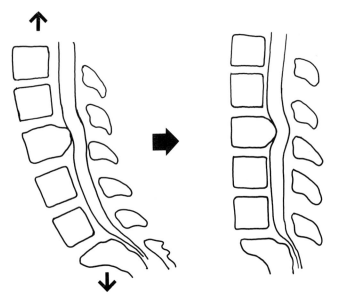

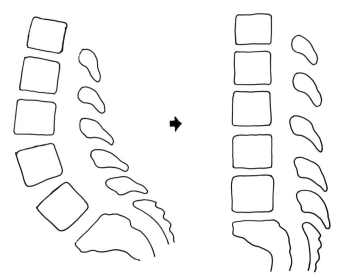

FIGURE 22-3 Isolated posterior spinal distraction forces may exaggerate segmental kyphotic deformation if superimposed on a region of the spine with an intrinsic lordosis. Note the flexion of the spine at the site of pathology.

FIGURE 22-4 A flattened back (loss of lordosis) may result from the application of an isolated posterior distraction force.

CLINICAL EXAMPLES

Simple posterior distraction is uncommonly applied clinically. The application of distraction via Knodt rods may be the most common example of this force application (Fig. 22-5).

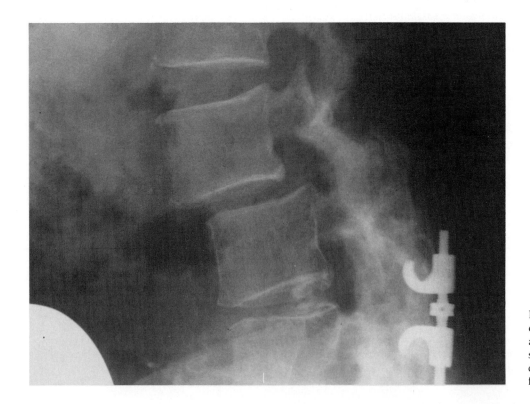

FIGURE 22-5 The application of distraction via a Knodt rod allows for the flexing of the spine about the intervening disk interspace; this results in a flattened back.

Chapter 23

Posterior Compression (Tension-Band) Fixation

INTRODUCTION

Short-segment fixation constructs, such as those applying *tension-band fixation* forces to the spine, result in less spinal stiffness than longer constructs, on account of the shorter segment of spine immobilized. Furthermore, forces applied to the spine are smaller with short-segment fixation techniques than with longer constructs (see Chap. 15). There-fore, a shorter construct, appropriately employed, carries lower chances of early and late implant-bone interface failure.

Posterior tension-band fixation forces rely for their success on a "closing of the the fish mouth" principle (Fig. 23-1). If the "jaw" of the "fish" is intact, then simply forcing the fish's "mouth" into a closed position will result in a tight approximation of the teeth (and a solid construct). On the other hand, if the jaw of the fish is fractured, closing the fish's mouth will not ensure the approximation of the upper and lower teeth (Fig. 23-2*A*); in fact, it may further disrupt their alignment (Fig. 23-2*B*). The clinical correlate of the "fractured jaw" is the disruption of the lamina or spinous process (Fig. 23-2). Closing the "fish's mouth" with a ten-sion-band fixation construct may exaggerate the deformity while doing little to augment spinal stability.

Tension-band fixation constructs function by closing the fish's mouth. This force application, in order to give spinal stability, requires an intact hinge serving as the instantane-ous axis of rotation (IAR). Without this intact hinge, success cannot be expected.

Another relative requirement of the anatomic or pathoanatomic arrangement of the spine, prior to the appli-cation of posterior tension-band fixation, is the intrinsic or surgically created ability of the spine to resist over-com-pression. If, for example, the fish had no teeth, but the hinge of the jaw was intact, the forceful closing of the mouth would result in an "over-closure" of the jaw. In the case of

the spine, a similar mechanism could result in nerve root impingement at the level of the neuroforamina or in buck-ling of the ligamentum flavum into the spinal canal (Fig. 23-3).

If, on the other hand, the fish's tongue (our hypothetical fish has a tongue) were swollen and protruding into the mouth, the application of a tension-band fixation force would result in further protrusion of the tongue into the mouth cavity. Repositioning of the tongue, or reduction of its volume prior to jaw closure (implant placement), would be optimal (Fig. 23-4).

It has been emphasized in Chap. 10 that an adequate ven-tral neural element decompression must be performed prior to the application of a tension-band fixation construct to the spine. Obviously, the closing of the fish's mouth will wedge any mass that is dorsal to the hinge (IAR) toward the dural sac (Figs. 23-3 and 23-4). This phenomenon is a result of the redirection of the transmitted forces. Remember, a tension-band fixation technique only closes the fish's mouth. It does not stabilize the hinge of the jaw (Fig. 23-5).

The application of posterior compression forces (i.e., by a tension-band construct) with an accompanying interbody fusion enhances the bone-healing-enhancing forces, if the interbody fusion is positioned dorsal to the IAR. The under-lying principle is that of "load-sharing." The placement of the construct in a compression mode in this manner allows the axial load–supporting capacity of the ventral interbody fusion to be maximally exploited (Fig. 23-6).

A discussion of the forces applied to the spine by tension-band fixation constructs, as well as a comparison of such constructs to three-point bending fixation constructs, was presented in Chap. 14. The direction of the force applied to the spine by tension-band fixation constructs differs by 90 degrees from that of the force applied by three-point bend-ing constructs. The former is parallel to the long axis of the spine; the latter is perpendicular to this axis (Fig. 23-7).

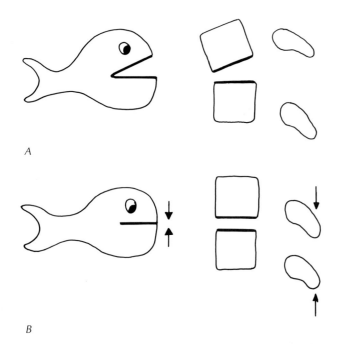

A

B

FIGURE 23-1 *A.* Analogy between an open mouth of a fish and a flexion deformity. *B.* The fish mouth can be closed, or the deformity reduced, by a tension-band fixation mechanism.

Because of the parallel orientation of the force application and the fact that the moment arm is perpendicular to this orientation, the length of the construct does not affect the bending moment applied at the termini of the construct. Therefore, the length of the construct does not affect the

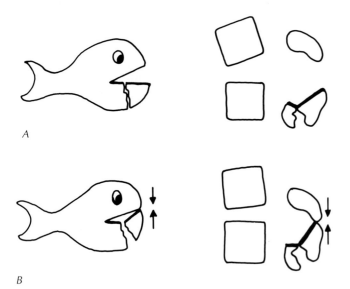

A

B

FIGURE 23-2 A fractured jaw (or spinous process) (*A*) will impede the approximation of the teeth (or reduction of the flexion deformity) by a tension-fixation mechanism (*B*).

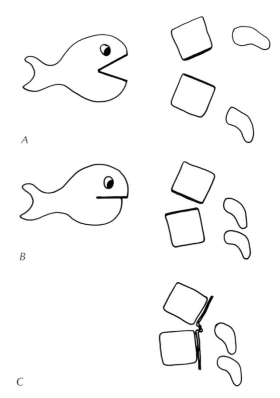

A

B

C

FIGURE 23-3 If the fish's jaw had an intact hinge (anterior and posterior longitudinal ligaments) but the teeth were missing (facet joint disruption or injury) (*A*), the application of posterior tension-band fixation forces could result in "over-closure" of the jaw, or overextension of the spine (*B*). This, in turn, could result in nerve root impingement or ligamentum flavum buckling (*C*).

efficacy of deformity correction. The only factor affecting the length of the moment arm is the distance from the IAR to the point of attachment of the construct (Fig. 23-8).

TECHNIQUES

The techniques of application of tension-band fixation vary widely. They range from cerclage wiring in the cervical spine (true tension-band fixation) to the use of cantilever beam fixation constructs in a compression mode. They all have one attribute in common: the application of a compression force complex at a point that is dorsal to the IAR and the neutral axis.

CLINICAL APPLICATIONS
Cervical Spine

As described in Chap. 10, posterior tension-band fixation techniques for application in the cervical region have one significant advantage that similar applications in the tho-

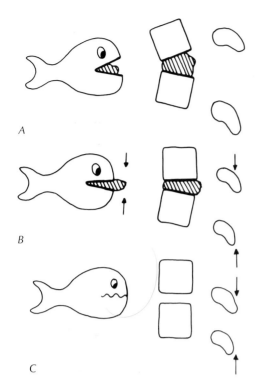

FIGURE 23-4 If the tongue were swollen (retropulsion of disk and/or bone into the spinal canal) (*A*), closure of the mouth (the application of posterior tension-band fixation forces) would result in further tongue protrusion (exaggeration of the dural sac compression) (*B*). Repositioning of the tongue or reduction of the volume of the tongue (removal of ventrally located bone and/or disk—i.e., ventral dural sac decompression) would eliminate this pathological dural sac compression (*C*).

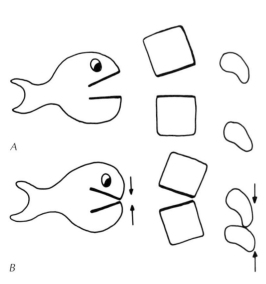

FIGURE 23-5 If the hinge of the fish's jaw is disrupted (anterior and/or posterior longitudinal ligament disruption) (*A*), the closure of the jaw (application of a tension-band fixation force) may not adequately stabilize the jaw or the spine (*B*).

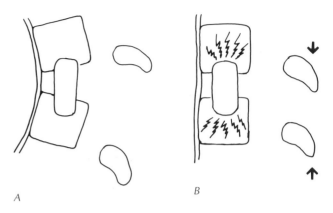

FIGURE 23-6 Assuming the presence of intact anterior ligamentous structures, the placement of a posterior tension-band fixation force complex may result in augmented application of compressive force to a ventral interbody bone graft strut.

racic and lumbar region do not: the orientation of the facet joints in the coronal plane (Fig. 23-9). If the integrity of the facet joints is left intact by the pathological process, the dorsal application of tension between two vertebral segments at the lamina or spinous process level (dorsal to the IAR) positions the involved facets so that flexion—and, more important, ventral translation—cannot occur (Fig. 23-9). These factors simplify the decision-making process and the application of posterior tension-band fixation spinal implants in the cervical region.

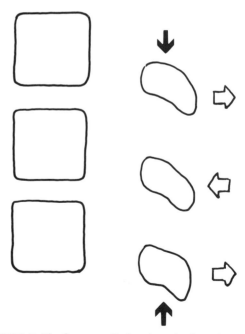

FIGURE 23-7 The forces applied to the spine by using a posterior tension-band fixation construct (*solid arrows*) are perpendicular to those applied by three-point bending constructs (*hollow arrows*).

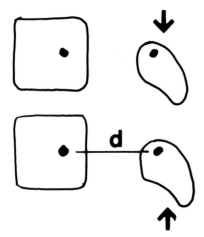

FIGURE 23-8 The length of the tension-band fixation construct does not affect the length of the moment arm (*d*), since the moment arm is perpendicular to the forces applied.

Thoracic and Lumbar Spine

In the thoracic and lumbar regions the facet joints are oriented in different planes. Hence, the forces applied to the spine by spinal implants and by normal and excessive spinal movements are much greater than in the cervical region. The evolution of devices and techniques for thoracic and lumbar instability has culminated in universal spinal instrumentation techniques for the treatment of posttraumatic spinal instability. These techniques allow the immediate acquisition of significant spinal stability. The degree of rigidity realized is substantial. Long spinal instrumentation rodding techniques frequently provide a more-than-adequate degree of spinal stability. Excessive stress shielding often results (which may limit healing and bony fusion). Terminal hook-bone interface failure may even be encouraged by the use of long rod–short fusion techniques (even following the acquisition of adequate bony fusion), necessitating the removal of instrumentation.

MULTISEGMENTAL FIXATION

Tension-band fixation can be applied in a multi-segmental manner. This can provide some advantages by distributing forces over multiple implant-bone interfaces. On the other hand, *terminal bending moments* may result, as with anterior tension-band fixation constructs (see Chap. 19). This usually occurs when too few intermediate fixation points have been used (Fig. 23-10).

When interspinous wiring techniques are to be used, multiple overlapping one-motion-segment cerclage wiring is best. When one long cerclage wire is used there is a tendency toward formation of terminal bending moments. This tendency is minimized by the multiple overlapping cerclage wiring technique (Fig. 23-11).

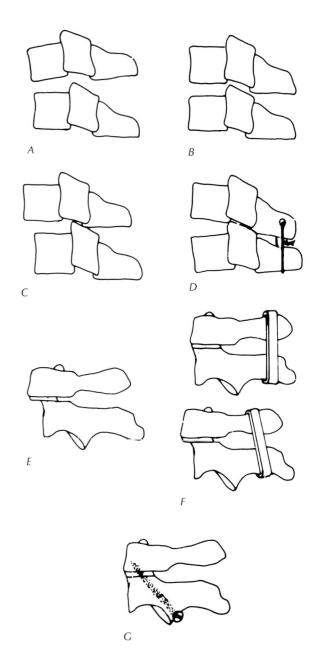

FIGURE 23-9 The coronal orientation of the cervical facet joints augments the efficacy of tension-band fixation in the case of flexion deformation (*A*). If the facet joints are intact, posterior compression facilitates their reapproximation (*B*). Whereas the lack of this close approximation of the facet joints does not protect against translation (*C*), forced approximation of the facet joints obstructs ventral translational deformation (*D*). The application of a tension-band fixation construct in a situation where C1-C2 sagittal plane translational stability has been disrupted (without coronally oriented facet joints) (*E*) may not adequately limit translation (*F*). A more rigid cantilevered construct may be required (*G*).

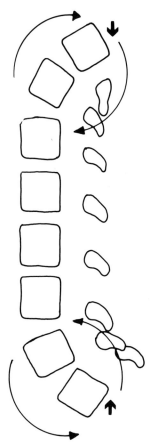

FIGURE 23-10 With multiple-level posterior compression fixation (*straight arrows*), terminal bending moments can occur (*curved arrow*).

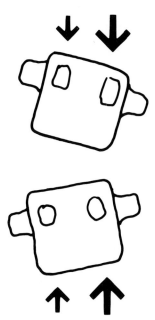

FIGURE 23-12 The application of asymmetric posterior tension-band fixation forces, or asymmetric resistance to the application of such forces, may exaggerate a scoliotic deformation.

COMPLICATIONS

Marked spinal deformities cannot be consistently reduced by posterior tension-band fixation techniques alone. Similarly, patients who have incurred a substantial loss of lateral translational stability or scoliotic curvature are poorly served by these techniques. Intervertebral ligamentous support, which is diminished after significant translational inju-

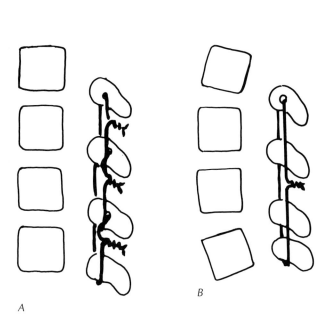

FIGURE 23-11 Multiple overlapping one-motion-segment cerclage wiring (A) helps prevent the terminal bending moments that might occur with a single-cerclage-wire technique (B).

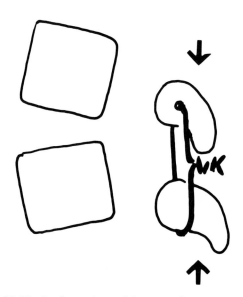

FIGURE 23-13 Cerclage wiring of the cervical spinous processes provides spinal extension via the application of posterior compression (tension-band fixation) forces.

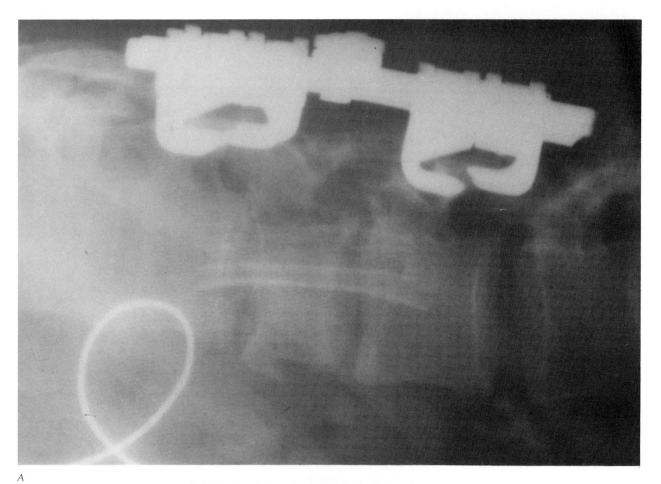

A

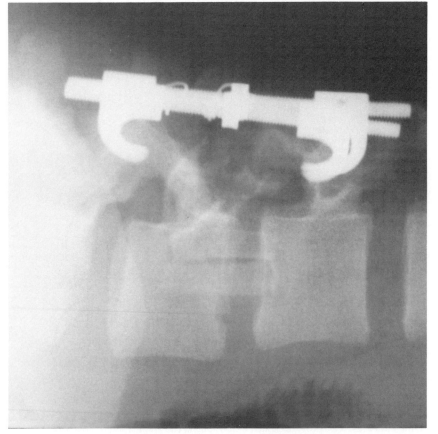

B

FIGURE 23-14 Various techniques can be applied with posterior tension-band fixation. Universal spinal instrumentation techniques (*A*) or Knodt rod in a compression mode (*B*) can apply compression (tension-band fixation) forces to the laminae.

ries, is often necessary to the success of tension-band fixation techniques.

Similarly, posterior tension-band fixation techniques have a poor ability to apply an effective lever arm for either the reduction of a scoliotic or kyphotic spinal deformity or the prevention of the development of a translational deformity when significant translational instability is suspected. The scoliotic deformation may be exaggerated following use of the posterior short-segment fixation compression techniques (Fig. 23-12). Wire cut-through may occur with any cerclage wiring technique.

CLINICAL EXAMPLES

Tension-band fixation constructs are commonly applied clinically. The prototype of this construct type is the interspinous wiring technique (Fig. 23-13). This provides for cerclage wiring of spinous processes. A variety of laminar clamps can be used to apply similar forces to the spine (Fig. 23-14).

Chapter 24

Posterior Three-Point Bending Fixation

INTRODUCTION

Three-point bending instrumentation is usually, but not always, applied in a complex manner with accompanying distraction—for example, by Harrington distraction rods or by universal spinal instrumentation techniques applied in a distraction mode. (Three-point bending instrumentation may also be applied in a neutral mode by universal spinal instrumentation or segmental sublaminar wiring constructs—see Chap. 15). It is usually the preferred mode of implant-derived force application for most posterior distraction techniques and many neutral techniques. Three-point bending constructs involve instrumentation application over multiple spinal segments (usually five or more) with accompanying dorsally directed forces applied at the upper and lower construct-bone interfaces and an equal ventrally directed force applied at the fulcrum (Fig. 24-1). This technique is often used following trauma to accomplish a ventral decompression of the dural sac by distracting the posterior longitudinal ligament. The desired resultant force should push the offending retropulsed bone and/or disk fragments ventrally and away from the dural sac. Because of the relative weakness of the posterior longitudinal ligament and/or the fixed nature of the retropulsed fragments, this technique may not always succeed (see Chap. 7). Sleeves around the rods that function as spacers may be used for spinal extension, enhancing force application (Fig. 24-2).

Posterior distraction nearly always applies a three-point bending force complex to the spine. Even if a three-point bending construct is not initially planned, the application of sufficient distraction will eventually result in enough spinal flexion that the construct makes contact with the spine at the level of the spinal deformity—that is, at an intermediate point along the construct called the *fulcrum*. Prior to engagement of the fulcrum, flexion occurs because of the application of the distraction force at points dorsal to the instantaneous axis of rotation (IAR). This is most common in the lumbar region, where a lordotic posture is present (Fig. 24-3).

CLINICAL APPLICATIONS

Posterior three-point bending constructs can be appropriately applied in many clinical situations. As mentioned above, they are usually applied in combination with distraction forces at the termini of the construct. Distraction aids in the acquisition of a solid construct and enhances the ability to reduce kyphotic deformities.

Although distraction is often applied simultaneously with three-point bending, segmental neutral fixation may offer significant advantages. Segmental fixation may be used to apply three-point bending force at multiple points on the spine (Fig. 24-4). It is a very solid construct and allows the graded intraoperative reduction of kyphotic deformities via use of the "crossed rod" technique (Fig. 24-4).

Terminal three-point bending fixation is achieved when the fulcrum of the three-point bending construct is situated near one end of the construct (see Chap. 15). It is applicable in situations where parallelogram deformation in the sagittal plane is likely to occur with shorter (tension-band) fixation techniques (see Chap. 15).

In the lumbar spine the use of sleeves may provide the advantage of bringing the fulcrum to the rod so that spinal extension can be realized (Fig. 24-2). The use of multiple intermediate points of fixation, cross-fixation, or rods that cannot rotate (such as square-ended rods) can also be used to obviate this problem (Fig. 24-5).

MULTISEGMENTAL FIXATION

Posterior three-point bending constructs, by definition, fixate multiple spinal segments. The spanning of at least three

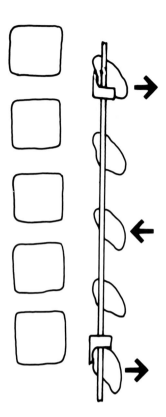

FIGURE 24-1 The dorsally and ventrally directed forces (*arrows*) applied by three-point bending constructs.

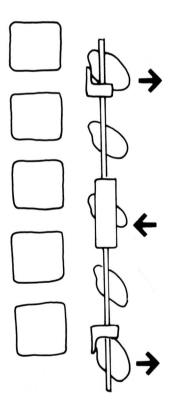

FIGURE 24-2 Sleeves may be used as spacers to provide an advantage in the form of ventrally directed force application at the fulcrum. Arrows depict the forces applied.

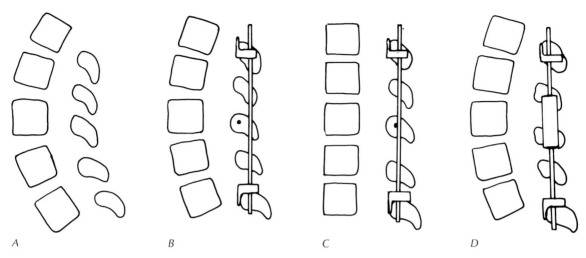

FIGURE 24-3 Posterior lumbar distraction (in the presence of the normal lumbar lordosis) (*A*) results in spinal flexion (*B*) until the fulcrum is engaged by the rod (*C*). Only after engagement of the fulcrum is a three-point bending force application achieved. (Up to that point, simple distraction is achieved.) Sleeve application (Fig. 24-2) facilitates the engagement of the fulcrum by the rod (*D*).

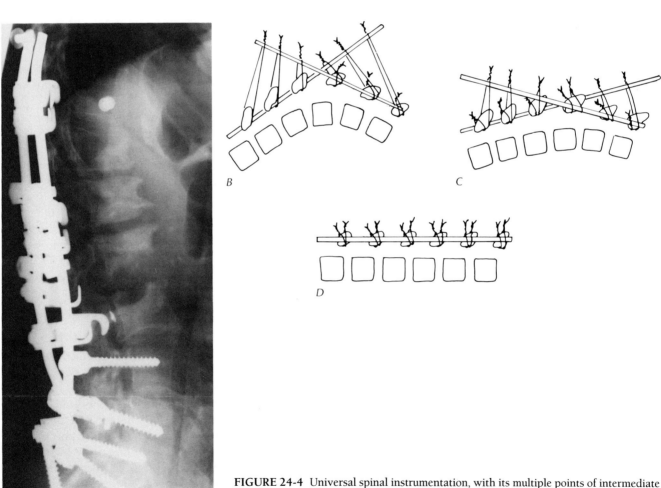

FIGURE 24-4 Universal spinal instrumentation, with its multiple points of intermediate fixation, may apply multiple dorsally or ventrally directed forces to the spine (*A*). This concept is effectively used in the "crossed rod fixation technique", where kyphotic deformity reduction is achieved in a sequential manner. In the case depicted here, sublaminar wires are used to gradually reduce the kyphotic deformity via sequential tightening of the wires at each end of the construct (*B*), (*C*), and (*D*).

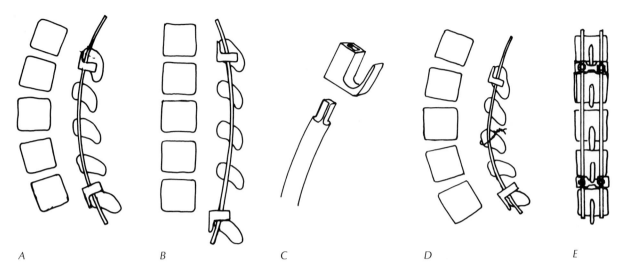

A   B   C   D   E

FIGURE 24-5 The lordotic curvature may be preserved by the use of sleeves, as shown in Fig. 24-2. Rod contouring alone (*A*) may not effectively preserve the lordotic posture of the spine, because the rods may rotate (*B*). Elimination of this rotation can be achieved via elimination of rod-hook interface mobility—for example, by the use of square-ended rods in square acceptance sites (*C*). This prevents rotation of the rod within the hook and thus minimizes the chance that the rod itself will rotate. Providing at least one additional intermediate rod-bone interface will also eliminate rotation (*D*). Finally, rigid crosslinking of one rod to the other will eliminate rotation of the rods (*E*).

vertebral levels (two motion segments) is mandatory if a three-point bending construct is to achieve its goal. For example, if a distraction construct is placed between two laminae (e.g., as is the case with one-motion-segment Knodt rod placement), three-point bending cannot be achieved, because there is no intermediate point for the application of the ventrally directed force (i.e., no fulcrum). In this case, simple distraction is all that is achieved (Fig. 24-6).

The use of multiple points of fixation adds to both construct complexity and construct utility in three-point bending force application. In many circumstances one can think of this type of construct as the application of three-point bending forces at multiple points on the spine (Fig. 24-4). This is the case if extension (dorsally directed force) is applied at each metal-bone interface site. If only the terminal metal-bone interface sites are applied in extension (e.g., the intermediate sites are applied in either a flexion or a neutral mode), the intermediate sites behave independently—as if they had been applied independently (Fig. 24-4).

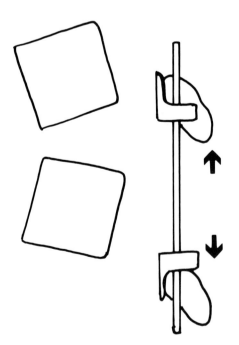

FIGURE 24-6 Distraction of a single motion segment (*arrows*), as is achieved with a Knodt rod, can result only in distraction, because no fulcrum is present or possible. Therefore, a three-point bending force complex application is impossible.

COMPLICATIONS

Three-point bending constructs are most likely to fail at either terminus. The upper implant-bone interface is usually the most vulnerable point (Fig. 24-7A). This is so because of the upper hooks' tendency to flex out of position and other factors addressed in Chap. 16. Compensation for this may be achieved via the lengthening of the upper portion of the construct by one or two segmental levels; this increases the length of the applied moment arm. This decreases the dorsally directed forces applied at the upper implant-bone interface ($M = F \times D$) (Fig. 24-7B and C).

The placement of a three-point bending construct over too few motion segments provides inadequate leverage for appropriate terminal metal-bone fixation. Either inadequate

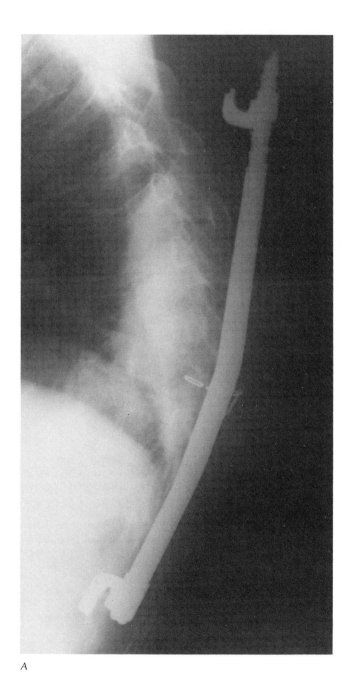

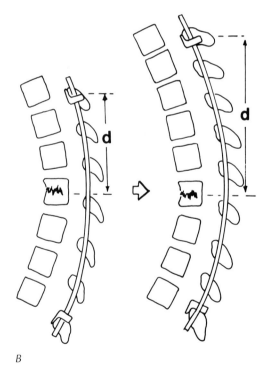

A

B

FIGURE 24-7 Three-point bending constructs commonly fail at a terminal implant-bone interface, usually at the upper terminus (*A*). Increasing the length of the upper portion of the construct increases the length of the moment arm applied, thus decreasing the dorsally directed force applied (*M* = *F* × *D*) (*B*).

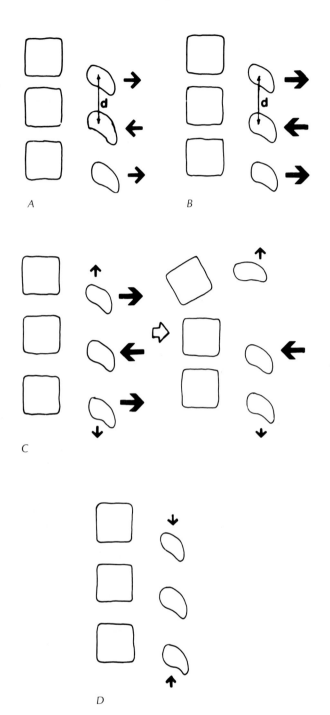

FIGURE 24-8 *A*. Short three-point bending constructs obligatorily apply a short moment arm. This may result either in inadequate force application or in the requirement for excessive dorsally directed force application at the termini of the construct. *B*. This is so because, assuming the bending moment (*M*) is constant, the force applied (*F*) is inversely proportional to the length of the moment arm (*D*) ($M = F \times D$). *C*. Especially with simultaneous application of distraction, the moment arm may not be long enough, and the applied forces not great enough, to prevent pivoting of a terminal motion segment. *D*. However, if the construct is placed in a compression mode, the construct shares the load with intrinsic spinal elements. In this case, excessive pivoting is much less likely to occur.

three-point bending forces are applied, or excessive ventrally and dorsally directed forces—applied at the fulcrum and terminal attachment sites, respectively—are required to compensate for short constructs (Fig. 24-8*A* and *B*). This, together with the exaggerated forces applied at the terminal metal-bone interface, allows only minimal opportunity to prevent sagittal angulation of vertebral bodies above and below the unstable segment. The use of too short a construct leaves the terminal metal-bone interfaces too near the unstable motion segments. Pivoting of the terminal vertebral segment commonly occurs in this situation (Fig. 24-8*C*). However, if the construct is placed in a compression mode, thus "asking" the intrinsic anterior spinal elements to "share" the load with the implant, this pivoting is less likely to occur (Fig. 24-8*D*).

One should bear in mind, then, that appropriately applied three-point bending constructs carry several advantages, such as ventrally directed force application at the ful-

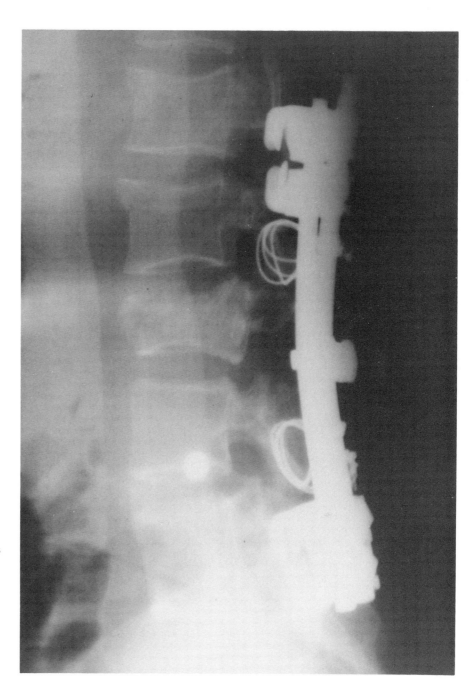

FIGURE 24-9 Three-point bending foces may be applied to the spine by the traditional Harrington distraction rod technique or via universal spinal instrumentation techniques, as depicted. With both techniques other force applications—such as distraction (particularly with the Harrington distraction rod) or compression—are almost always made.

crum and the opportunity to address relatively easily the problem of deformity (kyphosis) reduction. Excessive force application usually is not mandatory. The application of appropriate (not excessive) forces, however, may often result in long construct applications. These may result in unacceptable stiffness or pain, necessitating construct removal after the acquisition of bone fusion.

CLINICAL EXAMPLES

Posterior three-point bending forces are commonly applied in the thoracic and lumbar regions. They are commonly applied with accompanying distraction or compression forces. The Harrington distraction rod is the prototype of this type of fixation. It is being supplanted, however, by more complex universal spinal instrumentation systems (Fig. 24-9).

Chapter 25

Posterior Cantilever Beam Fixation

INTRODUCTION

Cantilever beam fixation provides a rigid (fixed or applied moment arm) or dynamic (nonfixed moment arm) fixation of the spine. As discussed in Chap. 14, both rigid and dynamic constructs may be applied in distraction, compression, or neutral modes. The variety of combinations thus allowed is represented by the five anterior and five posterior modes of application. Each of the three posterior cantilever beam construct types employs one or more of the five posterior modes of application (Fig. 25-1).

CLINICAL APPLICATIONS

Fixed Moment Arm Cantilever Beam Fixation

Rigid pedicle fixation techniques (such as rigid plate or screw-rod combinations) may compensate for a short moment arm by allowing a fixed moment arm cantilever beam construct to be applied. Although the initial application of such a construct may be in a neutral mode (no distraction, rotation, compression, or translational forces applied to the spine at the time of surgery), when a load is applied—for example, during the assumption of an erect posture—the construct must resist the axial load by its intrinsic fixed moment arm cantilever beam characteristics; that is, by rigidly buttressing the spine. One noteworthy feature of such a construct is its lack of requirement for a ventrally directed force at a fulcrum. This is compensated for by the buttressing effect, which places a significant stress at the point of maximum bending moment of the construct: the screw-longitudinal member interface. This stress, if excessive, may result in screw fracture.

Rigid cantilever beam constructs mimic, in a sense, three-point bending constructs. The forces and moments resisted by these constructs are similar to, but oriented differently from, their three-point bending counterparts (Fig. 25-2). A

major difference, however, is observed at the time of surgery. Usually, three-point bending constructs are inserted with the three-point bending forces applied at the time of surgery, whereas rigid cantilever bending constructs are usually (but not always) applied in a relatively neutral mode.

Nonfixed Moment Arm Cantilever Beam Fixation

Nonfixed moment arm cantilever beam constructs do not apply substantial axial load–resisting forces to the spine. The toggling of the screw on the plate allowed by this technique dictates that a minimal bending moment, if any, is applied to the spine at the termini of the construct. Therefore, these techniques are appropriate only when axial load–resisting capabilities of the spine are already present. Because of their biomechanical characteristics, their ability to resist screw pullout is diminished (see Chap. 15).

The axial load–resisting ability of a nonfixed moment arm cantilever beam construct is enhanced by the use of two points on the moment arm (screw) as fixation points—for example, bicortical purchase points—or by provision of an interbody buttress for axial load–resisting support (Fig. 25-3).

Nonfixed moment arm cantilever beam constructs can be used effectively in a tension-band fixation or three-point bending manner. If posterior compression forces are applied to the spine, then, because of the force vector's location at a finite dorsal distance from the instantaneous axis of rotation (IAR), a moment arm is applied that restricts movement in the opposite direction (Fig. 25-4). These effects are also similar, but opposite in direction, to those achieved with anterior constructs (see Chap. 20).

As with analogous anterior techniques (see Chap. 20), if screw-pullout resistance is substantial, nonfixed moment arm cantilever beam constructs may apply a three-point bending force complex to the spine (Fig. 25-5). It is precar-

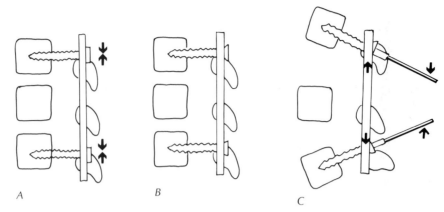

FIGURE 25-1 The cantilever beam fixation types and their associated possible modes of application. *A.* A fixed moment arm (rigid) cantilever beam construct can be applied in a distraction, neutral, or compression mode. *B.* A nonfixed moment arm (dynamic) cantilever beam construct can be effectively applied only in a neutral mode. *C.* An applied moment arm cantilever beam construct can be employed via the modes of application of its fixed moment arm counterpart. With an applied moment arm construct, one must keep in mind that the construct may be used to apply axial forces (distraction or compression) as well as bending moments (extension or flexion). Arrows depict applied-force vectors.

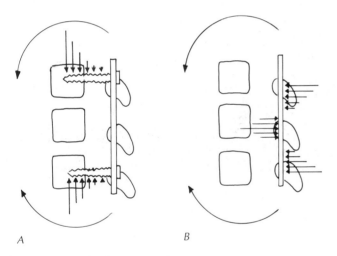

FIGURE 25-2 The forces (*straight arrows*) and bending moments (*curved arrows*) resisted by rigid cantilever beam constructs (*A*) and three-point bending constructs (*B*).

ious to rely on screw pullout resistance alone to maintain a desired spinal configuration. For this reason, three-point bending constructs are usually applied via hook, rather than screw-bone, interfaces.

Posterior nonfixed moment arm cantilever beam constructs that use a plate as their longitudinal member (e.g., Luque plates and a wide variety of lateral mass plates) provide an additional advantage: the ability of the construct to hold posteriorly placed bone graft into its desired fusion bed. Theoretically, this should encourage bone fusion by increasing bone-healing-enhancing forces (i.e., compression and close approximation of bone graft and its acceptance bed).

Applied Moment Arm Cantilever Beam Fixation

The use of a Schanz screw–like application technique allows the application of very complex forces at the time of surgery. These usually are either extension or flexion forces (Fig. 25-6).

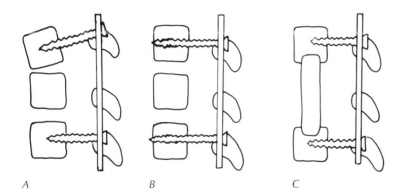

FIGURE 25-3 Nonfixed moment arm–associated toggling (*A*) may be minimized by the use of a bicortical purchase (*B*) and/or by the use of an interbody strut graft to assist in the buttressing of the spine (*C*).

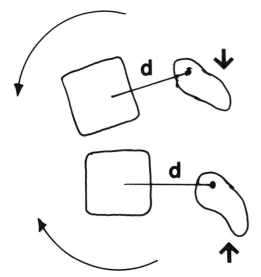

FIGURE 25-4 The moment arm (*d*) associated with the forces applied by posterior tension-band fixation construct (*straight arrows*) provides resistance to flexion. Curved arrows depict the resisted flexion bending moments.

MULTISEGMENTAL FIXATION

Cantilever beam constructs can be employed in a multisegmental manner. In situations where multiple spinal levels are to be fused and spanned by a posterior cantilever beam construct, there is no substantive evidence of any need to instrument all segmental levels, rather than just the terminal levels, of the construct (Fig. 25-7).

COMPLICATIONS

Pedicle fixation constructs may fail during axial loading, because of a parallelogram-like translational deformation. A

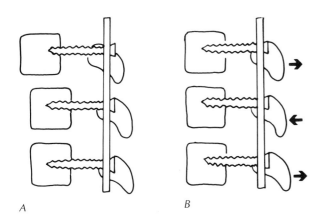

FIGURE 25-5 Nonfixed moment arm cantilever beam constructs can impart three-point bending forces to the deformed spine (*A*), thus reducing the deformity (*B*). Screw pullout is obviously a significant risk. Arrows depict forces applied.

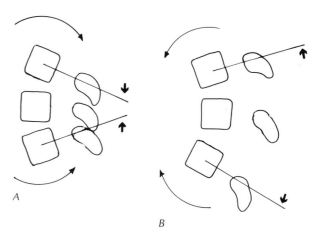

FIGURE 25-6 Applied moment arm cantilever beam constructs apply either an extension (*A*) or a flexion (*B*) bending moment to the spine (*curved arrows*). Straight arrows depict the forces applied to the Schanz-like screws required to create the bending moments.

simple toeing-in of the screws, or rigid cross-fixation, or both, should minimize the chance of this complication (Fig. 25-8).

The use of the terminology of biomechanics and physics in the literature of spinal surgery has often been confusing. Much of the confusion has been associated with the biomechanics of injury and instrumentation. The concept of the bending moment has been misrepresented and misunderstood.

Anterior and posterior cantilever beam constructs call for screws of different lengths. Anterior constructs use shorter screws, because of their closer proximity to the vertebral

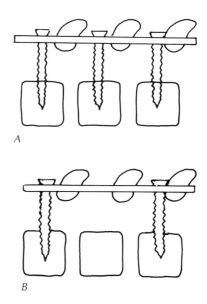

FIGURE 25-7 There is no substantive evidence that multiple-level rigid pedicle screw fixation (*A*) is better than terminal-level screw fixation (*B*).

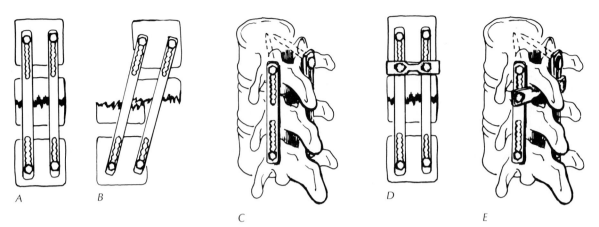

FIGURE 25-8 Pedicle fixation (*A*) may fail to prevent lateral translational deformation (*B*) because of a non-toed-in configuration of the screws (*A*). A toeing-in of the screws (*C*), or rigid crosslinking of the two longitudinal members (*D*), or both (*E*), assists in preventing this complication.

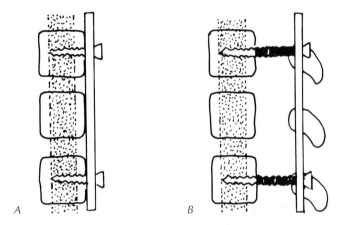

FIGURE 25-9 Otherwise-similar anterior and posterior screw-plate fixation constructs call for different screw lengths. *A*. The anterior construct applied the plate directly to the vertebral body and, hence, closer to the neutral axis (*stippled areas*). *B*. In posterior techniques the plate is situated farther from the neutral axis (by the length of the pedicle, *darkened areas*). As long as the screws span (cross) the neutral axis (*A* and *B*), the buttressing effect of the construct is, in theory, optimized with either approach. A shorter screw is associated with a lesser chance of screw fracture; thus the shortest screw with which this can be achieved is optimal.

body (Fig. 25-9). This results in a shorter moment arm that, in turn, results in a lesser force applied at the screw-plate or screw-rod interface. With shorter screws that span the neutral axis, the chance of instrumentation failure (screw fracture) is diminished, while axial load-bearing is not altered (so long as the screw passes the plane of the neutral axis) (Fig. 25-9).

The most common complications of cantilever beam constructs are screw fractures arising from the rigid nature of fixed and applied moment arm constructs, and screw pullout arising from the dynamic nature of nonfixed moment arm constructs. *Bone toggling* can occur with either type of construct (Fig. 25-10).

CLINICAL EXAMPLES

Posterior cantilever beam fixation forces can be applied to the spine via a variety of techniques. These include fixed, nonfixed, and applied moment arm constructs. The former and the latter are most commonly applied in the thoracic and lumbar regions (Fig. 25-11). Posterior nonfixed moment arm constructs may be readily applied in any region of the spine (Fig. 25-12).

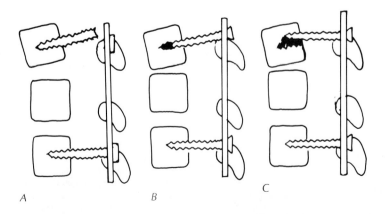

FIGURE 25-10 *A*. Fixed and applied moment arm cantilever beam constructs may fail via screw fracture at the screw–longitudinal member interface. *B*. Nonfixed moment arm constructs are most apt to fail at the screw-bone interface, via screw pullout. *C*. Either type is susceptible to failure via bone toggling (cutout).

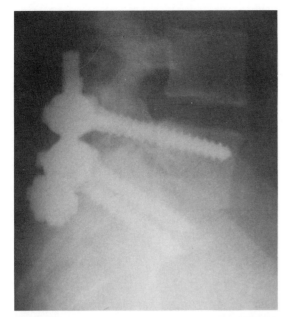

A

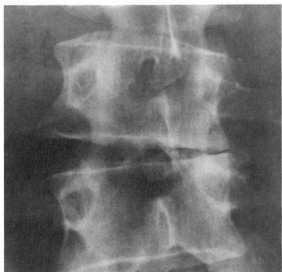

B

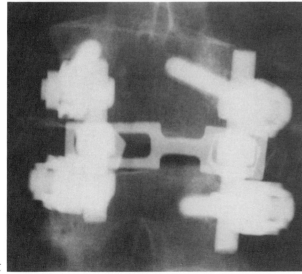

C

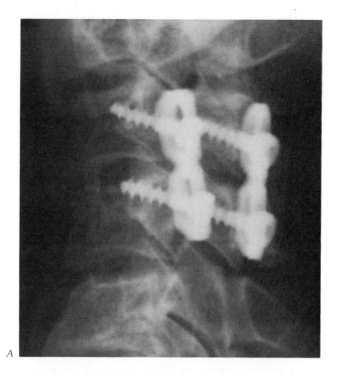

A

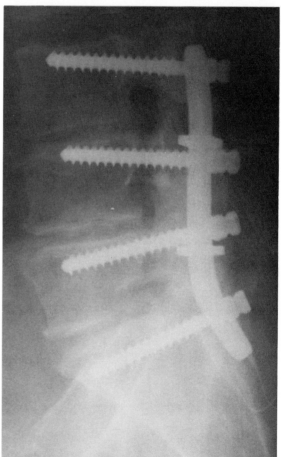

B

FIGURE 25-11 Fixed (*A*) and applied (*C*) moment arm cantilever beam construct types are most common in the thoracic and lumbar regions. A coronal plane deformity (*B*) was corrected by an applied moment arm via a cantilever beam construct (*C*).

FIGURE 25-12 Nonfixed moment arm cantilever beam (screw-through-the-plate) constructs may be applied via lateral mass plates in the cervical region as illustrated by an oblique x-ray (*A*) or via pedicle fixation in the thoracic and lumbar regions (*B*).

Part VII

Special Concerns

Chapter 26

Complex Instrumentation Constructs and Force Applications

In many respects most spinal implants, if not all, are complex. For the purposes of this chapter, however, *complex instrumentation constructs* include those that have not already been discussed and that employ multiple and/or complex force applications.

One or a combination of two fundamental techniques can be used for deformity correction: (1) implant force application via "bringing the spine to the implant" and (2) implant force application via in-vivo implant configuration alterations. A fundamental understanding of these techniques will provide the surgeon a greatly increased degree of surgical latitude and allow for an individualized customized implant "fit" for each patient.

This classification scheme is not always clearly applicable; a given construct may not fit clearly into one or another category. Nevertheless the scheme is used loosely herein, in order to facilitate an understanding of this often-confusing aspect of spinal instrumentation. Some implants discussed below are not used primarily for deformity reduction. Their occasional use as deformity prevention devices, however, warrants their inclusion here.

Implant forces applied via "bringing the spine to the implant" can be applied along any of the three axes of the Cartesian coordinate system. They are usually applied along the long axis of the spine or in the sagittal plane of the spine. Less commonly they are applied along the coronal axis of the spine (Fig. 26-1).

Implant force application via in-vivo alteration of implant configuration involves first the application of the implant to the spine, and then the alteration of the relationships between the implant-bone interfaces already achieved. This alteration of the relationships between the implant-bone interfaces is achieved via one or a combination of three fundamental types of implant manipulation: (1) implant contouring, (2) *intrinsic implant bending moment* application about the long axis of the spine (i.e., derotation),

and (3) the application of an intrinsic implant bending moment about an axially oriented axis of the spine (Fig. 26-2).

"BRINGING THE SPINE TO THE IMPLANT"

Various techniques can be used to bring the spine to the implant. As mentioned above, this is accomplished via the application of forces to the spine along one or a combination of the three axes of the Cartesian coordinate system. Forces applied along the long axis of the spine (e.g., distraction) can be used to correct compression deformations, as well as coronal and sagittally oriented translational deformations (Fig. 26-3). Rotatory torques (bending moments) applied in the sagittal plane generally are of a three-point bending nature; applied moment arm cantilever beam force complexes are also applicable (Fig. 26-4).

Although many of these techniques have already been described herein, some have not. Those that have not are described below. Particular nuances of certain others are also described.

Terminal Three-Point Bending Force Application

Three-point bending constructs were discussed in Chap. 15. The forces that they apply to the spine are common and, for the most part, well understood. They are the classic example of "bringing the spine to the implant" (Fig. 26-5).

Terminal three-point bending force applications are similarly common, but often are applied unknowingly by the surgeon. For example, a screw is usually judged on the basis of its ability to resist pullout. However, the screw commonly resists other forces in vivo, as evidenced by the incidence of screw fracture as a not-uncommon complication. For a screw to fracture, it must be subjected to forces (loads)

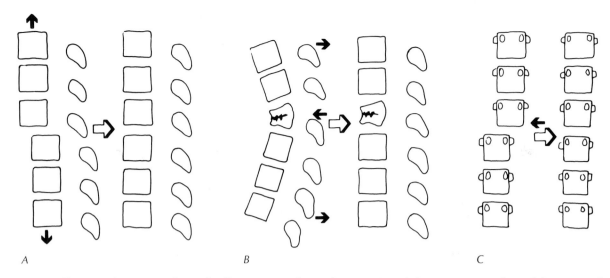

FIGURE 26-1 In "bringing the spine to the implant" one may use forces that are oriented along any axis or plane of the spine—along the long axis (*A*), the sagittal plane (*B*), and the coronal plane (*C*). Arrows depict forces applied by the implant.

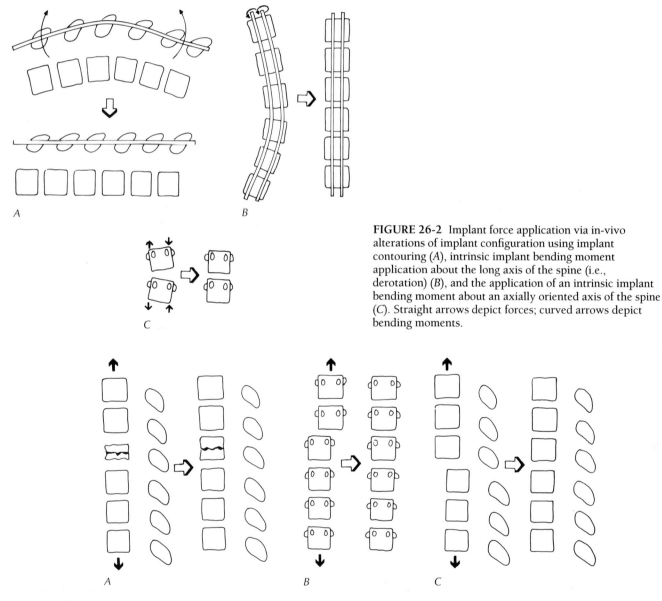

FIGURE 26-2 Implant force application via in-vivo alterations of implant configuration using implant contouring (*A*), intrinsic implant bending moment application about the long axis of the spine (i.e., derotation) (*B*), and the application of an intrinsic implant bending moment about an axially oriented axis of the spine (*C*). Straight arrows depict forces; curved arrows depict bending moments.

FIGURE 26-3 Distraction (a force applied along the long axis of the spine) can be used to correct compression deformations (*A*), coronal plane translational deformations (*B*), and sagittal plane translational deformations (*C*). Arrows depict applied forces.

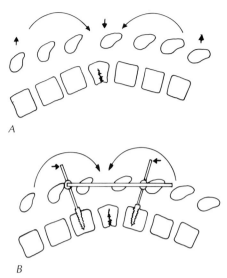

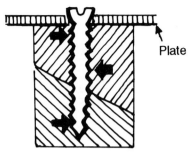

FIGURE 26-6 A depiction of three-point bending forces applied to a screw that transverses two mobile bone segments. Solid arrows depict the three-point bending forces applied to the screw.

FIGURE 26-4 Rotatory torques (bending moments) applied in the sagittal plane. *A*. Three-point bending. *B*. Applied moment arm cantilever beam. Straight arrows depict forces; curved arrows depict bending moments.

applied from its side—that is, *transverse loads*. These loads cause a shear-type stress if applied at different points on the screw and from different orientations. These asymmetrically applied transverse loads, by definition, apply three-point bending forces to the screw; hence the screw applies three-point bending forces to the bone (see Cantilevered Screw Techniques below). This is observed with fixed or nonfixed moment arm cantilever beam screw-plate or screw-rod constructs (Fig. 26-6).

Terminal three-point bending techniques can be used to "bring the spine to the implant" as well as to prevent the spine from "falling away from the implant" (Fig. 26-5). This technique can be applied to any spinal level. It is most commonly used in the cervical region, because of the lesser loads accepted by the implant and the relatively insubstantial design of the construct. It is most useful for the prevention or reduction of translational deformation (see Chap. 15). Note that if a ventral translation deformation is to be corrected or prevented, the long arm of the construct must be

situated caudal to the site of translation; whereas if dorsal translation deformation is to be corrected or prevented, the long arm of the construct must be situated rostral to the site of translation (Fig. 26-7).

Four-Point and Three-Point Bending and Reversed Four-Point and Three-Point Bending Fixation

Four-point bending of the spine, as defined by White and Panjabi, involves the loading of a long structure (i.e., the spine) with two transverse forces on one side and two on the other (Fig. 26-8A). The bending moment is constant between the two intermediate points of force application if all forces are equal—as opposed to three-point bending, where the bending moment peaks at the intermediate point of force application (Fig. 26-8A and B; see Chap. 15).[1] If the forces applied by a three- or four-point bending construct are oriented in the opposite direction, the technique is called *reversed three-point* or *reversed four-point bending fixation* (Fig. 26-9A and B). This technique has been used to reduce lumbar spondylolisthesis deformations.[2]

Applied Moment Arm Cantilever Beam Force Application

Applied moment arm cantilever beam constructs were discussed in Chap. 15. Applied moment arm cantilever beam

FIGURE 26-5 *A*. A three-point bending construct "bringing the spine to the implant." *B*. Terminal three-point bending constructs simply have a long and a short lever arm. Arrows depict forces applied.

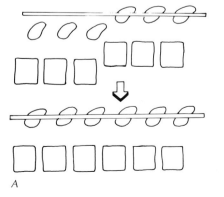

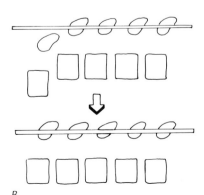

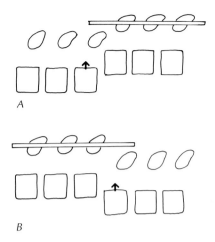

A

B

FIGURE 26-7 For terminal three-point bending constructs to be effective in reducing translational deformation, they must be applied properly. For example, the long arm of the construct must be placed caudally with ventral translational deformations (A), and rostrally with dorsal ones (B).

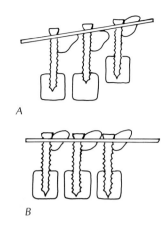

A

B

FIGURE 26-9 Reversed three-point bending forces can be used to reduce a spondylolisthesis. This subjects the screw to significant pullout stresses. Arrows depict forces applied.

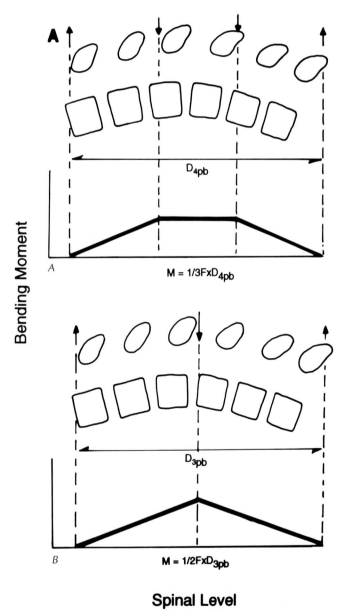

$$M = 1/3FxD_{4pb}$$

$$M = 1/2FxD_{3pb}$$

Bending Moment

Spinal Level

FIGURE 26-8 Four-point bending (A) and three-point bending (B) construct forces and associated bending moments. In the four-point bending construct depicted here, all forces (F_{4pb}) and the distance from the intermediate and terminal points of force application ($\frac{1}{3} \times D_{4pb}$) are equal. In this situation, the maximum bending moment, which is constant between the two intermediate points of force application, is defined by the equation: $M_{4pb} = F_{4pb} \times \frac{1}{3} \times D_{4pb}$. D_{4pb} is the length of the entire construct. Since the forces (F_{4pb}) are applied at points dividing the construct into thirds, the moment arm defining the bending moment is one-third of the entire construct length. In the three-point bending construct depicted here, the intermediate force is applied halfway between the terminal points of force application. Therefore, as demonstrated in Chap. 15, the maximum bending moment occurs at the point of intermediate force application and is defined by the equation: $M_{3pb} = 0.25 F_{3pb} \times D_{3pb}$. However, since F_{4pb} is the force applied at the terminal hook/bone interface and F_{3pb} is the force applied at the fulcrum, at the outset, F_{4pb} and F_{3pb}, by definition, vary by a factor of two. The force applied at the terminal hook/bone interface in this example is, thus, $\frac{1}{2} \times F_{3pb}$. This is defined here as $F_{\text{terminal 3pb}}$ and is equal to $\frac{1}{2} F_{3pb}$. Therefore $M_{3pb} = \frac{1}{4} \times 2 \times F_{\text{terminal 3pb}} \times D_{3pb}$. In order to compare three-point and four-point bending constructs, the following derivation is performed. Assume that a three-point and four-point bending construct, as depicted, are of similar length and that the bending moments applied are equal. The following derivation, thus depicts the comparison between the constructs: since $D_{4pb} = D_{3pb}$, and since $M_{4pb} = M_{3pb}$, $F_{4pb} \times \frac{1}{3} \times D_{3pb} = \frac{1}{2} \times F_{\text{terminal 3pb}} \times D_{3pb}$, $F_{4pb} = \frac{3}{2} \times F_{\text{terminal 3pb}}$. The forces applied at the terminal hooks by each construct are depicted by the above equations. The closer the intermediate forces are applied to the terminus of the four-point bending construct, the greater the numerator of the right half of the equation and the greater the forces required to achieve an equivalent bending moment (compared to a three-point bending construct of similar length). Conversely, the closer the intermediate forces of a four-point bending construct are placed to the middle of the construct, the more it biomechanically approximates a three-point bending construct, i.e., $F_{4pb} = F_{\text{terminal 3pb}}$.

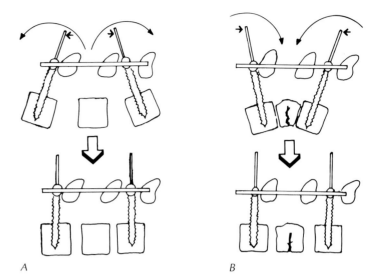

FIGURE 26-10 Applied moment arm cantilever beam forces may be applied with either flexion (*A*) or extension (*B*) bending moments. Straight arrows depict forces; curved arrows depict bending moments.

constructs are applicable in situations where short segment constructs are desired as the method of deformity reduction.[3,4] They are most applicable in the thoracolumbar and lumbar regions, for the reduction and fixation of wedge compression and burst fractures. The nature of their application dictates that the construct receives significant forces both at the time of insertion and later—for example, during ambulation.

They can be applied with either flexion or extension bending moments (Fig. 26-10). They can be used with or without distraction or compression or an accompanying

ventral dural sac decompression and/or interbody bone graft. These factors are important to consider if an optimal construct design, customized to a given clinical situation, is to be employed. For example, if extension and distraction without an accompanying interbody fusion are to be employed, large screws must be used in order to withstand the applied axial loads (Fig. 26-11*A*). In spite of this, construct failure may result.[5] Pedicle diameter or geometry may dictate the use of relatively small screws. In these situations the use of distraction and extension, followed by ventral decompression and the placement of an interbody weight-

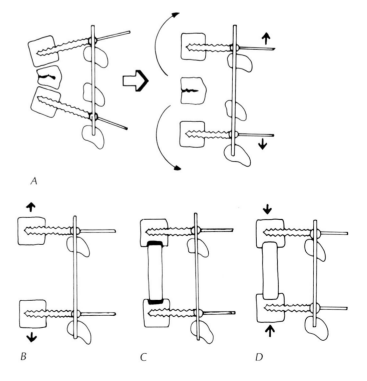

FIGURE 26-11 An applied moment arm cantilever beam construct that employs distraction and an extension bending moment, without an interbody fusion (*A*). This may be associated with a suboptimal success rate.[5] Load bearing–to–load sharing force application may minimize this complication by allowing sharing of the load between the implant and the spine (unloading the implant). In this case, the spine is distracted (with or without extension or flexion bending moment application) by the implant (*B*), followed by bone graft placement (*C*) and compression of the implant (*D*). This shares the load between the implant and the spine. Straight arrows depict forces; curved arrows depict bending moments.

bearing bone graft, and then compression of the construct onto the ventral graft and other intrinsic ventral weight-bearing spinal elements, results in the "sharing of the load" between the construct and the spinal elements and the interbody fusion—while simultaneously applying the desired extension bending moment for deformity reduction (Fig. 26-11B, C, and D).

The technique of sequentially applying distraction *(load bearing),* decompression of the dural sac, interbody fusion placement, and the compression of the construct, in order to share the load with the anterior spinal elements, is called *load bearing–to–load sharing* force application (Fig. 26-11B, C, and D). It provides biomechanical *(load sharing),* as well as clinical, advantages.

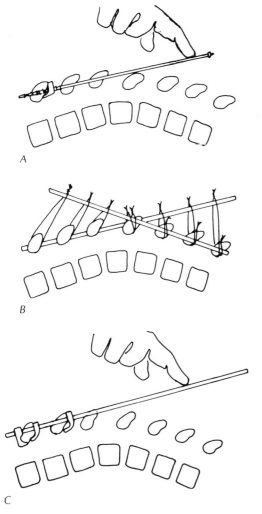

FIGURE 26-12 The crossed rod technique of thoracic and lumbar kyphotic deformity correction employed via the Harrington distraction rod (*A*), Luque sublaminar wiring (*B*), and universal spinal instrumentation (*C*). The latter technique is facilitated by the use of sequential hook insertion. *(From E.C. Benzel.[8])*

Crossed Rod Deformity Correction

The *crossed rod technique* is a well-established method of thoracic and lumbar kyphotic deformity correction. It was first used with Harrington distraction rods (Fig. 26-12A); later it was used more effectively with multisegmental sublaminar wiring (Luque) techniques (Fig. 26-12B).[7] Most recently it has been used with the *sequential hook insertion (SHI)* technique with universal spinal instrumentation constructs (Fig. 26-12C).[8] Regardless of the construct type employed, the technique involves the simultaneous application of kyphosis reduction forces to the spine via moment arms (longitudinal members) affixed at opposite ends and opposite sides of the spine. Gradual reduction is thus achieved (Fig. 26-13).

Short Segment Parallelogram Deformity Reduction

Short segment parallelogram deformity reduction is a rigid cantilever beam pedicle fixation technique that can be used in the thoracic and lumbar regions to reduce lateral translational deformities. This technique is best used in circumstances where short-segment fixation constructs are desired. The technique involves (1) placement of pedicle screws, (2) appropriate dural sac decompression, (3) attachment of the longitudinal members to the screws (i.e., rods), (4) application of rotatory and distraction forces to the rods, (5) maintenance of the achieved spinal reduction via rigid crossfixation, (6) placement of a fusion (interbody and/or lateral), and finally (7) compression of the screws so that load-sharing is achieved and the interbody bone graft secured in its acceptance bed (Fig. 26-14). This gives a load bearing–to–load sharing force application.

Short-segment parallelogram deformity reduction is best used in the low lumbar region, since sacropelvic fixation

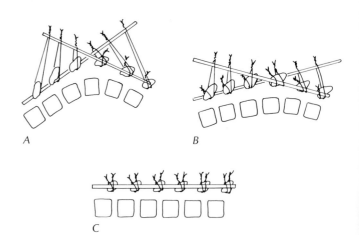

FIGURE 26-13 The crossed rod technique involves gradual reduction of the kyphotic deformity, as illustrated serially.

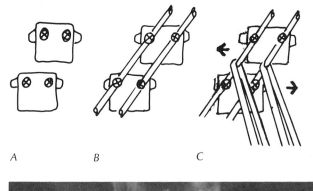

A   B   C

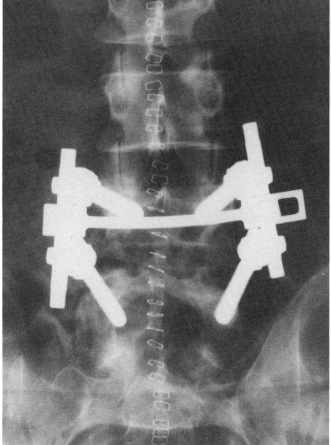

D

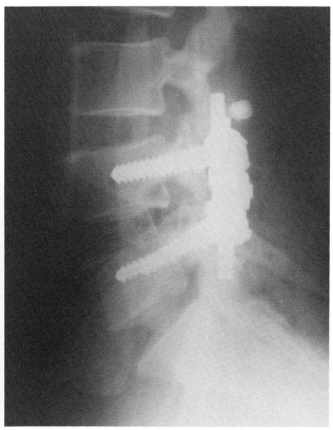

E

FIGURE 26-14 Short-segment parallelogram deformity reduction. A lateral translational deformity is observed and pedicle screws placed (*A*). Pedicle screws are placed and connected by rods (*B*). Rods are connected (friction-glide tightness) and a torque applied to both rods simultaneously via rod grippers (*C*). The reduction is maintained via rigid crossfixation (*D*). Distraction, followed by interbody bone graft placement and finally compression, is used to secure the bone graft in place (*E*).

points are often suboptimal. In addition, techniques like posterior lumbar interbody fusion (PLIF) can be used in this region to attain an anterior interbody fusion mass.

Crossed Screw Fixation

The *crossed screw fixation* technique is not designed primarily for deformity reduction, but can most certainly be used for same. It is a short-segment fixation technique applicable from the midthoracic region to the low lumbar region. It is

employed via the lateral extracavitary approach to the spine.[9] It is used as an alternative to other short-segment fixation techniques, such as pedicle fixation and hook-rod fixation constructs. It uses two large screws that bear axial loads and two ipsilateral smaller pedicle screws that attain reduction and prevent flexion or extension deformation. Screw triangulation optimally resists pullout.[10] Finally, the load bearing–to–load sharing technique affixes the interbody graft into the acceptance bed and reduces the load applied to the construct during ambulation. This allows the

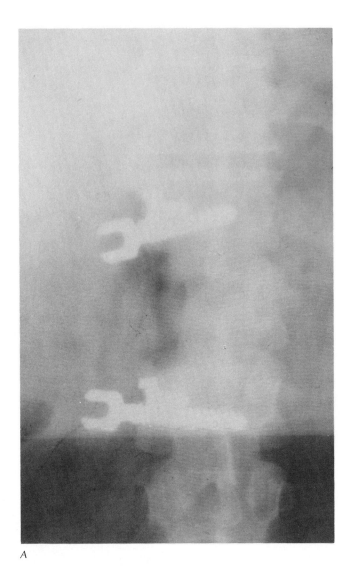

A

B

FIGURE 26-15 The crossed screw fixation technique. *A.* An intraoperative anteroposterior x-ray of two pedicle and two transverse screws in place. *B.* A lateral view of a crossed screw fixation construct. Note that the rigid crosslinking maintains the near-90-degree screw toe-in angle.

use of shorter constructs to achieve the same biomechanical advantage achieved with much longer constructs. It also obviates the need for blind pedicle screw insertion, since the screw is applied only under direct vision on the ipsilateral side of the exposure. Finally, large screws resist stresses much better than multiple smaller screws (see Chap. 13). This technique is employed with 7.5- to 8.5-mm diameter transverse screws (Fig. 26-15).[10]

Both sagittal and coronal plane deformity reductions may be achieved with this technique. The manipulation of the pedicle screw's relationship with the rod, via pivoting of the spine about the already placed transverse screws, can be used to reduce flexion deformation. With the use of variable angled screws, coronal plane deformities can also be corrected (Fig. 26-16).

IN-VIVO ALTERATION OF IMPLANT CONFIGURATION

In-Vivo Implant Contouring

The contouring of the longitudinal member, usually a rod, provides the opportunity to alter spinal segmental relationships. This is commonly used for the "fitting" of the implant to the contour of the spine. This is unfortunate, since the need for excessive in-vivo rod contouring for this purpose usually reflects inadequate pre-insertion rod contouring and poor planning.

In-vivo implant contouring to alter segmental relationships—for deformity reduction, for example—is often effective. A hook-rod universal spinal instrumentation system might be inserted so as to conform to a spinal deformity. Following insertion, the rods could be contoured, along with the attached spine, to achieve an improved alignment (Fig. 26-17). Adequate hook-bone interface security is mandatory. Implant contouring, by its nature, alters the relationships between the implant and the spine. In this case hooks may overtighten or loosen, infringe on the spinal canal, or migrate laterally or medially, depending on their orientation (rostral or caudal) and on the orientation of the applied contouring-related bending moment (Fig. 26-18).

Intrinsic Implant Bending Moment Application about the Long Axis of the Spine

The popularization of spinal derotation as a therapeutic maneuver is credited to Cotrel and Dubousset.[11] It can be used for very complex spinal deformations as well as for simple scoliotic curvatures of the thoracic and lumbar spine. With lateral bending spinal deformations (scoliotic deformations), there is usually a coexisting obligatory rotatory component. This is related to the phenomenon called *coupling* (see Chap. 2). This rotatory component must be borne

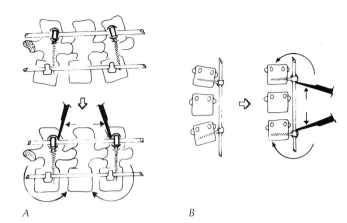

FIGURE 26-16 The crossed screw fixation technique can be used to alter sagittal plane angles (*A*) and coronal plane angles (*B*).

in mind continuously during implant application (see Chap. 4).

Spinal derotation essentially is a maneuver whereby a scoliotic curvature is converted to a kyphotic curvature. If the resultant kyphotic curvature is unacceptable, it is then reduced via rod contouring. In order to accomplish this task the rods are first inserted and attached to hooks, screws, or wires. These are attached loosely (*friction-glide tightness*) so that rotation can occur at the connection site. The hooks can then rotate about the rod as the rod is rotated. This allows the hooks to maintain their relationship with the spinal attachment site.

The rods are then simultaneously rotated 90°, in order to eliminate the scoliotic curve. If need be, the rods are then contoured to reduce any unwanted excessive resultant kyphotic curvature, and the hook-rod interfaces are tightened and secured. Finally, two crossmembers are usually inserted (Fig. 26-19).

One must take care to perform these maneuvers gradually. This allows continuous assessment and reassessment of the implant-bone relationships. For example, a hook may not be rotating on the rod during rotation of the rod; this places significant stress on the hook-bone interface (Fig. 26-20). Some implants, especially those using rods with rough surfaces, are prone to this untoward phenomenon.

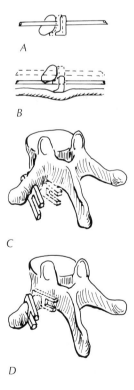

FIGURE 26-18 During rod contouring, implant-bone interface relationships must be watched closely. Some hooks may overdistract, while others may loosen (*A*). Infringement of a sublaminar hook upon the dural sac (*B*), and lateral or medial migration of pedicle hooks (*C*) or transverse process hooks (*D*), may also occur.

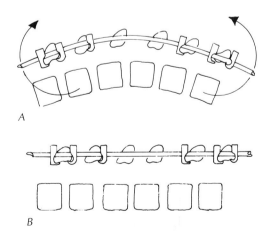

FIGURE 26-17 Rod contouring can be used to alter spinal alignment from a pathological kyphotic curvature, with the rods configured to match the curvature of the pathological spine (*A*), to a corrected alignment (*B*).

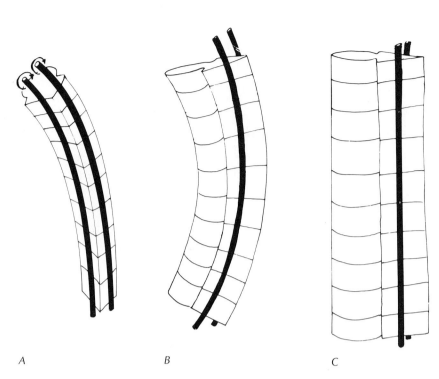

A   *B*   *C*

FIGURE 26-19 Spinal derotation is accomplished via careful simultaneous rotation of two rods that have been attached to the spine in its deformed scoliotic state (*A*). The rotation of the rods by 90° converts a scoliosis to a kyphosis (*B*). If the resultant kyphotic deformity is unacceptable, it may be corrected by rod contouring (*C*).

Intrinsic Implant Bending Moment Application about the Axial Axes of the Spine

Intrinsic implant bending moment application about an axial axis is usually employed in the thoracic and lumbar spine, in order to achieve the reduction of a rotatory deformation. This force complex can be applied in either the sagittal or the coronal plane.

One- or two-segment scoliotic (coronal plane) deformations, usually lumbar, can at least be partially corrected by this technique. Pedicle screws are inserted, with care taken to consider the rotatory component of the deformation. Then rods are attached to the screws, the screws on the concave side of the curvature are distracted (usually 1 to 2 cm), and the screws on the convex side of the curvature compressed. Crossfixation is usually used, to maintain the correction (Fig. 26-21). A similar technique may be used on the lateral aspect of the spine, to reduce a sagittal plane deformation (Fig. 26-22). The use of an applied moment arm cantilever beam construct also applies an intrinsic implant bending moment (Figs. 26-10 and 26-11).[3,4]

With distraction or compression of screws in any of the techniques mentioned here, the relationship of the screw to the rod must be carefully monitored in order to avoid untoward screw-rod relationships—for example, flexion of the screw on the rod. Only a few screw-rod interfaces allow this to occur [e.g., the Texas Scottish Rite Hospital (TSRH) variable-angle screw]. One should, therefore, consider carefully the type of screw-rod interface—that is, variable-angle versus fixed-angle. The application of distraction forces to fixed-angle screws results in simple distraction with no application of any bending moment to the spine. If, however, a variable-angle screw is used, simple distraction may result in screw flexion at the screw-rod interface, thus causing a bending moment to be applied to the spine. This can be prevented by tightening of the screw to a friction-glide tightness prior to the application of the distraction forces (Fig. 26-23).

MAINTENANCE OF CORRECTION

Crossfixation

The connection of posterior bilaterally placed constructs to each other may substantially augment the integrity of the construct. In general, short constructs do not significantly benefit from crossfixation. However, if the maintenance of deformity reduction depends, in part, on crossfixation (e.g., as depicted in Fig. 26-14), then crossfixation is mandatory.

With longer constructs, crossfixation is biomechanically useful. It allows the acquisition of a quadrilateral frame construct, with its associated effects of rotatory stabilization and augmentation of the integrity of implant-bone interfaces. In general, two crossmembers are better than one; but using more than two adds very little to the effect of two crossmembers. In general, the two crossmembers should be placed roughly at the junctions of the middle and rostral thirds and of the middle and caudal thirds of the construct—in other words, at the two ends of the middle third of the construct (Fig. 26-24).

An additional indication for crossfixation is the mainte-

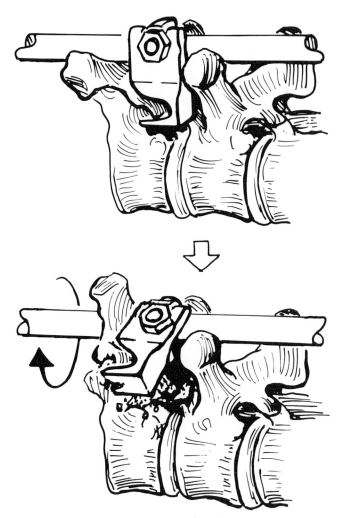

FIGURE 26-20 During derotation, if hooks are overly secured (not friction-glide tightness), they will rotate with the rod. This results in hook cutout.

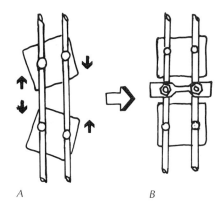

FIGURE 26-21 Intrinsic implant bending moment application. In this case, simple distraction of the concave side of the curvature and compression of the convex side (*A*) achieves the reduction of a scoliotic deformity. Crossfixation is usually employed to assist in maintenance of the reduction (*B*).

simple (translation), but the mechanism by which this is achieved is complex (Fig. 26-27).

Toggle, Cutout, Pullout, and Implant Fracture Prevention

Toggle, cutout, and pullout are undesirable movements at the implant-bone interface. Implant fracture usually occurs at the point of application of the maximum bending moment (Fig. 26-28). The occurrence of each of these complications is minimized by the application of the principles outlined in previous chapters. In general, toggle can be minimized by attempting to achieve a bicortical purchase and to optimize

nance of the desired inter-rod width. This may prevent pedicle hook migration, screw dislodgment from the ilium, and other problems (Fig. 26-25).

When crossmembers are employed with short constructs to maintain deformity reduction, very rigid crossmembers should be used. Substantial bending moments are applied at the crossmember-rod interface. These can be resisted only by the most rigid of crossmembers (Fig. 26-26).

Screw Toe-In

As depicted in Chap. 15, screw toe-in plays an integral role in the prevention of lateral translational deformation. So does crossfixation, though via a different mechanism (see above). As depicted in Fig. 26-14, screw toe-in may be used in conjunction with crossfixation to achieve, in a "belt and suspenders"-like manner, the maintenance of deformity reduction. The forces resisted by the toe-in technique are

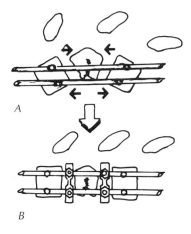

FIGURE 26-22 Intrinsic implant bending moment application. In this case, laterally placed transverse vertebral body screws are manipulated to reduce a kyphotic deformity (*A*). Compression of the two most dorsal screws and distraction of the two most ventral screws achieves reduction of this deformity. Crossfixation is usually employed to assist in maintenance of the reduction (*B*).

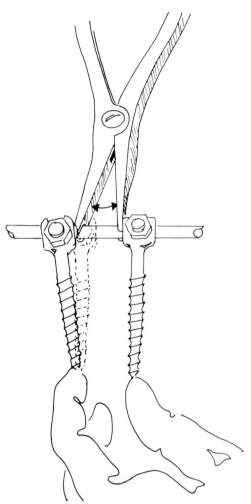

FIGURE 26-23 Screw flexion may occur during distraction if the screw-rod interface is of a variable-angle type. This untoward occurrence can be avoided by taking care to achieve friction-glide tightness at the interface prior to distraction. Arrows depict distraction forces applied by the distractor, and resistance to distraction exerted at the tip of the screw by spinal elements (or, in this case, fingers).

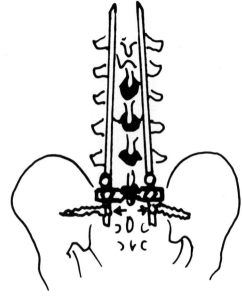

FIGURE 26-25 Besides giving a quadrilaterally framed construct, crossmembers provide the ability to maintain the desired inter-rod distance. This may be particularly useful in sacropelvic fixation, as depicted.

"load-sharing" principles (Fig. 26-29). Cutout can be minimized by avoidance of the untoward application of three-point bending forces with the use of appropriate-length screws (Fig. 26-30). Pullout can be minimized by the use of larger-diameter screws with an accompanying increased thread depth and pitch (see Chap. 13) (Fig. 26-31). The risk of implant fracture can be minimized by the use of implant components that are structurally sound at points of maximum bending moment application (Fig. 26-32). Implant contouring, obviously, weakens the implant by creating stress risers (Fig. 26-28D)

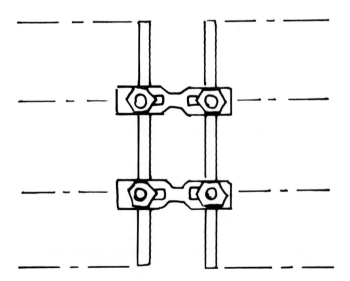

FIGURE 26-24 A depiction of crossmembers placed roughly at the junctions of the middle third with the upper and lower thirds of the construct.

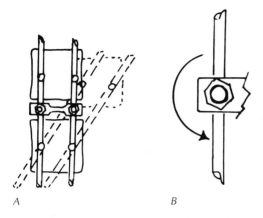

FIGURE 26-26 Rigid crossmembers are useful in deformity reduction via short constructs. The stresses placed at the crossmember-rod junction are often associated with a large bending moment. Only crossmembers that provide substantial torsional resistance capabilities can resist these stresses. In this case, the crossmember maintains the reduction of a translational deformity (*A*) by applying a torque to the rod (*B*).

HIGH CERVICAL AND OCCIPITOCERVICAL TECHNIQUES

Gallie, Brooks, and Related Techniques

The Gallie, Brooks, and combination techniques have been employed for C1-C2 fusions for decades (Fig. 26-33).[12–14] They all (especially the Gallie technique) minimally resist sagittal plane translation deformation. This deformation occurs in a parallelogram-like manner (Fig. 26-34). The Brooks and combination techniques[12,13] provide an

increased rigidity that the Gallie technique does not. However, they are still somewhat deficient in this regard. The combination technique, described by Sontagg and coworkers, provides a biomechanical advantage like that of the Brooks technique, without one of the latter's chief disadvantages: the risk associated with bilaminar sublaminar wire passage.[13]

C1-C2 Clamp Techniques

C1-C2 clamp techniques, such as the Halifax clamp,[15] provide a safety factor in their lack of need for sublaminar wire passage. However, they are prone to the same translation deformation complications as the above-mentioned wiring techniques (Fig. 26-35).

Cantilevered Screw Techniques

Cantilevered screw techniques may be applied in any region of the spine. For years they have been used for translaminar and facet fixation in the lumbar region (Fig. 26-36).[16] In recent years, however, they have been used mainly in the upper cervical spine, for anterior fixation of dens fractures,[17] and posteriorly, for C1-C2 transarticular fixation for C1-C2 instability.[18] They employ and withstand a combination of complex force applications; the predominant force complex application is three-point bending. *These constructs are usually placed in a neutral mode at the time of surgery.* However, they are asked to resist predominantly three-point bending forces during the activities of daily living.

The cantilevered screw technique is a classical application of terminal three-point bending forces. In this situation, cantilevered screws are used as implants in and of them-

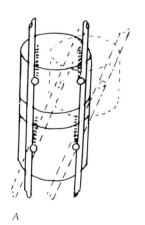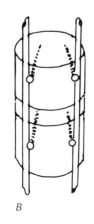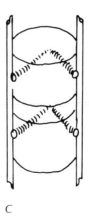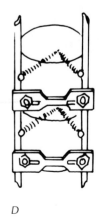

FIGURE 26-27 Screw toe-in maintenance results in much greater pullout resistance, translational deformity prevention, and construct security. Parallel screws cannot resist translation and resist pullout poorly (*A*). An intermediate toe-in provides moderate security in these respects (*B*). Significant toe-in results in even greater security (*C*). Crossfixation *plus* significant screw

toe-in provides the optimum in both pullout resistance and translational deformation resistance (*D*). This concept is applied by the crossed screw fixation technique (see Figs. 26-15 and 26-16). With this configuration, pivoting of the bone about a screw is prohibited by its toed-in counterpart. Similarly, pullout of a screw is prohibited by its toed-in counterpart.

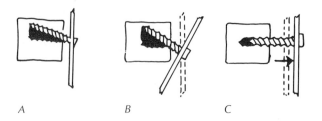

A   *B*   *C*

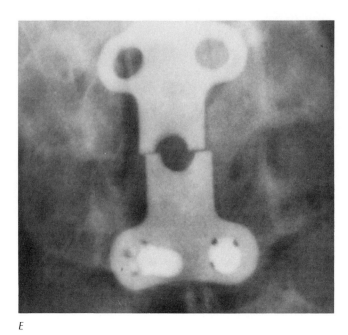

E

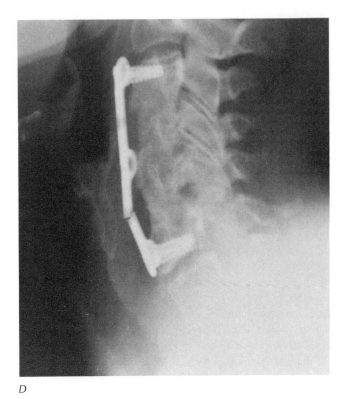

D

FIGURE 26-28 Screw-bone interface failure can occur via toggle (*A*), cutout (*B*), and pullout (*C*). Plate fracture can occur at the point of maximum bending moment application or at a weak point in the plate. The latter may occur at a stress riser caused by plate contouring. This is illustrated by x-rays (*D* and *E*).

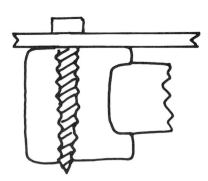

FIGURE 26-29 Screw toggle can be minimized by the use of bicortical purchase and load-sharing principles—that is, with an interbody bone graft.

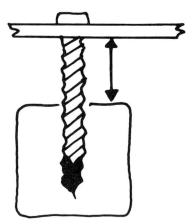

FIGURE 26-30 The minimization of three-point bending force application via a rigid screw-plate construct may prevent cutout.

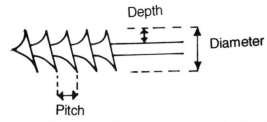

FIGURE 26-31 The risk of pullout can be minimized by the use of larger-diameter screws with a deep thread depth and pitch.

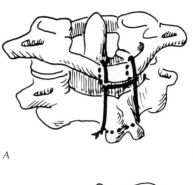

A

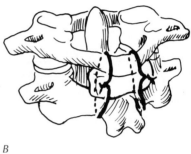

B

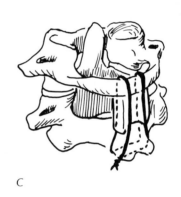

C

FIGURE 26-33 The Gallie (*A*), Brooks (*B*), and modified (*C*) techniques of C1-C2 wire fixation.

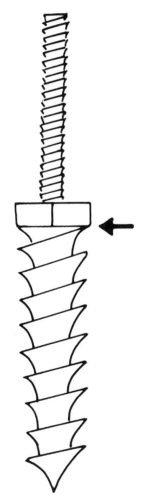

FIGURE 26-32 Implants, such as screws, may be designed so that they are of greatest structural integrity at points of maximal bending moment application—for example, in the region of the screw-rod or screw-plate interface.

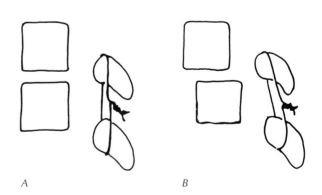

A　　　　　*B*

FIGURE 26-34 Posterior cervical wire fixation techniques may inadequately resist parallelogram-type sagittal plane deformation (*A* and *B*).

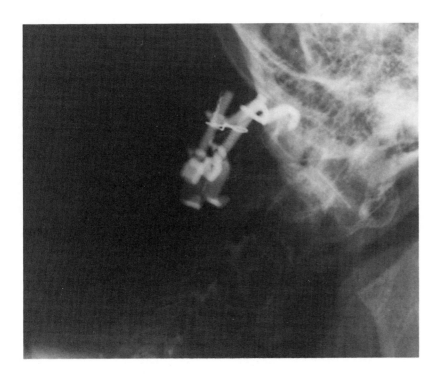

FIGURE 26-35 The use of clamps in the upper cervical spine may result in parallelogram-type sagittal plane deformation, as depicted.

selves. They usually apply neutral transverse forces to the spine during insertion, although significant tensile forces are usually applied, as mentioned above. During activity, significant transverse forces are applied to the screw. In some respects this type of force application is akin to a fixed moment arm cantilever beam (Fig. 26-37). However, they are most appropriately classified as terminal three-point bending force applications (Fig. 26-6).

An understanding of the loads to be withstood by such a construct is imperative to its appropriate employment. Both screw size and moment arm length need careful consideration. For example, a terminal 3-point bending force application to a thin cantilevered screw may be appropriate if the

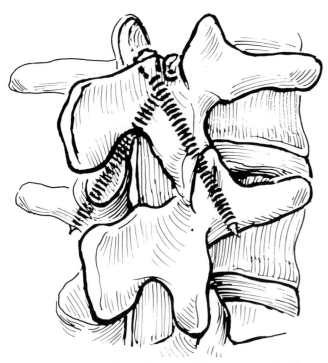

FIGURE 26-36 Cantilevered screw techniques are applicable to translaminar facet fixation.

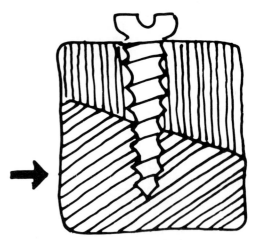

FIGURE 26-37 Cantilevered screw techniques withstand transverse loads in a manner akin to that of a fixed moment arm cantilever beam construct, as depicted. They also may be viewed as providing a three-point bending–like construct (see Fig. 26-6). Arrow depicts transverse force resisted.

FIGURE 26-38 If the transverse loads resisted by a cantilevered screw technique are substantial (*A*), the length of the moment arm should perhaps be shortened to decrease stress on the screw (*B*), or, more appropriately, a larger screw diameter employed (*C*). Arrows depict transverse forces resisted.

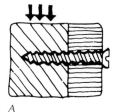 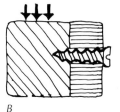 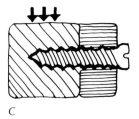

A   *B*   *C*

load is not great and the moment arm not long. If neither of these conditions holds, a larger screw or shorter moment arm should be considered (Fig. 26-38).

Occipitocervical Techniques

Various techniques have been used to stabilize the occipitocervical region. As outlined in Chap. 1, the occipitocervical region (defined by the occipital condyles, the occiput, and the C2 vertebra) is associated with complex movements and stress resistance modes. At the occiput-C1 segment, flexion occurs with very little rotation or lateral bending. At the C1-C2 segment, minimal lateral bending, moderate flexion and extension, and significant axial rotation occur (see Chap. 1). To put it more simply, the occiput-C1 joint functions predominantly in flexion and extension, while the C1-C2 joint functions predominantly in rotation and secondarily in flexion and extension (Fig. 26-39). It is imperative, therefore, that flexion-extension, lateral bending, and axial rotation be restricted.

The occiput provides limited security of implant fixation. Screws have only a short width of bone in which to anchor. Similarly, wires may easily pull through the thin bone of the occiput. Hooks pose similar dilemmas. This is compounded by the need for long fixation lever arms; thus it is often necessary to use a fixation to the mid- or low cervical spine.

One must assess what is expected from the construct. Is axial load-bearing required, or is simple prevention of translational deformation all that is required? Different forces are resisted by the implant in each of these circumstances. Consideration of the upper cervical spine as akin to a universal-like joint may assist one in understanding the complexities of upper cervical spine motion (Fig. 26-40).[18] These factors must be considered carefully.

Rotatory deformation at the C1-C2 segmental level (Figs. 26-39 and 26-40) may complicate occiput-C1 stabilization procedures by allowing relatively unrestricted C1-C2 rotation to weaken occiput-C2 fixation constructs. The elimination of this rotational deformation may allow the use of shorter constructs by providing a substantial platform for occiput-C1-C2 fixation (Fig. 26-41).

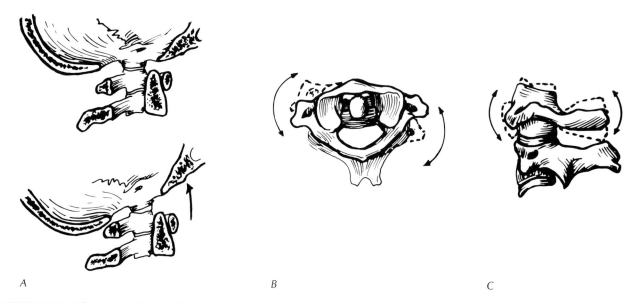

A   *B*   *C*

FIGURE 26-39 The occiput-C1 joint functions predominantly in flexion and extension (*A*); the C1-C2 joint functions predominantly in rotation (*B*) and secondarily in flexion and extension (*C*).

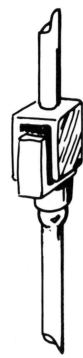

FIGURE 26-40 Envisioning the overall movements in the upper cervical spine as if they occurred about a universal-like joint, combined with a ball-and-socket joint may facilitate an understanding of the complex movements observed in this region. Flexion and extension and some lateral bending at the joint's rostral component (the occiput-C1 joint) and flexion, extension, and lateral bending with axial rotation about its caudal component (the C1-C2 joint) exemplify, though perhaps in an oversimplified manner, these movements.

LOW LUMBAR AND LUMBOSACRAL TECHNIQUES

The surgical management of low lumbar fractures is fraught with complications. Surgical management, therefore, should be entertained only if at least one of these two indications is present: (1) the presence of a neurological deficit in the presence of spinal canal compromise, and (2) the presence of an unstable fracture (both posterior and anterior elements disrupted).

If surgery is indicated, various options are available—and none of them is optimal. The confines of the lumbosacral region are prohibitive. Ventral decompression is possible via anterior, anterolateral, lateral extracavitary, and posterior approaches (the latter via transpedicular postlaminectomy anteropulsion of traumatically retropulsed bone and disk fragments) (see Chap. 8). Indeed, the placement of axial load–supporting instrumentation constructs is not without complications.

If adequate axial load–supporting capacity is already present or has been established by a ventral interbody operative procedure, the instrumentation aspect of the stabilization process is simplified. In this case, the provision of

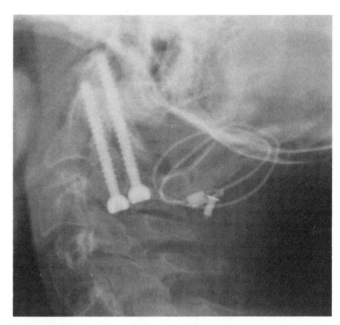

FIGURE 26-41 The optimization of an occiput–upper cervical fusion may be achieved by first eliminating C1-C2 rotation via a transarticular screw fixation technique. Then, the elimination of flexion-extension movements at the occiput-C1 junction is made simpler by the use of a simple cerclage wiring technique, as depicted.

simple compressive forces—or no posterior instrumentation construct whatsoever—may suffice.

If, on the other hand, adequate axial load–supporting capacity neither is inherent nor has been achieved surgically, the stabilization process becomes a complex one indeed. The available choices include pedicle fixation, complex lumbosacral-iliac fixation techniques, and multisegmental distraction fixation techniques.

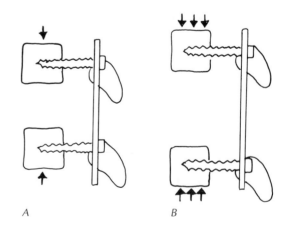

FIGURE 26-42 Distraction of a rigid implant loads the implant so that it bears a greater load than an implant placed in a neutral mode. Neutral (*A*) and distracted (*B*) implants are shown. Arrows depict the forces accepted (or resisted) by the implants.

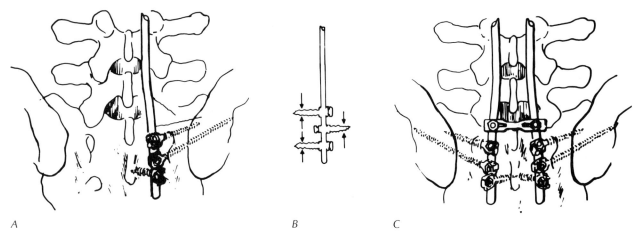

A   *B*   *C*

FIGURE 26-43 A tripod geometry of the implant for sacropelvic fixation is provided by bone screws placed in the sacrum (pedicles and/or ala) and iliac crest (*A*). This splayed configuration helps prevent migration of the implant much as does toeing-in of screws (*B*). An additional component of the splayed configuration is achieved if a rigid crossmember is placed (*C*).

The application of a pedicle fixation construct in the presence of inadequate axial load–resisting capacity perhaps asks too much from the instrumentation construct. Cantilever beam constructs (usually with fixed moment arms) that are required to support total torso weight are excessively stressed, as is the screw-bone interface. Repetitive loading of such a construct may produce failure at the screw-bone interface or the screw-plate or screw-rod interface (Fig. 26-42).[5]

Complex lumbosacral-iliac techniques, such as the slingshot and Galveston techniques,[19] are cumbersome. They affix to predominantly loose medullary bone and may provide inadequate implant-bone interface security. The leverage for the prevention of lumbosacral flexion and extension, therefore, may be inadequate. Iliac screw fixation techniques, using bicortical ilial fixation, are viable alternatives to these techniques.[20] They allow the acquisition of a tripodlike geometry for buttressing against the sacroilial segment and for the utilization of the splayed geometry of the implant-bone interfaces for improved resistance to implant-bone interface failure (Fig. 26-43). The anteromedial orientation of sacral screws appear to be superior to an anterolateral (alar) orientation, particularly when employed with rigid implant connections (constrained).[21] Greater bone density, and hence a stronger implant-bone interface, may be attained in the region of the sacral midline at the margin of the promontory (Fig. 26-44). The bone is more densely compacted in this region than in other regions of the sacrum.

Additional implant-bone interfaces for the prevention of lumbosacral flexion and extension include the first sacral lamina, the second dorsal sacral neuroforamina, and the dorsum of the sacrum itself (Fig. 26-45).[22] Lumbosacral fixation via multisegmental distraction offers the ability to distract the lumbosacral spine, restore height to the collapsed vertebral segments, allow two or more points of sacral fixation, and use the sacrum as a buttress for support of the torso against axial loads (Fig. 26-45).

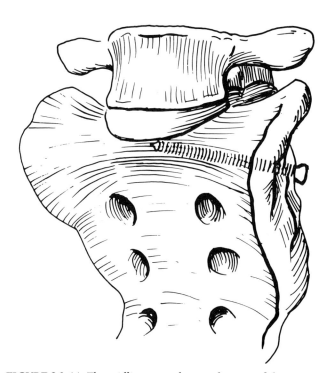

FIGURE 26-44 The midline, rostral, ventral aspect of the sacrum, near the promontory, consists of denser bone than that found in the rest of the sacrum. A screw placed in this region may achieve a stronger purchase than is available in other regions of the sacrum.

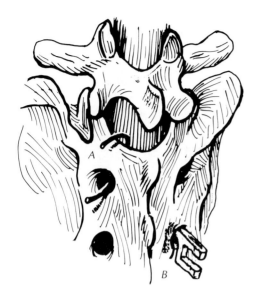

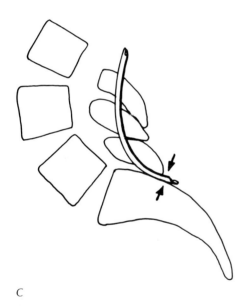

C

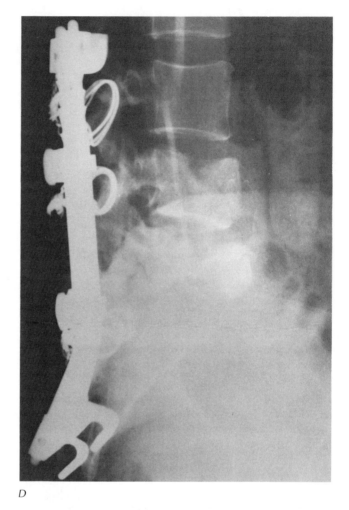

D

FIGURE 26-45 Additional implant-bone interfaces for the prevention of lumbosacral flexion and extension include the first sacral lamina (*A*), the second dorsal sacral neuroforamina (*B*), and the dorsum of the sacrum itself (*C*). The first sacral lamina is more substantial laterally than medially. A sublaminar wire (usually placed in a rostral-to-caudal direction from the L5-S1 interlaminar space through the S1 neuroforamina) engages the thickest portion of the S1 lamina (*A*). The caudal border of the second dorsal sacral neuroforamina is thick and accepts hooks readily (*B*).[22] The dorsum of the sacrum itself may function as a buttress for a contoured rod (*C*). A lateral x-ray depicts the utilization of these purchase points (*D*).

All of the techniques of lumbosacral fixation should take advantage of the *lumbosacral pivot point* described by McCord and coworkers.[23] This is defined as the point of intersection of the middle osteoligamentous column (region of the posterior longitudinal ligament) in the sagittal plane, and the L5-S1 intervertebral disk. Constructs that attempt lumbosacral fixation via bone screws are best able to resist flexion and extension deformation if the screws extend ventrally beyond the plane dictated by the location of this point (Fig. 26-46).[23]

ENHANCING BONE GRAFT SECURITY

Bone grafts can migrate or dislodge. Implants can be used to enhance the security of the bone graft and, thus, to augment

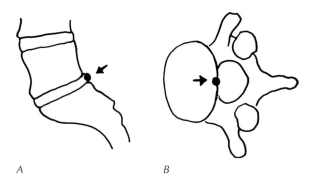

FIGURE 26-46 The lumbosacral pivot point is the junction of the middle osteoligamentous column (region of the posterior longitudinal ligament) in the sagittal plane, and the L5-S1 intervertebral disk, as depicted in sagittal (*A*) and axial (*B*) views. Ilial and sacral screws should pass ventral to this point if an optimal biomechanical advantage is to be achieved. *(From D.H. McCord et al.[23])*

fusion rates. Two techniques that find clinical utility are *interference screw fixation* (for enhancement of interbody bone graft security) and *cerclage and compression wiring* (for enhancement of posterior onlay bone graft security) (Fig. 26-47).[24,25] The efficacy of interference screw fixation is improved by the use of multiple (two versus one) and larger (3.5-mm versus 2.7-mm) screws.[25]

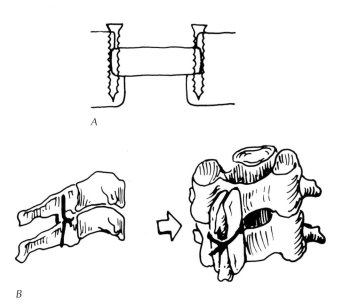

FIGURE 26-47 Interference screw fixation (*A*) and cerclage and compression wiring (*B*) enhance bone graft security for interbody and posterior fusions, respectively. Interference screw fixation does so by using the threads of the screw as extra points of friction between the bone graft and the vertebral body. Cerclage and compression wiring force the graft onto the spinous processes.

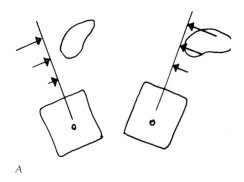

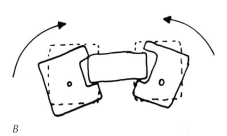

FIGURE 26-48 Posterior spinal compression force application compresses all points dorsal to the instantaneous axis of rotation (IAR) (*A*). An interbody bone graft placed posterior to the IAR prior to the application of the compression force will thus be impacted into the vertebral body and, therefore, accept a greater portion of the load during axial load-bearing (load bearing–to–load sharing) (*B*).

COMBINED TECHNIQUES

The use of posterior spinal compression with an accompanying anterior interbody (distraction) strut will compress the strut into the accepting vertebral bodies if the strut is behind the instantaneous axis of rotation (IAR)—which it usually is. The short rod–two claw technique uses this principle.[6] Essentially it uses the load bearing–to–sharing principle described above. By compressing the spine dorsally, the ventral interbody strut is forced to accept a substantial portion of the axial load (at rest and during weight-bearing). Similarly, rotatory movements and stresses may be shared by the construct (Fig. 26-48).

Various force complexes may be applied, at different levels, via long spinal implants. These force complexes may be difficult to understand and to predict fully. They may be associated with intrinsic aberrations of the individual's anatomy and the anatomic relationships created by the spinal pathology; some of these factors may not be obvious. This is exemplified by a long, complex construct that was applied to one patient's lumbar and lumbosacral region (Fig. 26-49). This case illustrates the combination of cantilever

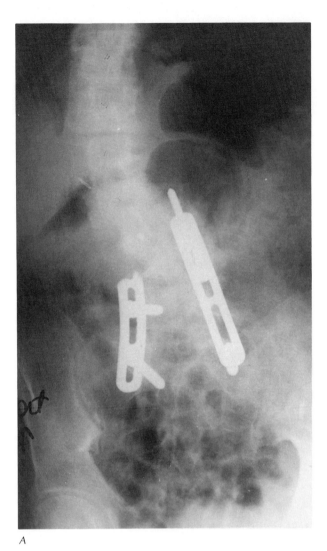

A

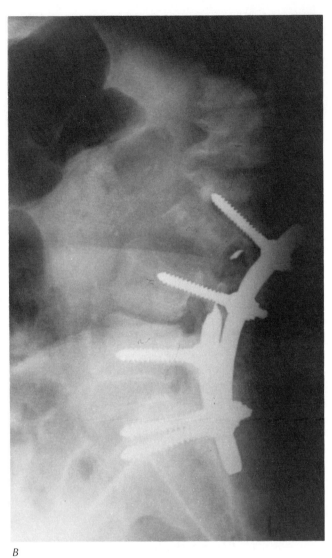

B

FIGURE 26-49 A variety of force complexes applied at different levels via a long spinal implant. The patient had previously undergone an L3-S1 fusion with instrumentation and subsequent partial implant removal. *A* and *B*. Preoperative anteroposterior and lateral x-rays showing partial implant removal and resultant scoliotic and kyphotic deformations. *C*. A line-drawing blueprint depicting the corrective forces to be applied by the planned construct. *D* and *E*. Postoperative anteroposterior and lateral x-rays showing insertion of planned construct after existing construct was removed. Note that individual portions of the construct apply fixed moment arm cantilever beam, three-point bending, distraction, and compression force complexes to the spine. Also note the use of bicortical iliac fixation purchase site.

beam, three-point bending, distraction, compression, and other forces in a single construct. These forces were successfully applied to achieve the desired results: stability, decompression, and pain relief.

COMPLICATIONS

Complications of construct applications designed to achieve spinal stability tend to increase with the complexity of the construct applied. Therefore, the risk-to-benefit ratio must be weighted as much as possible toward the patient's advantage. In other words, the complications associated with a more complex construct must be outweighed by the advantages it provides. Particularly with complex constructs, the application of segment-specific forces to the spine must be individually considered. *The foundation of appropriate construct design (see Chap. 16) is the surgeon's solid understanding of the biomechanical principles of both the pathological process and the planned surgical correction.*

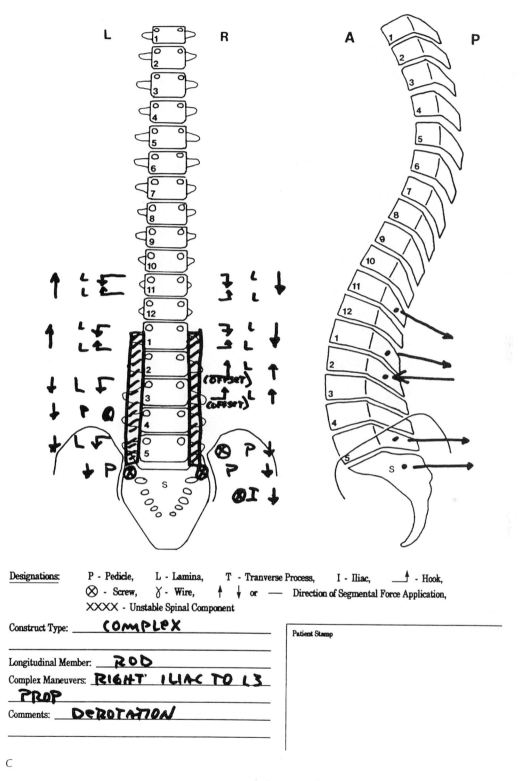

Designations: P - Pedicle,   L - Lamina,   T - Tranverse Process,   I - Iliac,   ⌐ᵀ⌐ - Hook,   ⊗ - Screw,   ɣ - Wire,   ↑ ↓ or — Direction of Segmental Force Application,   XXXX - Unstable Spinal Component

Construct Type: ___COMPLEX___

Longitudinal Member: ___ROD___

Complex Maneuvers: ___RIGHT ILIAC TO L3 PROP___

Comments: ___DEROTATION___

Patient Stamp

C

FIGURE 26-49 *(Continued)*

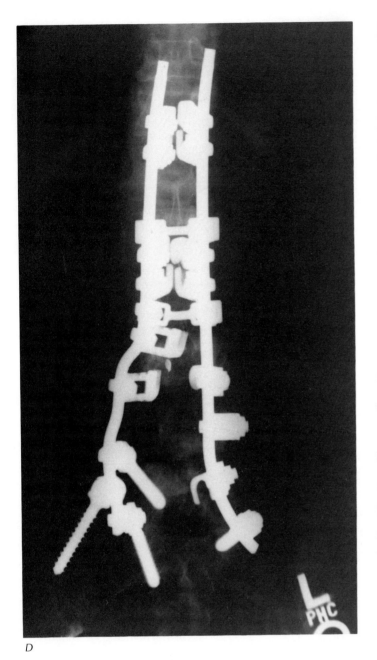

D

E

FIGURE 26-49 (*Continued*)

REFERENCES

1. White AA, Panjabi MM: *Clinical Biomechanics of the Spine* (2d ed). Philadelphia: Lippincott, 1990: 1–125.
2. Steffee AD, Biscup RS, Sitkowski DJ: Segmental spine plates with pedicle screw fixation. *Clin Orthop Rel Res* 1986; 203:45–53.
3. Dick W: The "fixatuer interne" as a versatile implant for spine surgery. *Spine* 1987; 12:882–900.
4. Krag MH, Beynnon BD, Pope MH, et al: An internal fixator for posterior application to short segments of the thoracic, lumbar, or lumbosacral spine. *Clin Orthop Rel Res* 1986; 203:75–98.
5. McLain RF, Sparling E, Benson DR: Early failure of short-segment pedicle instrumentation for thoracolumbar fractures: *J Bone Joint Surg* 1993; 75A:162–167.
6. Benzel EC: Short-segment compression instrumentation for selected thoracic and lumbar spine fractures: The short-rod/two-claw technique. *J. Neurosurg* 1993; 79:335–340.
7. Benzel EC: Luque rod segmental spinal instrumentation, in Rengachary SS, Wilkins RH (eds): *Neurosurgical Operative Atlas,* vol 1. Baltimore: Williams and Wilkins, 1992: 433–438.
8. Benzel EC, Ball PA, Baldwin NG, et al: The sequential hook insertion technique for universal spinal instrumentation application. *J Neurosurg* 79:608–611, 1993.
9. Maiman DJ, Larson SJ: Lateral extracavitary approach to the tho-

racic and lumbar spine, in Rengachary SS, Wilkins RH (eds): *Neurosurgical Operative Atlas*. Baltimore: Williams and Wilkins, 1992: 153–161.

10. Benzel EC, Baldwin NG: Crossed screw fixation of the unstable thoracic and lumbar spine. *J Neurosurg* (in press).

11. Cotrel Y, Dubousset J, Guillaumat M: New universal instrumentation in spinal surgery. *Clin Orthop Rel Res* 1988; 227:10–23.

12. Brooks Al, Jenkins EB: Atlantoaxial arthrodesis by the wedge compression method. *J Bone Joint Surg* 1978; 60A:279–284.

13. Dickman CA, Sonntag VKH, Papadopoulos SM, et al: The interspinous method of posterior atlantoaxial arthrodesis. *J Neurosurg* 1991; 74:109–198.

14. Gallie WE: Fractures and dislocations of the cervical spine. *Am J Surg* 1939; 46:495–499.

15. Holness RO, Huestis WS, Howes WJ, et al: Posterior stabilization with an interlaminar clamp in cervical injuries: Technical note and review of the long term experience with the method. *Neurosurgery* 1984; 14:318–322.

16. Jacobs RR, Montesano PX, Jackson RP: Enhancement of lumbar spine fusion by use of translaminar facet joint screws. *Spine* 1989; 14:12–15.

17. Apfelbaum RI: Anterior screw fixation for odontoid fractures, in Camins MB, O'Leary PF (eds): *Disorders of the Cervical Spine*. Baltimore: Williams and Wilkins, 1992: 603–608.

18. Panjabi M, Dvorak J, Duranceau J, et al: Three-dimensional movements of the upper cervical spine. *Spine* 1988; 13:726–730.

19. Allen BL, Ferguson RL: The Galveston technique for L-rod instrumentation of the scoliotic spine. *Spine* 1982; 7:276–284.

20. Baldwin NG, Benzel EC: Improved sacral fixation using iliac instrumentation and a variable angle screw device. *J Neurosurg* (in press).

21. Carlson GD, Abitbol JJ, Anderson DR, et al: Screw fixation in the human sacrum. *Spine* 1992; 17:S196–S203.

22. Ball PA, Benzel EC: Non-screw dorsal sacral fixation. (Submitted.)

23. McCord DH, Cunningham BW, Shono Y, et al: Biomechanical analysis of lumbosacral fixation. *Spine* 1992; 17:S235–243.

24. Benzel EC, Kesterson L: Posterior cervical interspinous compression wiring and fusion for mid to low cervical spinal injuries. *J Neurosurg* 1989; 70:893–899.

25. Vasquez-Seoane P, Yoo J, Zou D, et al: Interference screw fixation of cervical grafts: A combined in vitro biomechanical and in vivo animal study. *Spine* 1993; 18:946–954.

Chapter *27*

Spinal Orthotics

INTRODUCTION

The achievement of spinal stability is optimized by (1) appropriate decompression, (2) appropriate bone graft placement (fusion), (3) appropriately placed internal fixation constructs, and (4) appropriate use of external splinting techniques. The latter may not be necessary or may include such techniques as bed rest, traction, and spine bracing. General references regarding orthotics and bracing are available.[1-3]

Both bed rest, with or without traction, and spine bracing are fraught with difficulties. The duration of bed rest required to attain adequate bony healing is considerable. Furthermore, this time spent in bed is not without risk; possible complications include deep vein thrombophlebitis, pulmonary embolism, pneumonia, decubiti, joint contractures, and depression.

Spine bracing presents its own set of associated problems, the most significant of which is its relative lack of effectiveness in achieving its stated goal—that is, to minimize "excessive" spinal movement. The amount of soft tissue separating the spine and the brace itself minimizes the effectiveness of the brace. In fact, there is an inverse relationship between the thickness of soft tissue between the spine and inner surface of the brace and the effectiveness of the brace. Furthermore, a longer brace usually gives more spinal stability than a shorter one. Therefore, the *length-to-width ratio* of the brace plays a significant role in efficacy of stabilization (Fig. 27-1).

The goals of spinal bracing include (1) restriction of movement, (2) spinal realignment, and (3) trunk support. The achievement of these goals and the mechanisms by which they are achieved are of great importance. *The surgeon planning to use spinal bracing must understand the goals of bracing and must have the ability to realistically appraise, within reason, the properties of individual orthoses.*

Various external splinting techniques have been used to gain the advantage of early ambulation of the patient with an unstable spine. Spinal splints are made from various materials and combinations thereof. The splints generally are constructed of material that furnishes some minimal flexibility while simultaneously providing adequate structural support. Plastic polymer brace materials offer several advantages: less weight, the possibility of ventilation holes to allow increased comfort, relative ease in the doffing and donning of the brace, and ease of fabrication.

Splinting devices that do not closely conform to the torso (e.g., the Halo and the Jewett brace) have several disadvantages. The Jewett brace, for example, applies a dorsally directed force at the sternum and the pubic region. Because the pressure applied may be significant, it frequently causes discomfort. In the case of lumbar instability, it does not place the ventrally directed force in an appropriate location (i.e., in the low lumbar or lumbosacral spine). Furthermore, the Jewett brace and similar techniques do not promote the maintenance of the cylindrical body shell; that is, contact with the torso is made over a relatively small surface area (Fig. 27-2). The concept of the body shell has been previously addressed from several viewpoints.[4-7] The Jewett brace, however, does provide a three-point bending biomechanical advantage (Fig. 27-3).[3,6] This has been shown to be an important factor in the stability achieved with external splinting. The maintenance of the body shell also increases the stability of the anterior and posterior spinal elements (columns). Morris and coworkers have nicely shown and illustrated the significant role of the trunk as a stabilizer of the spine.[5] Last, the Jewett and similar braces do not significantly restrict lateral bending.

The conformation and close "fit" between the anterior and posterior halves of a brace are critical to the brace's ability to stabilize the spine. The lack of a close "fit" between halves allows parallelogram deformation of the bracing construct. This, in turn, diminishes protection. The halves of the brace should not only be secured so that the sliding of one past the other does not occur, but they should be rigidly attached to one another (Fig. 27-4).

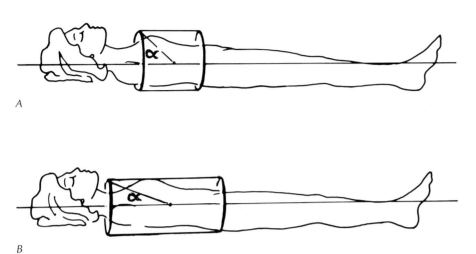

FIGURE 27-1 The effectiveness of spinal bracing is inversely related to the axial distance between the spine and the inner surface of the brace. This is *theoretically* defined by the following relationship: Efficacy of bracing is related to the cosine of α where α is the angle defined by the edge of the brace, the instantaneous axis of rotation (IAR) at the unstable segment, and the long axis of the spine. This angle is dictated by both the length of the brace and the thickness of tissue between the spine and the inner surface of the brace. *A.* A short brace (α = 15 degrees; cosine α = .966). *B.* A long brace (α = 45 degrees; cosine α = .707). Obviously, a significant reduction of efficacy comes with the use of a shorter, wider brace; that is, the length-to-width ratio of the brace is too small.

CERVICAL SPINE BRACING

The cervical spine is, perhaps, the region of the spine that is most effectively stabilized by external splinting techniques. This has to do partly with the lesser amount of soft tissue separating the brace from the spine itself. It has to do also with the substantial points of fixation available at the ends of the cervical region: the cranium and the thoracic cage.

Difficulty in preventing rotation and bending in all directions is variably associated with all techniques.[8-13] The extent of lateral bending is difficult to assess; one has to rely

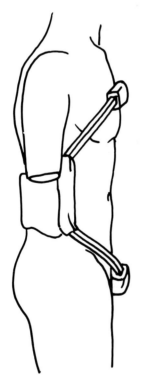

FIGURE 27-2 The design of the Jewett brace does not exploit the intrinsic advantage of the body shell. It minimizes contact area with the torso.

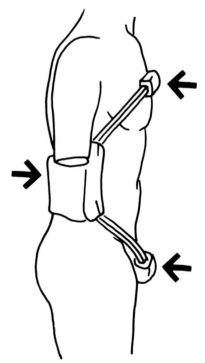

FIGURE 27-3 The three-point bending forces applied by the Jewett brace *(arrows)*. These forces are similar to those applied by spinal implants (e.g., Harrington distraction rod).

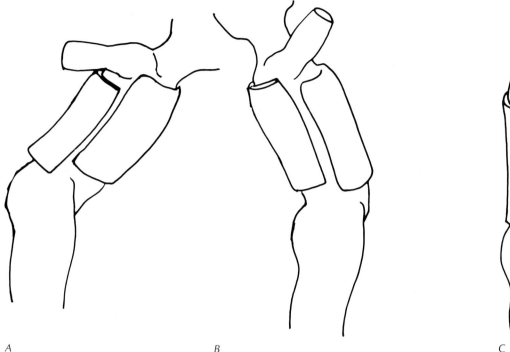
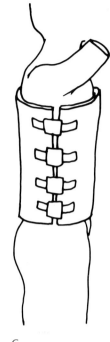

A   *B*   *C*

FIGURE 27-4 The disadvantage of a poorly fitted brace, where the anterior and posterior halves are allowed to slide past each other, is depicted. In this case, flexion (*A*) and extension (*B*) are not significantly restricted because of this phenomenon. The elimination of this sliding motion, and accompanying tight security between the halves (causing the brace to function as a single solid unit), minimize this problem. (*C*).

on anteriorposterior x-rays. These are inherently more difficult to assess than equivalent lateral x-rays. Rotation is even more difficult to assess. Maiman and coworkers and Johnson and coworkers used a goniometer scheme to assess rotation following cervical bracing.[13,14] These lateral and rotatory movements, however, usually are less important than sagittal plane movements with regard to clinical stability concerns.

The *parallelogram-like bracing effect* is a unique characteristic of the cervical spine. It is related both to the signifi-cant mobility of the cervical spine and to the lack of adequate fixation points in the mid-to-low cervical region. The extensive mobility of the upper cervical (atlantooccipital) and mid- and lower cervical regions combines the unique characteristics of both *capital and true neck flexion and extension* movements to exaggerate the parallelogram-like bracing effect (Fig. 27-5).

Braces that attempt fixation from the mandibular region to the base of the neck and shoulder often do not effectively prevent parallelogram-like movement (Fig. 27-6); in fact,

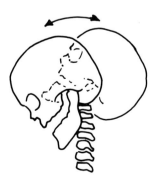
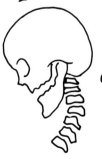
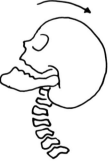

FIGURE 27-5 Capital neck flexion-extension is that movement associated with mobility between O-C1, C1-C2, and C2-C3 (*A*). True neck flexion-extension is that movement associated with mobility between the segments of the subaxial cervical spine (*B*).

A   *B*

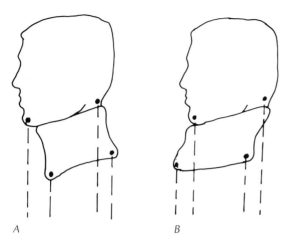

A   *B*

FIGURE 27-6 The parallelogram-like bracing effect is a unique aspect of cervical spine bracing that is associated with the combination of capital and true neck movements and the unique points of fixation available. When inadequate low cervical or thoracic fixation is attained, true neck flexion-extension is relatively unimpeded. Thus the compensatory relationship between the capital and true neck movements is not significantly thwarted. In this case low cervical flexion is accompanied by compensatory capital extension. This, in fact, may be encouraged somewhat by the brace itself (*A*). The converse is also true (*B*). The vertical dashed lines highlight these parallelogram movements.

they may encourage it. A review of published data on cervical orthotic effectiveness illustrates this point (Tables 27-1 and 27-2).[12] Devices using mandible fixation points without chest fixation points allow excessive movement at each motion segment. *The prevention of lower cervical spine movement via the attainment of solid points of chest fixation appears to provide significant reduction of segmental movement at all cervical spine levels. This may pertain to upper tho-*

racic spine segmental movement as well.[15] The combination of capital and compensatory true neck movements (or vice versa) can be controlled by limiting one or the other type of movement, since they are compensatory. Since capital (upper) cervical movement is, indeed, difficult to restrict, the most effective alternative is the minimization of true (mid-to-low) cervical neck movement. This is attained via the use of solid points of chest fixation (Fig. 27-7).

Another problem associated with cervical spine fixation is *snaking*. This phenomenon is defined as "a serpentine movement of the spine, whereby a simple overall movement (such as flexion or extension) is accompanied by an unexpected combination of flexion and extension movements at each intervertebral level."[8,12] Although overall movement from the head to the chest may be minimal, the cumulative segmental movement between these points may be substantial. Therefore, snaking can be defined quantitatively as the difference between the sum of all segmental movements between the head and the chest and the overall movement between the head and the chest.[8] Although one cannot fairly and objectively assess segmental movement of the spine, on account of inconsistent responses of the patient (see below), one can measure the difference between the observed overall movement and the sum of segmental movements. This, then, becomes a relatively objective assessment that relies only on each subject as his or her own control.[8]

The means used to assess the efficacy of cervical bracing techniques are somewhat artificial. Therefore, one must be careful not to rely too heavily on the published data. The movement measured in most studies is elicited by neck movement, the extent of which depends on the cooperativeness of the braced individual. Furthermore, and much more significant, it depends on a consistent submaximal attempt at flexion, extension, rotation, or lateral bending. This consistency is nearly impossible to attain and, more important, to quantitate. These factors are especially impor-

TABLE 27-1 Flexion and Extension Allowed at Each Segmental Level[a]

Test Situation	Motion	0-C1	C1-C2	C2-C3	C3-C4	C4-C5	C5-C6	C6-C7	C7-T1
Normal	Flexion	0.7 ± 0.5	7.7 ± 1.2	7.2 ± 0.9	9.8 ± 1.0	10.3 ± 1.0	11.4 ± 1.0	12.5 ± 1.0	9.0 ± 1.1
unrestricted	Extension	18.1 ± 2.1	6.0 ± 1.2	4.8 ± 0.8	7.8 ± 1.1	9.8 ± 1.2	10.5 ± 1.3	8.2 ± 1.2	2.7 ± 0.7
Soft collar	Flexion	1.3 ± 1.3	5.1 ± 1.9	4.5 ± 1.2	7.4 ± 1.5	8.4 ± 2.4	9.9 ± 1.7	9.7 ± 0.9	7.7 ± 2.5
	Extension	13.7 ± 3.5	1.9 ± 1.4	3.9 ± 1.0	5.8 ± 1.7	6.8 ± 1.6	7.8 ± 1.2	7.4 ± 1.4	2.8 ± 1.9
Philadelphia	Flexion	0.9 ± 1.0	4.0 ± 1.8	1.6 ± 1.0	3.1 ± 1.1	4.6 ± 1.8	6.2 ± 1.9	6.2 ± 1.6	5.5 ± 1.8
collar	Extension	6.8 ± 2.2	4.5 ± 1.5	1.8 ± 0.9	3.4 ± 1.0	5.8 ± 1.2	5.9 ± 1.2	5.8 ± 2.0	1.3 ± 0.9
Somi brace	Flexion	3.6 ± 1.8	2.7 ± 1.8	0.9 ± 0.7	1.6 ± 1.1	1.9 ± 0.8	2.8 ± 1.2	2.9 ± 1.6	3.1 ± 1.8
	Extension	9.1 ± 2.6	5.4 ± 1.9	4.4 ± 1.1	6.3 ± 1.4	6.0 ± 1.8	6.0 ± 2.0	5.6 ± 1.8	2.1 ± 1.1
Four-poster	Flexion	2.9 ± 2.0	4.4 ± 2.1	1.6 ± 1.0	2.1 ± 1.1	1.8 ± 0.9	3.0 ± 1.2	3.9 ± 1.6	2.8 ± 1.4
brace	Extension	9.3 ± 2.2	3.2 ± 1.4	2.0 ± 0.7	3.2 ± 1.2	3.4 ± 1.3	2.9 ± 0.9	3.1 ± 1.5	1.6 ± 0.8
Cervicothoracic	Flexion	1.3 ± 0.9	5.0 ± 1.9	1.8 ± 0.8	2.9 ± 1.2	2.8 ± 0.7	1.6 ± 0.8	0.7 ± 0.6	2.4 ± 1.0
brace	Extension	8.4 ± 2.1	2.5 ± 0.8	2.1 ± 0.7	1.6 ± 0.7	2.2 ± 0.9	2.8 ± 0.9	3.4 ± 1.1	1.7 ± 0.8

[a]Data are expressed as mean degrees and 95% confidence limits of the mean.

SOURCE: From R.M. Johnson et al.[12]

TABLE 27-2 Average Movement at Each Intervertebral Level from Maximum Flexion to Maximum Extension[a]

Stabilization Device	0–C1	C1–2	C2–3	C3–4	C4–5	C5–6	C6–7	Sum of Angles	Average Movement at Each Level	Sum of Angles 0 to C-6 or C-7	Measured Movement
Halo jacket	4.5 ± 2.7	1.3 ± 1.1	4.1 ± 2.6	4.1 ± 3.2	3.1 ± 2.6	3.0 ± 1.9	6.3 ± 5.7	23.4 ± 13.7	3.7 ± 3.1	23.4 ± 13.7	5.2
Minerva jacket	3.5 ± 2.1	2.1 ± 1.1	1.7 ± 1.7	1.9 ± 1.2	2.0 ± 2.1	2.5 ± 1.6	2.3 ± 1.8	14.8 ± 4.4	2.3 ± 1.7	14.8 ± 4.4	5.2

[a]Data expressed in degrees as means $\pm$ standard deviations. O = occiput; * = statistically significant difference ($p < .025$)
SOURCE: From E.C. Benzel et al.[8]

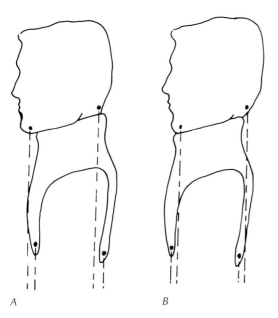

FIGURE 27-7 The parallelogram-like bracing effort depicted in Fig. 27-6 can be significantly diminished by the minimization of movement in the low cervical and cervicothoracic regions, via a three-point bending mechanism. This significantly restricts true neck flexion-extension (*A* and *B*).

tant in the cervical spine, but also play a role in the thoracic and lumbar spine.

Individual external cervical spine splinting techniques are discussed below with regard to the known data on their attributes and faults. *The techniques are grouped so as to facilitate the objective assessment of each technique.* These groupings are (1) limited cervical bracing techniques, (2) cervical-shoulder bracing techniques, (3) cervical-thoracic bracing techniques, and (4) cranial-thoracic bracing techniques.

Limited Cervical Bracing Techniques

Limited cervical braces have no neck base or shoulder fixation points. These points of fixation are important for the restriction of cervical motion. All of these techniques offer, to one degree or another, a mandibular point of fixation. They vary, however, in their ability to affix to the base of the neck, to the shoulder, or to the chest region. Collars that do not affix to the base of the neck, shoulder, or chest region are the least effective (Fig. 27-8*A*). They include the soft cervical semirigid collars. Flexion-extension movement is essentially unrestricted by these cervical collars (Table 27-1). Since these devices do not substantially restrict movement in any direction, they do not enhance the parallelogram-like bracing effect. Their overall ineffectiveness in restricting cervical movement, however, makes this a moot point.

Cervical-Shoulder Bracing Techniques

An extension of a limited cervical brace to include the mandible rostrally and the neck base or shoulder caudally (Philadelphia collar) provides some movement restriction (Fig. 27-8*B*). However, it simultaneously causes an exaggeration of parallelogram-like spinal movements (Figs. 27-5 and 27-6). These two points are obviously a tradeoff. The parallelogram-like bracing effect cannot be quantitated. The relative extent of its presence, however, can be assessed (subjectively, to be sure) by observation of flexion- and

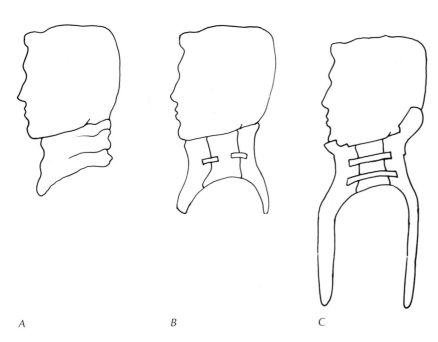

FIGURE 27-8 Limited cervical bracing techniques provide little cervical spine stabilization (*A*). Their length-to-width ratio is insufficient, and their points of contact with the torso are not solid. Cervical-shoulder bracing techniques provide a slight advantage over limited cervical bracing techniques, via extension of the brace to include the neck base–shoulder region. This, however, minimally influences movement in the low cervical region (*B*). This, in turn, has significant impact on upper cervical segmental movement (Figs. 27-5 and 27-6). Cervical-thoracic bracing techniques provide a biomechanical advantage by limiting low cervical and cervicothoracic motion and, hence, compensatory higher cervical segmental movements. They are typified by the SOMI, four-poster, and cervicothoracic braces (*C*).

extension-induced motion in the upper cervical region (capital flexion and extension). Note, in Table 27-1, that capital and true cervical flexion-extension movements are relatively unimpeded by cervical-shoulder bracing techniques (e.g., the Philadelphia collar).

The advantage of this technique is that it provides some degree of movement restriction (Table 27-1). The significance of this movement restriction, however, is difficult to assess.

Cervical-Thoracic Bracing Techniques

The extension of a cervical brace caudally to include the chest region provides a three-point bending biomechanical advantage, whereas the previously discussed devices provide lesser restrictions of movement or exaggerate the parallelogram-like bracing effect (Figs. 27-5 through 27-7). These splinting techniques (e.g., SOMI, four-poster, and cervicothoracic brace) (Fig. 27-8C) provide substantial restriction of movement in the mid- to low cervical region (Table 27-1).

Cranial-Thoracic Fixation Techniques

For years the Halo device has been the "gold standard" of cervical bracing.[16] Other orthoses, however, have recently been used in its stead. Rigid (Halo) and semirigid (Minerva) techniques for fixation of the cranium to the chest provide the greatest restriction of segmental cervical spine movement. As mentioned above, this may be due largely to their shared ability to limit mid-to-low cervical movement. This type of fixation considerably limits segmental movement while simultaneously minimizing the parallelogram-like effect (as is evidenced by the diminished segmental movement observed in the upper cervical region—see Table 27-2).

It has been observed that there is a significant difference between (1) the overall movement between the head and the chest from flexion to extension and (2) the summation of segmental movements between these two regions.[8,12] This difference can be quantitatively derived from x-rays (Fig. 27-9). It provides an objective measure of snaking.[8] Much more important than overall movement between the head and the chest, obviously, is the movement allowed at each segmental level, since instability is almost always a segmental (not a global) phenomenon.

The rigid cranial fixation afforded by the Halo considerably restricts capital flexion and extension movements; hence the parallelogram-like bracing effect is minimized. This occurs, however, at the expense of an exaggeration of the snaking of the mid-to-low cervical spine (Table 27-2).[8] This correlates with clinical data showing an unexpected deficiency of Halo efficacy in patients with unstable cervical spine injuries.[17-19]

The Minerva jacket provides similar minimization of the

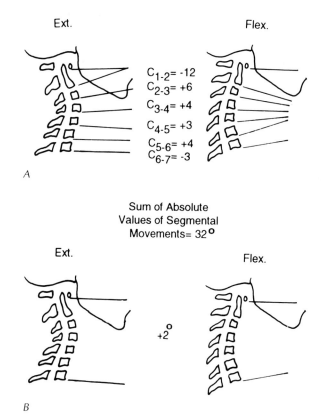

FIGURE 27-9 The assessment of segmental movement at each individual level (in degrees) can be measured and calculated from flexion and extension x-rays. The total movement is the sum of angles. The overall movement between the cranium and the low cervical region (lowest segment assessed) is the measured movement. The difference is an objective assessment of snaking.[8] The differences at segmental levels are depicted in this hypothetical example (*A*). *Ext.* identifies the extension intersegmental angles, and *Flex.* the flexion intersegmental angles. The sum of angles is 32 degrees. The overall movement between the cranium and the lowest segment assessed is 2 degrees (*B*). Therefore, in this case, the objective measure of snaking is 30 degrees.

parallelogram-like bracing effect. The Minerva's advantage in this regard is due mainly to the extent of chest fixation, which provides a three-point-bending biomechanical advantage (Fig. 27-7). The Minerva jacket, however, does not allow substantial control of capital flexion and extension. Therefore, it cannot be used effectively to provide these force applications. The major advantage of the Minerva jacket is its minimal amplification of snaking.[8,12,14]

If one compares Halo and Minerva data, it is apparent that the Minerva jacket controls subaxial sagittal plane segmental motion better than the Halo. On the other hand, the Halo is obviously much better able to control capital flexion and extension.[8,12,14] The degree of control of capital flexion and extension (via manipulation of the degree of tilt of the halo ring), combined with its additional ability to manipulate true neck flexion and extension (by movement of the

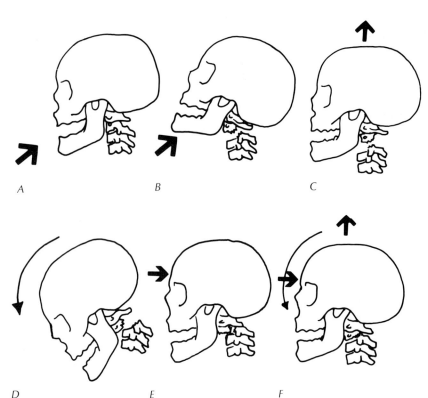

A   B   C

D   E   F

FIGURE 27-10 A very unstable hangman's fracture can be managed by application of a complex set of forces to the unstable segment. The fracture itself is a result of a hyperextension loading to failure (*A*). This usually results in a subluxation of C2 on C3 and disruption of the pars interarticularis of C2 (*B*). Neither simple distraction (*C*), capital flexion (*D*), nor true neck extension (*E*) alone provides adequate reduction. However, a combination of slight simple distraction, moderate capital flexion, and moderate true neck extension provides an optimal force complex application for reduction (*F*). Arrows depict forces and moments applied.

ring ventrally or dorsally) makes the Halo unique as the only technique that provides the ability to manipulate craniocervical translational *and* flexion-extension movement. The three-point-bending biomechanical advantage provided by chest fixation assists in this regard (Fig. 27-7). These points are especially important in dealing with such situations as the very unstable hangman's fracture (Fig. 27-10).

The cranial extension of the Minerva jacket (occiput and forehead) appears to be of minimal significance (unpublished data of E. C. Benzel). Therefore, a significant portion of the Minerva jacket's efficacy is provided by the mandible, occipital, and chest points of attachment. This is not unexpected (Fig. 27-7). The significance of the cervical points of attachment, however, should not be underestimated. They minimize spinal snaking via maintenance of the cervical shell (Fig. 27-11) (see also Lumbar and Lumbosacral Spine Bracing, below). The Halo does not offer this advantage. Therefore, the greater segmental movement restriction provided by the Minerva jacket may be due partly to this phenomenon. The relatively minimal amount of soft tissue separating the external splint (Minerva jacket) and the spine allows relatively thorough maintenance of the body shell (Fig. 27-1).

The extent of thoracic and lumbar extension of the external cervical splint is important. A principal goal in long bone splinting is the immobilization of the fractured bone from

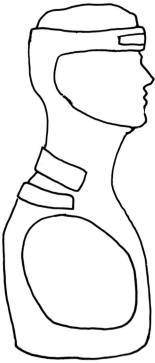

FIGURE 27-11 The Minerva jacket's significant area of contact with the torso helps it to maintain the body shell and prevent snaking.

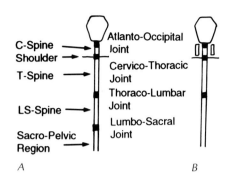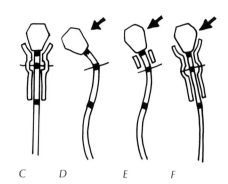

FIGURE 27-12 The consideration of the axial skeleton as consisting of five segments. The segments are depicted and defined (*A*). A cervical collar (*B*) and a brace embracing the mandible and the thoracic regions (*C*) are depicted. Responses to externally applied forces are depicted for the unbraced (*D*) and the collar- (*E*) and extensively braced (*F*) spines. Note the relative augmentation of protection provided by longer braces. This concept is also depicted in Fig. 27-1.

one joint above to one joint blow the site of injury. If one considers the axial skeleton as composed of five segments that might each be considered a long bone (cranial, cervical, thoracic, lumbar, and sacropelvic), then one might similarly consider the external splinting of an unstable motion segment in one of these regions as subject to the normal principles of long bone splinting (Figs. 27-1 and 27-12). By traditional dictum, cervical and lumbosacral immobilizations by external splinting are inadequate. The creation of a rigid cantilever-like construct via rigid attachment of the skull to the external splint (halo) (Fig. 27-13) and the use of three-point bending construct properties in the cervical-thoracic region (Fig. 27-7) compensate somewhat for this inadequacy. In the lumbar and lumbosacral regions, a hip-spica brace may function similarly (see below). Unfortunately, the efficacy of splinting in the thoracic and lumbar regions is compromised by the relatively large thickness of soft tissue separating the spine and the splint. This may explain the lack of correlation between length of brace and bracing efficacy observed by Triggs and coworkers.[20]

Nevertheless, the extension of a Minerva or halo brace to a lower chest or lumbar attachment increases the lever arm available for three-point bending force application. As was demonstrated in Chap. 10, the length of the construct is proportional—theoretically—to its efficacy (as assessed by its ability to resist bending moments at the unstable segment).

Most splinting techniques cause little compression or distraction, of the cervical spine. Furthermore, axially oriented force application generally is difficult to quantitate. However, Koch and Nickel assessed distraction and compression forces with the halo by inserting a transducer in the stabilizing bars of the halo. A surprising variation of axial forces (a variation of nearly 22 lb total) was observed during the assumption of several positions of normal daily activity.[15] These data were corroborated by Lind and coworkers.[22] In fact, the Lind group's conclusions were:

1. Great flexion-extension motion occurs in each motion segment of the cervical spine in spite of the halo-vest fixation.

2. The motion pattern of the cervical spine stabilized with a halo-vest is like a curling snake.

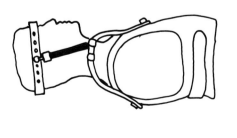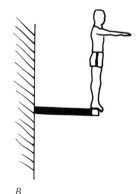

FIGURE 27-13 The halo ring is rigidly attached to the calvarium. This provides a rigid cantilever (fixed moment arm cantilever beam) construct (*A* and *B*).

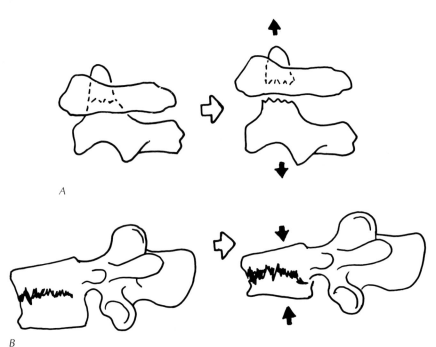

FIGURE 27-14 The distraction and compression force transmission to the cervical spine may be problematic in the face of a dens fracture, where overdistraction may decrease chances of union (*A*), or a subaxial wedge compression fracture, where further compression could exaggerate the deformity (*B*).

3. The motion is greatest in the upper part of the cervical spine and decreases further down.

4. The halo-vest provides distraction across the neck during the whole treatment period (3 months).

5. There are large variations of force across the neck depending upon type of exercise performed or position of the body (mean maximal variation: 175 N).

6. A tightly fitted vest exaggerates the variations of force across the neck.

7. Large distraction force across the neck of the patient in the supine position results in large variation of force and great motion in the motion segments of the cervical spine.[21]

These factors may affect stability adversely. For example, an interbody fusion or a dens fracture would heal less well if repetitively subjected to distractive forces. Conversely, a wedge compression fracture–related deformity could be exaggerated by compressive axial force application (Fig. 27-14).

Finally, pin site complications with the halo are not infrequent. These include dislodgment, calvarial penetration, and cosmetic problems. Many cannot be eliminated. However, it behooves the surgeon to affix the device most effectively to the calvarium. Appropriate torque and technique, obviously, are imperative. In this regard, a perpendicular insertion of halo pins into the skull maximizes the structural integrity of the interface.[22] The application of this consideration alone may reduce the incidence of pin site complications.

CERVICOTHORACIC SPINE BRACING

The external splinting of the cervicothoracic region can be effectively accomplished via either the extension of a thoracic brace to include the cervical region (by attaining a mandible point of fixation) or the use of the halo technique with a caudal extension of the brace to include the thoracolumbar or lumbar region. Koch and Nickel have furnished interesting data that demonstrate the gradual increased efficacy of the halo technique in limiting flexion and extension movement as the cervical spine is descended into the cervicothoracic region (Fig. 27-15).[15] Extrapolating this information into the upper thoracic spine with a caudally extended halo technique, one might expect to achieve a substantial splinting advantage with the halo technique in this region.

THORACIC SPINE BRACING

The thoracic spine is unique in that it is the only segment of the spine to which traditional external splinting principles can be applied [by virtue of the fact that it has two axial segments above (cranial and cervical) and two axial segments below (lumbar and sacropelvic)]. This allows the attainment of adequate points of fixation. The thickness of soft tissue separating the spine and the external splint is relatively unimportant in this region, because of the relatively firm rib cage.

Restriction-of-movement data for segmental external splinting in this region of the spine are lacking. Neverthe-

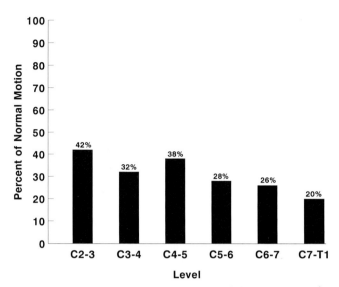

FIGURE 27-15 Koch and Nickel determined the percentage of normal cervical spine motion allowed in a halo. The average was 31 percent; the range was from 42 percent in the upper cervical spine to 20 percent in the low cervical spine. The restriction of segmental motion increased as the spine was descended, as depicted. *(From R.A. Koch and V.L. Nickel.[15])*

less, bracing can be assumed to be at least somewhat effective.

LUMBAR AND LUMBOSACRAL SPINE BRACING

The lumbar, and particularly the low lumbar, region is difficult to splint externally, on account of the limitations created by an inadequate caudal fixation point. For adequate fixation, two points that are at least four or five vertebral levels proximal and distal to the unstable segment, and that are amenable to immobilization by an external splint, are required. The pelvic region does not provide such an advantage; there is insufficient distance from the unstable segment to the pelvic points of fixation. In addition, hip flexion, even with hip spica application, allows unacceptable movement that may result in inadequate protection. Partial compensation for this can be achieved via the lengthening of the brace. This is accomplished either by the addition of an extension to a single lower extremity, in the form of a hip spica, or by the extension of the brace downward to the inguinal region, over the iliac crests. However, for effective stabilization of this region, sitting must be virtually eliminated. These braces generally are not well tolerated. Their efficacy, furthermore, is suspect.[23]

Objective data on the efficacy of external lumbar and lumbosacral splints are lacking. Such data as are available suggest that the comments of Sypert are rational and objective.[24] As Sypert cogently states, "the effectiveness of the various lumbosacral orthoses in lumbosacral immobiliza-

tion (excluding the spica type devices) is related more to their discomfort than to the actual magnitudes of the forces (abdominal compression, three-point fixation) transmitted from the appliance to the body. Thus, the function of most lumbosacral orthoses are to remind and to irritate the patient so that he restricts movements, to support the abdomen to alleviate some of the load on the lumbosacral spine, to provide some movement restriction of the upper lumbar and the thoracolumbar spine by three-point fixation, and to reduce excessive lumbar lordosis to provide a straighter and more comfortable low back."[3] An understanding of these principles is of the utmost importance; the spine surgeon must not harbor unreasonable expectations of external spinal splinting techniques.

COMPLICATIONS

Complications of orthoses include, but are not restricted to, (1) pain, (2) pressure, (3) psychological dependence, (4) poor hygiene, (5) axial muscle weakness and disuse atrophy, (6) restriction of activity, (7) aggravation of spinal symptoms, (8) vascular (venous) compromise, and (9) ineffective stabilization. Halo bracing is associated, in addition to the above complications, with pin site complications that include cosmetic problems, osteomyelitis, brain abscess, and other soft tissue and wound-healing problems. Therefore, spinal orthoses should be judiciously employed. Furthermore, they should be employed only as long as they offer a therapeutic advantage.

An uncommonly observed, but potentially fatal, complication of spinal bracing is the *body cast syndrome*. This syndrome is a manifestation of duodenal obstruction following the application of a body cast. Acute gastric dilatation with vomiting may be followed by aspiration, airway compromise, cardiac arrest, or gastric perforation and peritonitis. Removal of the brace and other symptomatic therapy may be urgently required.[25,26] The rarity of this syndrome is due to the rarity of extremely tight application of lumbar braces, and to the infrequent use of casts that are not removed or loosened.

REFERENCES

1. Benzel EC, Larson SJ: Postoperative stabilization of the posttraumatic thoracic and lumbar spine: A review of concepts and orthotoxic techniques. *J Spinal Disord* 1989; 2:47–51.
2. Redford JB: *Orthotics Etcetera* (3d ed). Baltimore: Williams and Wilkins, 1986.
3. Sypert GW: External spinal orthotics. *Neurosurgery* 1987; 20:642–649.
4. Morris JM: Spinal bracing, in Wilkins RH, Rengachary SS (eds):*Neurosurgery.* New York: Mcgraw-Hill, 1985: 2300–2305.

5. Morris JM, Lucas DB, Bresler B: Role of the trunk in stability of the spine. *J Bone Joint Surg* 1961; 43A:327–51.

6. Norton PL, Brown T: The immobilizing efficiency of back braces. *J Bone Joint Surg* 1957; 39A:111–138.

7. Waters R, Morris J: Effects of spinal supports on the electrical activity of muscles of the trunk. *J Bone Joint Surg* 1970; 52A:51–60.

8. Benzel EC, hadden TA, Saulsbery CM: A comparison of the Minerva and halo jackets for stabilization of the cervical spine. *J Neurosurg* 1989; 70:411–414.

9. Hart DL, Johnson RM, Simmons EF, et al: Review of cervical orthoses. *Physical Therapy* 1978; 58:857–860.

10. Hartman JT, Palumbo F, Hill BJ: Cineradiography of the braced normal cervical spine. *Clin Orthop Rel Res* 1975; 109:97–102.

11. Johnson RM, Hart DL, Owen JR, et al: The Yale Cervical Orthosis. *Spine* 1968; 58:865–871.

12. Johnson RM, Hart DL, Simmons BF, et al: Cervical orthoses: A study comparing their effectiveness in restricting cervical motion in normal subjects. *J Bone Joint Surg* 1977; 59A:332–339.

13. Jones MD: Cineradiographic studies of the collar-immobilized cervical spine. *J Neurosurg* 1960; 17:633–637.

14. Maiman D, Millington P, Novak S, et al: The effect of the thermoplastic Minerva body jacket on cervical spine motion. *Neurosurgery* 1989; 25:363–368.

15. Koch RA, Nickel VL: The halo vest. An evaluation of motion and forces across the neck. *Spine* 1978; 3:103–107.

16. Nickel VL, Perry J, Garrett A, et al: The halo. *J Bone Joint Surg* 1968; 50A:1400–1409.

17. Anderson PA, Budorick TE, Easton KB, et al: Failure of halo vest to prevent in vivo motion in patients with injured cervical spines. *Spine* 1991; 16:S501–S505.

18. Kelly EG: Frequent lateral films key to control cervical displacement in halo cast. *Surgical Practice News* 1981; 10:21.

19. Whitehill R, Richman JA, Glaser JA: Failure of immobilization of the cervical spine by the halo vest. *J Bone Joint Surg* 1986; 68A:326–332.

20. Triggs KJ, Ballock T, Byrne T, et al: Length dependence of a halo orthosis on cervical immobilization. *J Spinal Disord* 1993; 6:34–37.

21. Lind B, Sihlbom H, Nordwall A: Forces and motions across the neck in patients treated with halo-vest. *Spine* 1988; 13:162–167.

22. Triggs KJ, Ballock T, Lee TQ, et al: The effect of angled insertion on halo pin fixation. *Spine* 1989; 14:781–783.

23. Axelsson P, Johnsson R, Stromqvist B: Lumbar orthosis with unilateral hip immobilization. *Spine* 1993; 18:876–879.

24. Axelsson P, Johnsson R, Stromqvist B: Effect of lumbar orthosis on intervertebral mobility. *Spine* 1992; 17:678–681.

25. Berk RN, Coulson DB: The body cast syndrome. *Radiology* 1970; 94:303–305.

26. Schwartz DR, Wirka HW: The cast syndrome. A case report and discussion of the literature. *J Bone Joint Surg* 1964; 46A:1549–1552.

Chapter **28**

Surgical Indications

INTRODUCTION

The determination of surgical indications is the most difficult and yet the most important aspect of every surgical discipline. This may be most evident in spine surgery, especially with regard to the indication for spinal fusion. In the interest of furthering understanding of this extremely complex field, the author's opinions on surgical decision-making are presented below. *There are no official rules to guide patient management.* Confusion and misinformation often prevail. Nevertheless, the use of a logical patient management scheme should optimize the outcome for any given patient.

This chapter focuses on a small segment of the overall patient population (but perhaps the most difficult segment, so far as managment is concerned): the low back pain patient. Perhaps what is learned from this patient subpopulation may be extrapolated to other subpopulations.

The following pages present a scheme used by the author. This scheme is based largely on opinion. Each surgeon may or may not appropriately choose to incorporate all or part of this scheme into his or her own management scheme.

INDICATIONS FOR LUMBAR FUSION

Spinal fusion is indicated when excessive or abnormal spinal motion causes refractory pain that significantly interferes with the activities of daily living of a patient who is motivated and who is *actively* participating in his or her pain management program. This surgical indicator scheme is difficult, if not impossible, to quantitate. General rules of thumb, however, can be established on a surgeon-specific basis. Each surgeon should determine his or her own well-defined and clearly conceived criteria. In the author's opinion, spinal fusion is indicated if, and only if, these four conditions are clearly established: (1) that excessive or abnormal spinal motion exists, (2) that this motion is related to pain, (3) that this pain significantly interferes with the

activities of daily living, and (4) that the patient has demonstrated his or her commitment to the recovery process.

Excessive or Abnormal Spinal Motion

Proving that a spinal motion segment is the cause of a pain syndrome (pain generator) is difficult, if not impossible. Plain x-ray, MRI, CT, bone scanning, and diskography have been used as imaging criteria for this purpose. Internal disk degeneration or disruption (IDD) is often touted as a cause of pain of spinal origin. Its diagnosis by diskography or MRI, however, has not been shown to correlate with clinical outcome in randomized clinical series. CT, similarly, does not surpass other modalities regarding clinical correlation. Bone scanning, although appealing for its ability to define regions of "inflammation," similarly has not been shown to significantly correlate with surgical outcome.

Since surgical outcome is not correlated with traditional "outcome assessment parameters," the surgeon should perhaps seek surgical indicators that shrink, rather than expand, the indications for surgery. Theoretically, the painful motion segment that is unstable, excessively mobile, or excessively degenerated should become painless if immobilized. These joints can be effectively identified by plain x-ray (including flexion and extension views). Their relation to pain can be gleaned from the patient's history and clinical assessment (see below).

The x-ray findings associated with painful motion segments are (1) excessive mobility, (2) fixed subluxation or other segmental deformity, and (3) significant degenerative changes. A fixed spinal deformity or degeneration in and/or around the disk interspace indicates that abnormal segmental motion exists or has existed. Therefore, even in the face of an inability to demonstrate excessive motion by flexion and extension views, these findings may be associated with pain of spinal origin (pain generator). This pain, for lack of a better term, is called *mechanical back pain*. It results from *mechanical instability* and *"dysfunctional segmental motion."* Note that the painful motion segment cannot be

259

clearly localized, nor can it be distinguished from other similarly radiographically involved motion segments.

Clinical Assessment

Clinical assessment is the most important aspect of determination of surgical indications. It includes the establishment of the patient's history and the performance of a physical examination. The patient's history is important on two accounts. First, it establishes the history to date and the chronicity of the process. More important, it elucidates the *character* of the pain. The establishment of the character of the pain is a key concept in surgical indication determination.

Pain associated with mechanical instability is identifiable by three criteria: (1) Deep agonizing pain not associated with paraspinous muscle spasm, neurological deficit, or radicular or myelopathic symptoms; (2) association of the pain with activity or with placement of stresses on the allegedly painful motion segment; and (3) diminution or elimination of the pain upon minimization or elimination of stresses on the allegedly painful motion segment.

Before one can establish the presence of pain associated with mechanical instability (mechanical back pain), other components of the patient's pain syndrome must be either eliminated or "accounted for" by the surgeon. Paraspinous muscle spasm may be treated by muscle relaxants, exercises (mostly stretching), and other symptomatic therapy. Neurological deficits can be "accounted for" via both clinical means and imaging techniques.

Extent of Pain

The extent of pain is difficult to quantitate. Usually it cannot be effectively assessed in only one office visit. The surgeon must take adequate time to "get to know" the patient and his or her family. Scales and questionnaires may be useful in disability assessment and the establishment of guidelines.[1]

Patient Motivation

Identification of a motivated patient is easier than quantitation of the extent of the patient's pain. In fact, the extent of motivation may be objectively assessed, albeit indirectly. Several parameters can be monitored periodically, in order to assess progress: (1) cessation of smoking, (2) weight loss, (3) flexibility parameters, and (4) exercise tolerance and conditioning. Midlevel health care providers (nurse practitioners, physician assistants, and physical therapists) can play a central role in this, as well as in the patient education process.

THE LAST HURDLE BEFORE SURGERY: AGGRESSIVE NONSURGICAL MANAGEMENT

Four separate management techniques (making up a four-point program) are integral to the nonsurgical management process for mechanical back pain: (1) augmentation of physical well-being, (2) aerobic exercise, (3) stretching exercise, and (4) strengthening exercise. Each of these requires patient education by the surgeon, by the midlevel health care providers, or, more appropriately, by both.

Augmentation of Physical Well-Being

Augmentation of physical well-being makes the patient a better surgical candidate (if, indeed, surgery is deemed appropriate) and simultaneously brings about a physiologically and biomechanically improved clinical status. Programs for the cessation of smoking and for weight loss are imperative. Both can, and should, be objectively assessed and recorded on a periodic basis. If the patient *cannot* demonstrate progress in these areas, his or her motivation *may* be insufficient to warrant surgery.

Aerobic Exercise

Aerobic exercise can similarly be quantitated (at least by patient history) and recorded. The sense of well-being and accomplishment acquired from a planned aerobic exercise program (e.g., walking, running, swimming, or cycling) creates a positive internal physical and psychological milieu and further establishes the extent of the patient's motivation.

Stretching Exercise

The lack of flexibility is an integral component of the pain associated with mechanical instability. The spine of a patient with mechanical instability should be thought of as akin to a "frozen joint" arising from long-term immobilization. Flexibility can be improved, and progress quantitatively monitored. Toe-touching can be monitored by asking the patient to reach for his or her toes, with knees locked, and hold the lowest position achievable for 20 seconds. The distance from the floor is measured and recorded. "Bouncing" is discouraged. Progress is encouraged. In fact, lack of progress may very well be a manifestation of a lack of adequate motivation. Other exercises include "extension" and the "foot on stool" exercises. These, however, are not so easily quantitated and monitored (Fig. 28-1). Less aggressive exercises may be more appropriate at first.

Strengthening Exercise

Often, much of the pain of spinal origin associated with mechanical instability may be reduced by an appropriate

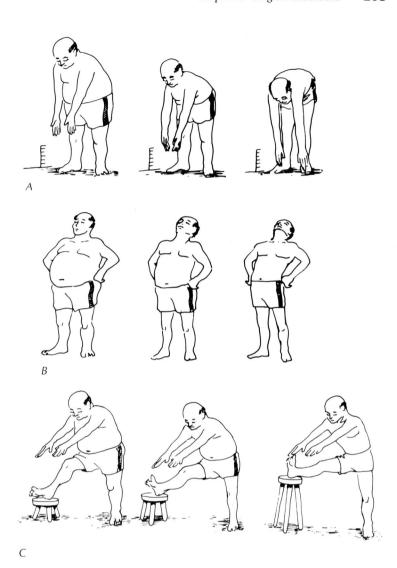

FIGURE 28-1 Stretching exercises. *A*. Toe touching. Note the method of measuring and monitoring progress. *B*. Back extension. *C*. "Foot on stool" exercise. This augments both flexion and rotation flexibility.

strengthening program. The supporting muscles of the spinal column can be thought of as such—as *supporting muscles*. These muscles assist in activities of daily living, provide support, and prevent excessive spinal movement. If asymmetry of muscle strength exists, excessive stresses may be placed on the spine or on its supporting muscles. Strengthening of the muscles that *stress* the spine, such as by weight-lifting or running, without strengthening of the muscles that *support* the spine (abdominal and paraspinous muscles), may result in a muscle strength imbalance. This, in turn, may result in an excessive "spinal stress force application–to–spinal support muscle strength" ratio. This may augment the dysfunctional nature of a "dysfunctional motion segment."

The muscle groups to be specifically exercised include the dorsal paraspinous muscles and the abdominal muscles. Specific exercises include supine leg lifts, progressing to

situps, for abdominal muscle strengthening; and prone leg lifts, progressing to the "airplane" or "rocking chair" exercise, for paraspinous muscle strengthening (Fig. 28-2). Less aggressive exercises may be more appropriate at first.

The surgeon cannot divorce him- or herself from this program of exercise and education. Without active involvement of both the patient and the surgeon, the chance of failure of the management plan will assuredly increase.

PATIENT EDUCATION

Patient education is critically important. If the patient understands the need for his or her active participation in the management of his or her problem, active participation is more likely. Documentation of the patient's progress is also imperative, for longitudinal monitoring purposes. A

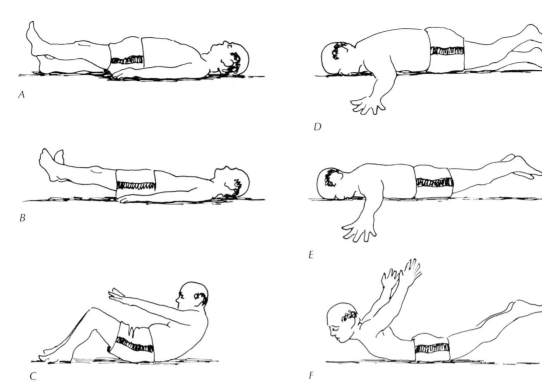

FIGURE 28-2 Strengthening exercises. Abdominal muscles can be strengthened by leg lifts, beginning with one leg at a time (*A*) and progressing to both legs (*B*) and, finally, to situps (*C*). Paraspinous and other dorsal low back muscles can be strengthened by prone leg lifts, beginning with one leg at a time (*D*) and progressing to both legs (*E*) and, finally, to the head, chest, and both legs (the "airplane" or "rocking chair" maneuver) (*F*).

patient who cannot participate or refuses to participate has demonstrated his or her relative inability to succeed in a program as outlined above. Such patients probably should seek relief elsewhere.

Two final points deserve emphasis. First, narcotics play a limited role in the management of chronic back pain. Dose reduction and withdrawal play an integral role in this management scheme. Second, contractual arrangements between the patient and the surgeon (written or verbal) regarding pain medication management and participation in the four-point program outlined above allow an honest and objective relationship between the patient and the surgeon. This assists both parties in their quest to defeat their mutual enemy: the patient's pain syndrome.

OPERATION SELECTION

Once the patient has met the clinical criteria for surgery and demonstrated the will to participate actively in his or her pain management program, consideration of surgery is reasonable if pain persists. However, three points still require addressing: (1) the level(s) to be fused, (2) the fusion technique to be employed, and (3) the need for instrumentation placement.

The level(s) to be fused are determined via lumbar spine x-rays (including flexion and extension views). The fusion technique to be employed is determined by the surgeon's armamentarium and his or her biases (obviously this needs to be based on sound biomechanical principles). The latter, obviously, are based on the clinical situation, the surgeon's clinical judgment, and his or her assessment of the literature. The need for instrumentation placement is similarly determined. Lumbar fusion is often supplemented by instrumentation placement. Other considerations, however, may prevail. Consider, for example, the performance of an isolated L5-S1 fusion in a young patient with less than 50 percent subluxation. This patient has a high likelihood of fusion acquisition without instrumentation supplementation. Therefore, the possible benefits of instrumentation placement in this patient may not warrant its risks and cost.

Finally, other factors may dictate the type of operation employed. The presence of neurological deficit and/or neural element compression may oblige the surgeon to do a surgical spinal decompression that further destabilizes the spine or that destabilizes the spine over additional motion segments. Such factors, obviously, complicate the surgical decision-making process.

REFERENCE

1. Fairbanks JCT, Couper J, Davis JB, et al: The Oswestry low back pain disability questionnaire. *Physiotherapy* 1980, 66:271–273.

Glossary

This glossary is a guide both to the definition of terms and to the locations of specific topics within the text. The numbers in parentheses following the definitions refer to the chapter(s) in which each term is introduced and/or used at length.

amphiarthrodial joint: A joint without a synovial membrane. (4)

anodic breakdown potential: An indirect measure of corrosion resistance, to which it is approximately proportional. (11)

anodizing: An electrolytic process that increases the thickness of a naturally occurring oxide surface layer. This is used to increase stability and corrosion resistance. (11)

annealing: A metallurgical treatment process designed to alter microstructure. The material is heated and cooled by a predetermined specific cycle. This creates a softer, weaker metal. (11)

applied moment arm cantilever beam fixation: A cantilever beam construct that applies a bending moment; either flexion or extension. (15)

axial ligamentous resistance: Resistance to deformation related to intrinsic elasticity of ligaments. (14)

bending moment (M) (also known as torque): The product of an applied force and the length of the moment arm through which it acts. (2, 15)

bulk modulus: The elastic deformation of a solid when squeezed (stress/strain). (2)

cantilever: A large projecting bracket or beam supported at one end only. (15)

cantilever beam fixation: The application of cantilever biomechanical principles to a spinal implant. (15, 20, 25)

cantilevered screw technique: A method of bone-to-bone fixation via a screw. A combination of complex force applications are employed and withstood by the construct. (26)

capital neck flexion and extension: Flexion and extension of the neck, centered in the upper cervical spine region. (27)

center of rotation (COR): The geometrically determined axis of rotation. Similar to the *instantaneous axis of rotation (quod vide).* (2, 3)

cerclage wiring: A method of fixation wherein a wire or cable is passed circumferentially around projecting spinal elements (e.g., spinous processes). This is a method of applying forces via a tension-band fixation mechanism. (26)

coincident: Occupying the same position and/or acting along the same axis or line. (6)

cold working: A metallurgical teatment process wherein the material is deformed at room temperature. This creates a harder, stronger material. (11)

complete myelopathy: The complete loss of function below a spinal level of injury. When this occurs, no motor or sensory function is present. (7)

compression wiring: A method of securing an onlay bone graft wherein a wire or cable is used to affix the bone graft to the acceptance site. (26)

"coronal bowstring" effect: The tethering of the spinal cord axially over a mass, in the coronal plane. (7)

couple: A pair of forces applied to a structure that are of equal magnitude and opposite direction, having lines of action that are parallel but not coincident. (2)

coupling: The phenomenon wherein a movement of the spine obligates a separate movement about another axis. (2, 26)

crevice corrosion: Corrosion that occurs within crevices and small cavities on a metal's surface. (11)

crossed rod deformity correction: A technique for reduction of kyphotic deformation that employs the simultaneous application of kyphosis-reduction forces to the spine via moment arms (longitudinal members) affixed at opposite ends and opposite sides of the spine. Gradual reduction is thus achieved. (26)

crossed screw fixation: A short segment fixation technique that is applicable from the midthoracic to the low lumbar region. It is employed via the lateral extracavitary surgical approach to the spine. It uses two large transverse vertebral body screws and two smaller unilateral ipsilateral pedicle screws. The screws are rigidly attached to rods, and the rods rigidly crossfixed. (26)

crossfixation: The fixation of bilaterally placed posterior fixation devices to each other in a rigid or semirigid manner, so as to add a quadrilateral-frame attribute to the construct. (12, 16, 26)

cutout: A type of implant-bone failure wherein the implant sweeps through the bone during failure. (26)

degenerative disk disease: A biomechanical and pathological condition of an intervertebral segment caused by degeneration, inflammation, or infection. (4)

derotation: An intraoperative maneuver wherein a scoliotic curvature is converted to a kyphotic curvature via simultaneous and gradual 90° rotation of all longitudinal members (rods) of an implant that has been applied to a scoliotic spine. (26)

diarthrodial joint: A joint lined with synovium. (4)

distraction fixation: Application of an implant-derived distraction force to the spine. (15, 18, 22)

dysfunctional segmental motion: Instability related to disk interspace or vertebral body degenerative changes, to tumor, or to infection, resulting in the potential for pain of spinal origin. Also called *mechanical instability*. (3, 28)

"effective" cervical kyphosis: A configuration of the cervical spine in which any part of the dorsal aspect of any of the C3-C7 vertebral bodies crosses a line drawn in the midsagittal plane from the dorsocaudal aspect of the vertebral body of C2 to the dorsocaudal aspect of the vertebral body of C7. (4)

"effective" cervical lordosis: A configuration of the cervical spine in which no part of the dorsal aspect of any of the C3-C7 vertebral bodies crosses a line drawn in the midsagittal plane from the dorsocaudal aspect of the vertebral body of C2 to the dorsocaudal aspect of the vertebral body of C7. (4)

elastic limit: During the deformation of a solid, the point at which the deforming force departs from its initial linear relationship with the extent of deformation. This is the upper aspect of the *neutral zone (quod vide)*. (2)

elastic modulus: The physical property of a material that describes the stress (*quod vide*) per unit of strain (*quod vide*) in the elastic region (i.e., stress/strain). Three types exist: Young's modulus, shear modulus, and bulk modulus. (2, 11)

elastic zone: That portion of the physiologic range of motion that begins with the onset of resistance incurred from adjacent joints and terminates at the end of the physiologic range of motion. (1)

fatigue: The process of progressive, permanent structural change occurring in a material subjected to repetitive alternating stresses. (1)

fixed moment arm cantilever beam fixation: A cantilever construct that employs a rigid attachment of the screw to the longitudinal member. (15)

flat back syndrome: A painful clinical syndrome related to implant-derived straightening of the normal lumbar lordosis. (22)

four-point bending fixation: A modification of three-point bending fixation (*quod vide*) wherein two intermediate forces are applied (i.e., wherein two fulcrums exist). (26)

fretting corrosion (corrosion wear attack): A form of corrosion that can occur when the protective passive film (e.g., oxide surface layer) is mechanically disrupted. (11)

friction-glide tightness: The tightening of a component-component interface to such an extent that the interface can still be manipulated (e.g., distracted or rotated) but is not freely mobile. (26)

fulcrum: The intermediate point of force application of a three-point or four-point bending construct (*quod vide*). (15, 24)

galvanic corrosion: An accelerated form of corrosion that can arise in a mixed-metal system on account of the difference in electrochemical potential between the two metals. (11)

glacial instability: A type of spinal instability that is not overt and does not demonstrate a significant chance of rapid development or progression of kyphotic, scoliotic, or translational deformities; but, like a glacier, progresses gradually with time, while substantial external forces do not cause movement or progression of deformity. (3)

helical axis of motion (HAM): That component of motion that is translational when rotation is superimposed upon translation; e.g., the translational component of a screw's movement during tightening. (2)

implant contouring: The contouring of the longitudinal members of a spinal implant, usually rods, in order to alter spinal segmental relationships. (26)

instability: The inability to limit excessive or abnormal spinal displacement. (3)

instantaneous axis of rotation (IAR): The axis about which a vertebral segment rotates. (1, 2, 3, 6, 15)

interference screw fixation: A method of securing an interbody bone graft wherein screws are inserted into the graft-acceptance site interface. (26)

instrumentation-fusion mismatch: The discrepancy between the number of spinal levels incorporated within an instrumentation construct and the number of spinal levels fused (i.e., the fusion of fewer spinal segments than are instrumented). (16)

intrinsic implant bending moment: The bending moment achieved by the application of forces in opposite directions (distraction and compression) to each half of a spinal implant, or by the application of torques in the same direction to the longitudinal members of the two halves of an implant. (20, 26)

knurling: Machining or other treatment of a surface to render it coarse or rough. Used on both surfaces of an interface in an implant, this creates a high-friction component-component interface. (11)

lead: The distance that a screw advances axially in one turn. This is roughly equal to the pitch (*quod vide*) of the thread. (13)

ligamentotaxis: The employment of spinal distraction to reduce displaced bone and/or disk fragments via the stretching of ligaments. (7, 9, 15)

limited instability: The loss of ventral or dorsal spine integrity, with the preservation of the other. (3)

load-bearing: Weight- or force-bearing by an implant. An implant usually bears a load during the assumption of the upright posture or, in a sense, when placed in a distraction mode (surgical load-bearing). (15, 26)

load bearing–to–load sharing: A method of serial complex spinal loading via implant-derived force application. First distraction is employed, then an interbody fusion is placed, and finally a compression force is applied by the implant. Thus sharing of the load between the spinal implant and the intrinsic spinal elements is achieved. (26)

load-sharing: The distribution of an applied load between multiple components of an implant system and/or between the implant itself and intrinsic spinal elements. (14, 15, 26)

longitudinal member: That aspect of a spinal implant that connects implant-bone interface components to each other along one side of the spine; e.g., rod or plate. (14)

lumbosacral pivot point: The point of intersection of the middle osteoligamentous column (region of the poste-

rior longitudinal ligament) in the sagittal plane, and the L5-S1 intervertebral disk. (26)

mechanical instability: The instability associated with dysfunctional segmental motion. (3, 28)

moment arm: The perpendicular distance between a force vector and the instantaneous axis of rotation (IAR) (*quod vide*) of the body on which it acts. (2)

moment of inertia (I): An indicator of an object's stiffness. It is a measure of an object's distribution about its centroid (e.g., the center of a rod). For a rod of uniform density, it is proportional to the fourth power of the diameter of the rod. (2)

momentum: The product of mass and velocity. (2)

motion segment: Two adjacent vertebral bodies and the intervening ligamentous soft tissue. (2)

multisegmental fixation: Fixation by spinal implants that employ implant-bone interfaces at intermediate points, in addition to the terminal points of fixation. (14, 24)

neural element: Nerves, cauda equina, and spinal cord. (14)

neutral axis: The longitudinal region of the spine within which no points significantly extend or compress during flexion or extension of the spine; i.e., that region of the spine where flexion or extension does not result in significant displacement of points located within its limits. (6, 10, 15)

neutral zone: A portion of the range of motion of a vertebral segment that begins with the neutral position and terminates with the onset of some resistance contributed by the adjacent joints. (1, 2)

noncoincident: Not occupying the same position; not acting along the same axis or line. (6)

nonfixed moment arm cantilever beam fixation: A cantilever beam construct that employs a dynamic or semi-constrained connection of the screw with the longitudinal member. (15)

notching: An injury to the surface of an implant that adversely affects its structural integrity. (11)

osteointegration: The direct bonding of bone to an implant. (11, 13)

overt instability: The inability of the spine to support the torso during normal activity. (3)

paradoxical spinal motion: Unexpected and potentially untoward segmental spinal movement (e.g., snaking) that occurs during the application of flexion, extension, or rotation stresses to the involved spinal segment and adjacent segments. (2)

parallelogram distraction: A phenomenon wherein a translational deformity is reduced by the application of distraction forces to the spine. This is accomplished via the distraction of diagonal (with respect to the long axis of the spine), but parallel, fibroligamentous structures (e.g., the anterior and posterior longitudinal ligaments) so that their diagonal relationship with the long axis of the spine is eliminated. (10)

parallelogram-like bracing effect: A unique characteristic of the braced cervical spine. In this case the brace functions as a fulcrum around which parallelogram-like movements can occur. The four points of the parallelogram are usually the submental region, the occiput, and the anterior and posterior neck base or shoulder region. (27)

permanent set: During the deformation of a solid, the exceeding of the elastic limit results in the solid's inability to retain its pre-deformation configuration. The new configuration is the permanent set. (2)

physiologic range: The displacement observed between extremes of movement. It comprises the neutral zone and the elastic zone. (1)

pitch: The distance from any point on a screw thread to the corresponding point on the next thread. This is roughly equal to the lead (*quod vide*). (13)

point of failure: In the deformation of a solid, the point at which failure occurs. (7)

pullout: A mechanism of implant-bone failure wherein the implant backs out of the bone during failure. (26)

reversed three-point (or four-point) bending fixation: A three- or four-point bending construct using a dorsally oriented force applied at the fulcrum(s). In most three- and four-point bending constructs the fulcrum applies force from a ventral orientation. (26)

"sagittal bowstring" effect: The tethering of the spinal cord along its long axis over a mass, in the sagittal plane. (7)

screw core: The shaft of a screw, which imparts the majority of screw fracture resistance; the minor diameter of a screw. (13)

screw head: The widened following edge of a screw, which resists the translational force created by the rotation of the thread through the bone at the termination of screw tightening. (13)

screw outside (major) diameter: Diameter of a screw as measured from thread crest to thread crest; major diameter. Proportional to pullout resistance. (13)

screw thread: The spiral ridge about the core of a screw. Its depth is half the difference between the core diameter and the outside diameter of the screw. (13)

screw tip: The leading edge of a screw. (13)

section modulus (Z):   An indicator of the strength of an object (e.g., a screw). For a screw, it is proportional to the third power of the core diameter of the screw. (2, 13)

sequential hook insertion (SHI) technique: A technique of universal spinal instrumentation insertion wherein the hook-bone interfaces are secured and the hook attached to the rod in a sequential manner. (26)

shear modulus: A measure of the shear deformation experienced by a body subjected to transverse forces of equal and opposite direction, applied at opposite faces of the body (stress/strain). (2)

short-segment fixation: The use of short implants that incorporate only the spinal segments fused. (16)

short-segment parallelogram deformity reduction: A rigid cantilever beam pedicle fixation technique that can be employed in the thoracic and lumbar regions for the reduction of lateral translational deformities. It involves (1) the placement of pedicle screws, (2) an appropriate dural sac decompression, (3) the attachment of the longitudinal members (i.e., the rods) to the screws, (4) the application of rotatory and distraction forces to the rods to achieve reduction, (5) the maintenance of the achieved spinal reduction via rigid cross-fixation, (6) the placement of a fusion (interbody and/or lateral), and finally (7) compression of the screws so that load-sharing between the implant and the intrinsic spinal elements is achieved and the interbody bone graft is secured in its acceptance bed (if placed). (26)

shot peening: An implant surface treatment whereby small hard pellets are shot against the surface of a metal. This results in compression deformation of the surface of the metal. (11)

snaking: A serpentine movement of the spine wherein a simple overall movement (such as flexion or extension) is accompanied by an unexpected combination of flexion and extension movements at each intervertebral level. The sum of the movements of individual spinal motion segments is greater than the overall spinal movement observed. (2, 27)

spinal segment: Vertebra. (2)

spondylosis: Vertebral osteophytosis secondary to degenerative disk disease. (4)

strain: The change in unit length or angle in a material subjected to a load. (2)

stress: The force per unit area applied to a structure. (2)

stress reduction osteoporosis: The result of stress shielding (*quod vide*) secondary to the transfer of stress away from bone by a rigid implant. (13, 14)

stress riser: A weakened portion of a structure that results from the focal application of stress, resulting in distortion (i.e., bending or contouring). (11)

stress shielding: A situation created by rigid implants wherein the spine is protected from the transfer of normal stresses of weight-bearing. This may result in weakening of the bone via stress reduction osteoporosis. (11, 13, 14)

surgical load-bearing: The bearing of a load at the time of surgery by the implant. If the implant is placed in a distraction mode, the surgical load borne is positive. If the implant is placed in a compression mode, the surgical load borne is negative. If an implant is placed in a neutral mode, no load is borne at the time of surgery (i.e., surgical load-bearing = 0). (15)

tension-band compression fixation: Application of implant-derived compression force at a perpendicular distance from the instantaneous axis of rotation (IAR) (*quod vide*). (15, 19, 23)

tension-band distraction fixation: Application of implant-derived distraction force at a point dorsal to the instantaneous axis of rotation (IAR) (*quod vide*). (15)

terminal bending moments: Bending moments (usually not desirable) applied at the termini of a long spinal implant that are segmental in nature, and separate from the desired implant-derived force application. (23)

terminal three-point bending fixation: A three-point bending construct in which the fulcrum is situated near one end of the construct (15, 26)

three-point bending fixation: Implant-derived force application via three forces, two of which are opposite in orientation to the third (the middle of the three forces, applied at the fulcrum). (15, 24, 26)

toe-in: The application of screws on opposite sides of an implant in such a manner that they converge at their tips. This provides both translation and pullout failure resistance. (26)

toggling: Wobbling at an implant-bone or implant-implant interface. The latter situation may be desirable; an implant that uses it is called *semiconstrained* or *dynamic* implant. (25, 26)

transverse loads: Force vectors applied to a cantilever strut (as in a cantilevered screw technique) from the side (transverse force application). (26)

true neck flexion and extension: Flexion and extension of the neck, centered in the mid-to-low cervical region. (27)

universal spinal instrumentation (USI): An implant that uses multisegmental implant-bone interfaces with the potential for multiple implant-bone interface types, applied in any mode. (14)

vector: For the purposes of this text, a force oriented in a fixed and well-defined direction in three-dimensional space. (2)

work hardening: A process wherein a metal is permanently deformed, resulting in increased hardness and decreased ductility. (11)

yield strength: Tolerable stress (to failure). The ultimate tensile yield strength is the highest tolerable stress. The 0.2 percent tensile yield strength is that stress that causes a linear deformation of 0.2 percent. (11)

Young's modulus: A measure of the elastic properties of a body that is stretched or compressed (stress/strain). (2)

INDEX

Note: Page numbers in italics indicate figures; page numbers followed by t indicate tables.